Cortex and Mind

CORTEX
AND
MIND
Unifying Cognition

Joaquín M. Fuster, M.D., Ph.D.
Neuropsychiatric Institute
and
Brain Research Institute
University of California, Los Angeles

OXFORD
UNIVERSITY PRESS
2003

OXFORD
UNIVERSITY PRESS

Oxford   New York
Auckland   Bangkok   Buenos Aires   Cape Town   Chennai
Dar es Salaam   Delhi   Hong Kong   Istanbul   Karachi   Kolkata
Kuala Lumpur   Madrid   Melbourne   Mexico City   Mumbai   Nairobi
São Paulo   Shanghai   Singapore   Taipei   Tokyo   Toronto

and an associated company in Berlin

Published by Oxford University Press, Inc.
198 Madison Avenue, New York, New York, 10016
http://www.oup-usa.org

Oxford is a registered trademark of Oxford University Press

Library of Congress Cataloging-in-Publication Data
Fuster, Joaquin M.
Cortex and mind : unifying cognition / Joaquín M. Fuster.
p. ; cm.
ISBN 0-19-514752-9
1. Cognition. 2. Cerebral cortex. I. Title.
[DNLM: 1. Cerebral Cortex—physiology. 2. Cognition—physiology. WL 307 F995c 2002]
QP395.F88 2002
612.8'25—dc21
2002017077

2 3 4 5 6 7 8 9

Printed in the United States of America
on acid-free paper

To my son Mark

Preface

....

*B*y all appearances, the neuroscience of the mind is entering the twenty-first century with a confident, expansive, and eclectic outlook. In unexpected new ways and places, different or even opposite views of the relation between brain and mind are finding a measure of mutual accord. In the quest to clarify that relation, widely diverse methodologies encounter increasing support from one another. Judging from their progress, we are getting closer to a solution of the brain–mind problem with every passing day. Yet profound uncertainty is in the air.

Indeed, despite the spectacular progress of neuroscience, many of us share the growing sense that we are not getting closer to that solution, but further away from it. Despite the relentless rise of analytical power, the object of our study seems to become ever more elusive. The more facts about the brain that we know, the less we feel we know about the cerebral substrate of the mind, which seems to be disappearing in a downward spiral of reductionism. Even the so-called integrative neuroscience drifts toward the fragmentation of systems and mechanisms. Of course, some analysts of the very small rationalize their efforts as a quest for foundation, to be able to build the mind from the bottom up. Nobody, however, seems able to put together the small building blocks they produce in any way that might help us understand the physical foundation of the mind. At the opposite end—or perhaps, rather, at a "higher level"—many attempt to reach that understanding by abstracting principles of cognitive function from the study of cognitive dysfunctions in brain injury. This second form of reductionism (*upward reductionism*) is hardly more conducive than the first to the solution of our problem. Altogether, it seems a classic crisis of scientific paradigm (Kuhn, 1996).

This book is an attempt to portray an emerging paradigm of neural cognition that seems more viable and more plausible than many of the models currently favored. To be sure, the new paradigm incorporates elements of the old ones, and thus in some sense it could be considered the outcome of their evolution. With regard to almost all of them, however, the new paradigm requires a Copernican shift in the way we construe how the cognitive code is represented and processed by the brain.

Before presenting the new paradigm, I should like to dwell briefly on some of the reasons for the limited value of the current paradigms. One reason, no doubt, is the inevitable failure of neuroscience to yield causal relations between brain and mind. Having sensibly rejected any conceivable brain–mind dualism, we are left with two independent, though presumably parallel, lines of causality: the causality of brain mechanisms and the causality of cognitive processes, however these processes may be treated by various schools of thought, from psychoanalysis to connectionism. A cognitive order, no matter how it is construed, cannot be causally reduced to a brain order. Only a semblance of causality can be indirectly inferred, for example, from the psychological effects of brain lesions or chemicals.

There are, of course, evident correlations between the brain and the mind. In the domains of scientific empiricism, however, where causality reigns supreme, correlation is the Cinderella. Yet correlation is the only logical relationship we can substantiate empirically between the brain and the mind. We must comfort ourselves by thinking, I believe justifiably, that correlation is all we need for upholding the indissoluble unity of cortex and mind. In order to use correlations properly to that end, however, we first have to change fundamentally our current functional models of the cortex, which is not a simple endeavor. A brief reference to sensory neuroscience will illustrate the magnitude of our problem.

In the past 50 years, anatomy and physiology have firmly estab-

lished certain patterns of organization in sensory cortex that correspond to—that is, correlate with—patterns of sensation, as determined behaviorally and psychophysically. We are beginning to identify in the cortex the spatial–temporal maps of what we see, hear, or
touch. What we see, hear, or touch appears represented in those maps
by discrete structural modules of interconnected cell assemblies. We
can even surmise how those maps are modified while the animal directs attention to different sensations or holds them in short-term
memory. Further, the maps in those conditions seem to resonate at
certain oscillatory electrical frequencies, the would-be expression of
their *binding* properties. All of that seems a logical first step toward
understanding the neural basis of perception and memory. It is a
small step on a road without much promise, however, because only
the sensory aspects of perception and memory can be mapped. It is
becoming increasingly evident that cognitive information transcends
any of the traditional subdivisions of the cortex by structural or functional criteria (e.g., column, cytoarchitectonic area, thalamic projection, or receptive field). Thus, whereas the modular paradigm has
been most helpful to clarify the neural basis of sensations, it is inadequate to clarify the central substrates of perception or memory. Simply extrapolating principles of modular representation to larger cortical modules does not lead to the identification of those substrates.
This is one of those situations in science where the acquisition of
more knowledge with a tested and successful paradigm does not lead
to the solution of a crucial problem, as it may have been expected to
do by simply extending the paradigm's field of application. A radically
new paradigm seems needed for cortical cognition.

There is probably no more profound root of our present crisis
than the inveterate Aristotelian tendency to consider cognitive functions as separate entities. Surely we all recognize the common properties and interdependencies of perception, attention, memory, language, reasoning, and intelligence. Because of them, the psychologist
who studies any of those functions is under the imperative to select
the behavioral variables that best measure it and to control the others in some manner. This methodology, which is the foundation of experimental psychology, has been eminently successful. Thus, cognitive functions can be methodologically separated at the psychological
level. It does not follow, however, that they have separate neural substrates, although this is precisely the unfounded assumption that has
spilled into cortical neuroscience. Here that assumption resonates

well with some of the established evidence of localized sensory and motor functions that are essential components of cognition. The result of that encounter between unproven assumption and partial evidence is the notion that there is a cortical region, or module, for every cognitive function. This notion has caused endless confusion. It is a serious impediment to the study of the brain mechanisms of cognition. The neuropsychology literature first, and now the neuroimaging literature, are full of conflicting results and interpretations that derive from that dubious idea.

Nonetheless, a welcome change is underway. This change is the transition from the modular model to the network model of cognition. With this change, the network model retains some of the essential features of the modular one, in part because arguably networks are made up of modules. Most importantly, however, whereas the functional units of the module are assembled in a small parcel of cortical tissue, those of the network—which may be modules—are noncontiguous, widely dispersed in the cerebral mantle.

That transition from the modular model to a large-scale, widely distributed view of cortical cognition began many years ago on theoretical grounds and with scanty empirical evidence. Concepts of distributed cortical function were introduced by theoreticians and by neuropsychologists; the latter were driven by the failure of empirical attempts to localize memory in discrete cortical areas. The more concrete idea of the *neural network* originated outside of neurobiology, in the field of artificial intelligence, and reached full development with the doctrine of so-called connectionism. Only recently has the network concept begun to be recognized by some neurobiologists as a suitable paradigm of cognitive information and thus has begun to gain empirical momentum. Contributing to that momentum are numerous neuroimaging and microelectrode studies that advance our understanding of the topography and dynamics of cognitive networks in the cerebral cortex. Especially contributory is the microelectrode research in monkeys performing cognitive tasks, as this research is helping us elucidate network mechanisms.

This book is a chronicle of that shift of paradigms and of the new rules of discovery that it entails. It is, I dare say, the chronicle of an ongoing revolution, for the shift is nothing less than a revolution in contemporary neuroscience. In the following pages, I defend ideas that today have little currency. Here are the most salient among them: (*1*) cognitive information is represented in wide, overlapping, and interactive neuronal networks of the cerebral cortex; (2) such networks develop on a core of organized modules of elementary sensory and motor functions, to which they remain connected; (3) the cognitive code is a relational code, based on connectivity between discrete neuronal aggregates of the cortex (modules, assemblies, or network nodes); (4) the code's diversity and specificity derive from the myriad possibilities of combination of those neuronal aggregates between themselves; (5) any cortical neuron can be part of many networks, and thus of many percepts, memories, items of experience, or personal knowledge; (6) a network can serve several cognitive functions; and (7) cognitive functions consist of functional interactions within and between cortical networks.

In this book, the reader will find a critical review of the evidence supporting those ideas. My ultimate objective is to substantiate the correlations between a neural order and a phenomenal order, the isomorphism of cortex and mind. Essentially, this is an agenda of practical dualism that, in my opinion, allows us to get as close as we can by experiment to the unity, indeed identity, of the two. It is a difficult and ambitious agenda. It is also an exciting one, where scientific rigor must be used to temper speculation every step of the way. Unavoidably in these pages, the admissions of ignorance are bound to outnumber the speculative insights. Nevertheless, I make every effort to describe what we do know in terms that are understandable to an educated but not necessarily specialized readership. Above all, I make every effort to avoid unfalsifiable statements.

The history of this book is in some respects the history of my research on the cognitive functions of the primate brain. From its beginning, 45 years ago, when it dealt with the issue of attention in the brain of the monkey, this research has been informed, if not formed, by concepts derived from human psychology and psychophysics. In recent years, my data from microelectrode studies of the monkey's cortex have been increasingly supporting the large-scale network view of cognition, a holistic idea that clearly agrees with some of the tenets of Gestalt and cognitive psychology. Here I cannot refrain from quoting a 1975 statement by J. Z. Young: "Addiction to holistic concepts is indeed an occupational disease of neuroscientists (especially psychologists). But it is a curable disease from which one recovers by patient therapy with microscopy, microanalysis or microelectrodes." In this neuroscientist, I am afraid, the remedy has not worked; in fact, it has aggravated the disease!

Where does this book fit in the context of contemporary efforts by philosophers and scientists to understand the natural foundation of the human mind? The question is especially relevant now in view of the recent proliferation of books on the brain–mind issue. Most these books are written from the point of view of cognitive psychology or computer science. Some are exceedingly attractive, notably for their style, erudition, and wit. Unquestionably my approach differs considerably from that of their authors. For one thing, whereas their emphasis is on the mind side of the equation (equation indeed!), mine is on the brain side. I believe the time has come when the facts of cortical function have finally caught up with theory and when we can judiciously liberate mental functions from real or imaginary cortical geometries.

Analogies between developments in different sciences are usually contrived. Here, however, an analogy with physics seems eminently appropriate. I believe it is not farfetched to compare the transition from modular to network cognition with the transition from Newtonian to Einsteinian physics. The two transitions, I should say revolutions, resemble each other in more ways than one. For one thing, both are based on an expansion of the frame of reference. Curiously, *relativity* is at the root of both, though with different meanings of this term. Any neural element of cognition derives its meaning from its context and its relations to others. It is in this sense that the cognitive code is essentially a relational code. In modern physics, the essential relativity is that of physical phenomena to spatial–temporal frames. To follow the analogy further, modular cognition is a special case of network cognition, much as Newtonian physics is a special case of Einsteinian dynamics. Plausible as the analogy may seem, however, it should not be stretched too far. Neurocognition and modern physics deal with phenomena in vastly different scales and orders of probability.

Many helped me in my effort to bring these pages to light. In this effort, I benefited immeasurably from discussions with fellow scientists—too many for me to name here—who share my fascination with the subject matter. I owe special thanks to those respected friends among them who took the time to read and comment on various passages of the manuscript: Luciano Barajas, Jean-Pierre Changeux, Gerry Edelman, Keith Holyoak, Pasko Rakic, and John Schumann. My gratitude extends to those who attend the regular gathering of our BRI-sponsored affinity group on higher cognitive functions (cohosted by Arne Scheibel and me), and to the students there, as well as in my lab and elsewhere, who insist on defying conventional wisdom for the good of us all. I also wish to thank Mary Mettler for helping me with the references and Carmen Cox for the long and exacting job of preparing the manuscript for publication, which she did with unflagging enthusiasm from start to finish. To conclude this preface, I acknowledge with deep appreciation the help and advice of Fiona Stevens, of Oxford University Press, in this my second publishing project with her.

Contents

....

1 Introduction, 3

The Problem, 3

Cognitive Networks: Theory, 4

Cognitive Networks: Neuroscience, 11

The Cognit, 14

2 Neurobiology of Cortical Networks, 17

Phylogeny of the Cortex, 18

Ontogeny of the Cortex, 24

Cognitive Network Formation, 36

Extracortical Factors, 45

Basic Structure of Cognitive Networks, 49

3 Functional Architecture of the Cognit, 55

Structure of Knowledge in Connectionist Models, 56

Categories of Knowledge, 59

Cortical Modularity, 62

Cortical Hierarchy of Perceptual Networks, 67

Cortical Hierarchy of Executive Networks, 74

Heterarchical Representation in Association Cortex, 80

4 Perception, 83

Perceptual Categorization, 84
Gestalt, 87
Cortical Dynamics of Perception, 91
Perceptual Binding, 99
Perception-Action Cycle, 106

5 Memory, 111

Formation of Memory, 112
Short-Term Memory, 117
Perceptual Memory, 121
Executive Memory, 127
Retrieval of Memory, 132

6 Attention, 143

Biological Roots of Attention, 144
Perceptual Attention, 149
Working Memory, 155
Executive Attention, 164
Set and Expectancy, 167
Execution and Monitoring, 172

7 Language, 177

Neurobiology of Language, 178
Hemispheric Lateralization, 184
Neuropsychology of Language, 190
Functional Architecture of Semantics, 195
Cortical Dynamics of Syntax, 206

8 Intelligence, 213

Development of Intelligence, 214
Anatomy of Intelligence, 220
Reasoning, 224
Problem Solving, 231
Decision Making, 236
Creative Intelligence, 242

9 Epilogue on Consciousness, 249

References, 257

Index, 285

Cortex and Mind

1

Introduction

T hree categories of facts are in the purview of natural science: the physical reality, the brain, and the mind. Philosophers busy themselves attempting to determine whether these three categories of facts are reducible to two or perhaps just one; see Feigl (1967) for sharp discussion of the issue. However, from the perspective of the natural scientist, the structures, events, and processes within each category are arranged in a certain order that is known or knowable, and each is accessible to a different scientific methodology: physics, neuroscience, and cognitive science. The physical order and the neural order are unquestionably related to each other by causal links, for the second is part of the first. Whether there are causal links between the brain and the mind is an open question and will always remain so. This is not, however, a question that I pose to myself or to the reader of these pages.

The Problem

What I ask and try to answer here is whether the mental order corresponds to the order of structures, events, and processes in one part of the neural order, namely, the cerebral cortex. A priori, I would characterize that potential relationship as *isomorphic,* though I hesitate

to use this term because it has different connotations for different
people, and in this book I want to avoid what Roger Sperry called the
"semantic gymnastics" that the brain–mind problem ordinarily generates. For clarity and simplicity, here I shall define my agenda as the
search for a spatial and temporal order in the cerebral cortex that
matches the cognitive order in every respect. By this match I mean
that the spatial or temporal constituents of the cortical order occupy
the same relative place with respect to one another as the corresponding constituents of the cognitive order. Thus, a change or difference
in the cortical order corresponds to a change or difference in the
mental order. The relations between the two might be linear or nonlinear, on continuous or on ordinal scales. In any case, neural measures would correlate with behavioral or psychophysical measures of
cognitive variables or changing states. From the aggregate of such relations, if demonstrable, we could legitimately conclude that the two
orders are identical, and so are the structures, events, and processes
in them.

Because neither the cortical nor the cognitive order is well known,
however, we need working models of both to conduct our quest. The
cortical model should accommodate as much scientific evidence as we
now have on the cerebral cortex. The cognitive model should do the
same with psychological evidence. On cursory review of the literature,
it becomes readily apparent that such models already exist, at least in
rudimentary fashion. Some of them now thrive in their respective
fields, cortical neuroscience and cognitive psychology. The most plausible among them have a *network structure*. Thus, our principal endeavor in the ensuing chapters will be to map cognitive networks onto
cortical networks. Before undertaking this endeavor, however, it seems
useful to briefly review, with a historical perspective, the epistemology
of cognitive networks in the cerebral cortex.

Cognitive Networks: Theory

The cortical network model utilized in subsequent chapters matches
to a considerable degree some of the connectionist models in current
cognitive psychology. The match is fragmentary, however, in part because the two lines of network modeling have developed independently of each other as a reaction to questionable or untenable positions in their respective fields. The cortical network model is a
reasonable alternative to the anatomical reductionism of cognitive

functions fostered by sensory and motor neurophysiologists—and also, to some extent, by neuropsychologists. The connectionist models grew out of dissatisfaction with abstract and computer-like cognitive models.

Whereas the cortical network model has taken over a century to develop after the discovery of its basic elements (neurons, fibers, and synapses), the connectionist models have taken much less time, products as they are of the computer revolution. There are other reasons for the different developmental periods of cortical and cognitive models and for their uneven race to what I see as their contemporary convergence. Despite early evidence for the distributed nature of cortical representations, the cortical network model has long been held back by a wealth of anatomical discoveries and neurological findings that seem to endorse modular or localizationist views of cognition. By contrast, connectionism has a much narrower base and has developed mostly on theoretical grounds—impatient, we might say, with the ignorance of neuroscientists and studiously eluding their debate on cortical representation.

That debate has been going on for more than a century and a half. Two sharply different schools of thought have engaged in it. On one side are those who advocate the *localization* of cognitive functions in different cortical regions. Their pioneers were Gall (1825) and Broca (1861), who made much of the apparent cortical localization of speech—the first for a spurious reason, the second for a sound one. Since the early stages of the debate, the localizationists have held the empirical high ground. They support their position with evidence that the cortex is divided into many areas of differing microscopic structure, each with separate connections. If the cortex supports cognition, and if different cortical areas have different structure and connections, it seems reasonable to think, as they do, that each area has a different cognitive function. Besides, there is the indisputable physiological specialization of certain areas in sensory and motor functions that are the foundation of cognition, the *primitives* of perception and of other cognitive functions. Then there are the neurologists' countless observations of the special disorders of perception, attention, memory, and speech that result from certain cortical lesions.

On the other side are those who think that cognitive functions are based on widely *distributed* cortical systems of interconnected neurons, systems that transcend anatomical areas and modules, however defined. The position of these *holistic* neuroscientists has been consis-

tently weaker because of the localizationist evidence against their
ideas and the lack of conclusive evidence to support them. In any case,
their argument goes somewhat as follows. Yes, in the cortex there are
separate areas and physiological modules, each with its connections
and special computational algorithms. They specialize in myriad
forms of sensation and movement. But those areas and modules simply constitute the lower stages of neural processing hierarchies *toward*
cognition. The cognitive functions of perceiving, remembering, recognizing, reasoning, and understanding, as well as language, rest on
vast territories of cortex that include, but certainly extend well beyond, those specialized areas and modules.

From early on in the history of neuroscience, the holistic concept
of cortical cognition had many distinguished proponents, such as Von
Monakow (1914) and Jackson (1958). They found a powerful ally on
the psychological side in the school of *Gestalt psychology* (Köhler, 1929;
Koffka, 1935; Wertheimer, 1967). The Gestalt psychologists' principal
area of interest was perception, especially visual perception. They argued that any perceived object (a *segregated whole*) has an organized
structure that transcends its physical components. This tenet is what
is meant by the common assertion that the whole, the percept, is
"more than the sum of the parts," a vague statement that begs a number of questions, for example, What are the parts that could conceivably be summed and how would they be summed? A more telling
statement is that the entire object of perception emerges from the
binding of elementary sensory parts; that what matters to the organism is the organization, the *relations* between those parts, and that
those relations cannot be undone without the object losing its identity. The Gestaltists maintained that the object was inborn, *given* in its
entirety, and, according to some of them, represented by some kind
of electric field in the cerebral cortex. There is not a hint of evidence
to support that nativist notion or the neuroelectrical substrate of
Gestalts (forms or structures) other than possibly in the primary visual
cortex. Yet the notion of the emergence of perception out of relations
between sensory elements (Chapter 4) has an enormous importance
in cognitive science and will remain a lasting contribution of Gestalt
psychology to the cognitive neuroscience of the cerebral cortex.

It was not until recent years that holistic views began to gain momentum in cognitive neuroscience. The first to challenge experimentally the old—but today still prevalent—views of cognitive localizationism was Karl Lashley (1950), a neuropsychologist. His careful analysis

of the effects of lesions of discrete cortical areas failed to reveal any deficits in discrimination or memory. With his negative results and the inferences he drew from them, and despite his puzzlement ("I sometime feel, on reviewing the evidence on the localization of the memory trace, . . . that learning just is not possible," he writes), Lashley helped to establish the groundwork for an integrative view of discrimination and memory, and of cognition in general. Throughout the article cited, he speculated about patterns of integrated neurons and about broad cortical systems of organized functions. Even more relevant to our theme are his conjectures that "the engram is represented thoughout a cortical region" and that "the same neurons which retain the memory traces of one experience must also participate in countless other activities." Thus, Lashley established the experimental foundation for distributed representation in the cerebral cortex and for the notion that its neuronal substrate serves assorted cognitive functions.

It was up to theoreticians of the brain to transform a conceptual undercurrent in favor of distributed representation into the concept of *cortical network*. Hebb (1949) proposed the idea in a structurally and dynamically limited sense by postulating that short-term memory consisted in the reverberation of excitation in discrete cortical nets or cell assemblies with the assistance of feedback loops. Further, he postulated certain principles of plasticity in synaptic contacts that would be the basis for the formation of memory. One of them is the principle of the temporal coincidence of sensory inputs. Two sensory inputs arriving in a neuron at the same time, he wrote, will induce permanent synaptic changes, such that the neuron's subsequent response to either of them *alone* will have been facilitated. Those changes would lead to the formation of net-like assemblies that represent the features of repeatedly coincident stimuli.

Friedrich Hayek (1952) was the first to propose the representation of percepts and memories in large-scale cortical networks of the kind proposed in this book. That was a curious intellectual development in several respects, for one thing because Hayek was neither a brain scientist nor a psychologist. He was an eminent economist (Nobel Prize, 1978) with a broad and profound interest in complex systems, including the economy of nations (his ideas have profoundly influenced modern governments). In addition to the economy, society of course is a complex system; another is the brain, and yet another is the cerebral cortex within it. All were the objects of Hayek's intense study. His sociological writings, like his economic writings, are very well known (his *Road to Serfdom*, 1944, is a towering classic). Much less well known is *The Sensory Order* (1952), his psychological essay. Yet this is one of the most scholarly contributions ever made to the understanding of the cerebral foundation of perception and memory. Its intellectual roots can be traced to the works of Müller (Johannes), Mach, Boring, Lashley, Hebb, Klüver, and the Gestalt psychologists, with all of which Hayek was thoroughly familiar. By and large, therefore, psychology was the ground on which his thinking developed, though with a view of the cerebral cortex that was highly advanced for his time.

The essence of Hayek's theory is the proposition that all of an organism's experience is stored in network-like systems (*maps*) of connections between the neurons of its cerebral cortex. Those connections—as Hebb also postulated in a limited sense—have been formed by the temporal coincidence of inputs from various sources (including the organism itself). In their strength, those connections record the frequency and probability with which those inputs have occurred together in the history of the organism *or of the species*. Perception is an act of classification of objects by those network-like systems of connections formed by prior experience with those objects. A key point, in terms of the representational properties of Hayek's model, is that there is no basic core of elementary sensation; that each sensation derives from experience and from other sensations with which it has been temporally associated in the past, including the past of the species. Thus, throughout the cerebral cortex, association becomes the essence of sensation, perception, and memory. Of course, to postulate in the human cortex representation networks as broad as those envisioned by Hayek presupposes extensive and intricate systems of connections between distant cortical neurons. It was an insightful supposition that he made long before such systems were anatomically demonstrated in the brain of the primate.

Twenty-five years later, with a better understanding of cortical connectivity and the physiology of sensory areas, Edelman and Mountcastle (1978) developed their concept of cortically distributed functions, which also assumes a cortical network-like structure. Extrapolating to the entire cortex the anatomical and physiological modularity of sensory areas, they theorized that learning, memory, and perception are widely distributed in interconnected cortical modules or cell-columns. Furthermore, Edelman (1987), largely based on analogies with evolution and immunology, launched an elaborate theory of learning that he named the theory of *group selection*. According to it, groups of cortical neurons are "selected" from an inborn repertoire by contact with the environment, thus becoming organized to perform a variety of representational functions. At the same time, unutilized groups recede and disappear (in accord with the evidence of postnatal recession of initially overproduced neurons and synapses). Essential for the selection and dynamics of those groups is the principle of *reentry*, which is an almost universal rule of neural connectivity. In analogy with immune-system processes, Edelman introduced in the cortex the principle of *degeneracy*, which states that there are several more or less effective ways for an assembly of neuronal groups to recognize an object and to act upon it.

While these developments in brain theory were taking place, cognitive and computer scientists also arrived at the network concept of information representation and processing. They did it through the route of artificial intelligence (AI). From its beginning, it was AI's avowed purpose to construct models of Turing machines, computers and robots that performed cognitive functions like those of the human brain. Among the most interesting early efforts were those produced by Pitts and McCulloch (1947), who constructed what now would be interpreted as network models of neural circuitry to perform perceptual and abstract functions. Though mistakenly attributing binary properties—fire or not fire—to real neurons, they effectively simulated those cognitive operations artificially and computationally. In theirs, as in all artificial models of the brain and "thinking machines" (Ashby, 1948; McCulloch, 1948; Wiener, 1948; Braitenberg, 1996), feedback was an essential mechanism. Indeed, feedback is the essence of cybernetics and a critical feature of all those machines that appear to conduct purposeful behavior. The principle of recurrence or reentry, which had been anatomically substantiated in the cerebral cortex (Lorente de Nó, 1938) and which Hebb (1949) used in order to construe the reverberation of short-term memory, emerges again here, in AI, as an essential component of artificial networks.

Connectionism developed from AI by further adopting neurally plausible network concepts. It applied those concepts hypothetically, and in some cases computationally, to the functions of neural structures such as the cerebellum, the retina, and the hippocampus, in addition to the neocortex (Marr, 1970; Grossberg, 1980; Palm, 1982). Especially applicable to my approach are the contributions by Kohonen

(1977, 1984). The central idea in his work is that of *self-organizing* associative memory networks in the neocortex, especially in the so-called
cortex of association. His thinking originates in hebbian concepts,
such as those of the cell assembly and the association of inputs by temporal coincidence. Cell assemblies, representing partial features of
sensory experience, would constitute the "nodes" of a memory network. Instead of presupposing a central agency to organize learning,
Kohonen proposes that the self-organization by hebbian principles
suffices for the acquisition of learning and memory (*unsupervised learning*). Memory would be acquired by the opening of new paths, that is,
by synaptic facilitation and autonomous expansion of cortical networks
as a result of sensory experience. Perception and recognition would
essentially be processes of completion by association: a part of a memory (e.g., a face, part of a picture) would, by association, activate the
entire network and thus evoke all of its associated components (e.g.,
the name, the place).

The acquisition and retrieval of memory, as well as perception
and other cognitive functions of a cortical network, do not have to be
serial processes, as in most modern computers. It is reasonable to suppose that in the real brain those processes take place to a very large
extent in parallel—and, as we will see, largely outside of consciousness. That line of reasoning gave rise to the concept of *parallel distributed processing* (PDP), which is the core of modern connectionism, first
described in two well-known volumes (McClelland and Rumelhart,
1986; Rumelhart and McClelland, 1986). Parallel networks with feedforward and feedback processing have become the hallmark of many
connectionist models of cognitive science.

Although connectionism has borrowed many neurobiological
concepts, it has not yet absorbed the full impact of recent neuroscience. So far, connectionism is a useful way of thinking about how,
in principle, neural networks could develop and do their job in cognitive function, but it does not solve any specific neural problem—
despite the use (rather, misuse) of the term *neural* for many of its constructs. Both the modeling and the computation that connectionism
offers will remain plausible but not definitive until real neural constraints are fully known and applied to its models. This is especially
true with regard to the cerebral cortex, where so much was unknown
50 years ago, when connectionism got started, and where so much still
remains unknown.

Cognitive Networks: Neuroscience

Three general fields of neuroscience are contributing significantly to our knowledge of the structure and functions of cortical networks, and thus to the applications of connectionism to cognitive neuroscience. The first, historically, is the field of cortical axonal *connectivity*. The connections of the cortex with subcortical structures, notably the thalamus, have been essentially well known for a long time. However, the old dictum that "the thalamus is the key to cortical functions" does not seem to apply to the cortex of association, which performs the major share of any cognitive function. Of course, the sensory functions of primary sensory cortical areas are best understood when inputs from specific sensory thalamic nuclei are taken into account. Not much is known, however, about the role of thalamic projections to associative cortex or about the nuclei in which they originate. In any case, it is the connectivity between cortical associative areas that appears most essential to any model of cortical network cognition and to the physiology of cortical networks in cognition.

Although the study of connections between cortical areas started long ago with axon-degeneration and neuronography methods, it did not take off as a major methodology until the advances in silver-staining methods of the 1960s. Later it received a major impetus with the extensive application of axon-transport methods (which had been discovered much earlier, in 1945, by Paul Weiss and his colleagues). These methods were later complemented by immunological and molecular methods, which have decisively clarified cortical synaptic transmitters and modulators. In the past three decades, a wealth of information has been acquired about the intrinsic and extrinsic connections of practically every region and subregion of the primate's cortex. Especially worthy of mention are the contributions by the laboratories of Nauta, Jones, Pandya, Goldman-Rakic, Jacobson, Reinoso-Suárez, and Barbas.

Electrophysiology is the second source of empirical support for elucidating cortical cognitive networks and their functional architecture. Since the discovery of the electroencephalogram (EEG) by Berger (1929), cortical field potentials have been extensively used as a means of assessing correlations between the activity of cortical neurons and cognitive states or functions. The EEG of the cortex, whether recorded from the surface of the scalp or from the cortex itself, is the time-honored method for determining global conditions of consciousness, such as the depth of sleep, the level of arousal, and the intensity of attention. However, more focused views of the topography and operations of cognitive networks are provided by the study of field evoked potentials, also called *event-related potentials* (ERPs). Changes in ERPs reflect cognitive operations—on the stimuli that elicit them— in discrete areas of the cortex. The method has proven useful in both humans and animals.

Especially contributory to the concept of cognitive network is the microelectrode study of the electrical discharge of cortical neurons in monkeys performing cognitive tasks. It appears paradoxical that the study of single cells could contribute to our understanding of the functions of vast cortical networks interconnecting myriad neurons. Indeed, having worked for many years with microelectrodes, I am often asked such questions as "How can anyone hope to draw inferences about the architecture and functions of cortical networks from such a narrow empirical base as the single cell?" The answer, in part, lies in the repeated application of the microelectrode method to multiple areas of cortex under controlled experimental conditions. For example, after recording active cells in several cortical areas in monkeys memorizing the same visual stimulus in the same memory task, the idea dawned on us that the active memory of that stimulus was distributed in those areas. In any case, microelectrode records provide us with the only tool now available for exploring *mechanisms* of cognitive function in cortical networks. It seems that only such records allow us to explore the algorithms of cognition and to develop realistic models of it.

The third source of network evidence is *neuroimaging*. A priori, it seems that *if* we were able to visualize neuronal activity continuously in the entirety of an individual's cortex, we would be able to figure out the extent of cortical networks and how they work in cognition. That *if* looms large, however, for there are daunting problems in the imaging methodology that remain unresolved. Among them is the problem of limited spatial and temporal resolution, though considerable progress has lately been made in increasing both. More fundamental and difficult to solve is the problem of the biophysical relationships, still largely unknown, between cerebral blood flow, metabolism, and neuronal activity. The issue is critical, because the blood-flow or metabolic image is a derivative of neuronal change, though with a different time course, which probably takes the image out of the temporal range of many cognitive changes and differences. For discussion of some of these methodological problems, the reader is referred to Raichle (1994) and Logothetis et al. (2001). Despite the difficulties, neuroimaging, especially by positron emission tomography (PET) and functional magnetic resonance imaging (fMRI), has contributed decisively to our understanding of the topography of cortical networks in certain cognitive functions.

Let us briefly reconsider our problem, as I stated it at the beginning of this introduction, in the light of the empirical methods just mentioned. It is my purpose, I said, to study relationships between structures, events, and processes in two spheres, neural and cognitive. Clearly, to achieve that purpose, the issue of *scaling* is going to be important. The establishment of isomorphism or topology between the two orders, neural and cognitive, requires brain scales with ranges and resolutions commensurate to those of cognitive phenomena, whether the latter occur on ordinal or continuous scales. Structurally, the brain space of cortical networks can be reasonably defined in metric coordinates, both in depth and in surface. Suitable resolutions of measurement should range from the size of cortical cell assemblies (e.g., cortical columns) to the length of cortico-cortical connections in the corpus callosum and the uncinate fasciculus. The matching of cerebral and cognitive times also requires appropriate scales and resolutions. The time scale of cortical processes and events should be commensurate with that of cognitive processes and events.

To sum up in general terms, the cortical network paradigm of cognition requires that both scales of measurement, spatial and temporal, be expanded beyond those that the sensory or motor physiologist is familiar with. In primitive organisms and in lower levels of the mammalian nervous system, single cells and single action potentials are functionally consequential. In the electric fish, the length of the interval between succeeding potentials is relevant down to the millisecond. None of this seems to apply to the cerebral cortex. Here hundreds or even thousands of cells may be lost without loss of function. Moreover, signals are not encoded by individual spikes but, instead, by groups or trains of spikes in cell populations. Of course, if large areas are damaged, function is compromised, in some cases dramatically. The same is true if neuron activity is depressed for substantial periods of time. Some of the available network models of cognition provide a suitable structure to match a cortical network, and thus they are in principle suitable to test relationships between neural and cognitive orders. The functional architecture of those models allows them to classify knowledge into specific combinations of physical and symbolic attributes, as required for perceptual and memory functions. Some of the models (propositional and semantic networks) can perform logical or linguistic operations (Anderson, 1995). Still, however, most of the published models lack the spatial or temporal constraints that would make them plausible in terms of neural or cognitive function.

The Cognit

To characterize the cognitive structure of a cortical network, I use the term *cognit,* a generic term for any representation of knowledge in the cerebral cortex. A cognit is an item of knowledge about the world, the self, or the relations between them. Its network structure is made up of elementary representations of perception or action that have been associated with one another by learning or past experience. These smaller units of representation constitute the nodes of the network, which themselves may also have a network structure at a more simple level (thus cognits within cognits). In any case, a cognit is defined by its component nodes *and* by the relations between them. In neural terms, the cognit is made up of assemblies of neurons and the connections between them. Any cortical cell assembly can be part of many cognits or networks. Inasmuch as cognits and cognitive networks coincide, the individuality of human knowledge derives from the practically unlimited possible combinations of neurons or subsets of them in a reservoir of 10 billion cortical neurons.

Cognits are the structural substrate of all cognitive operations— their raw material, so to speak. Arguably, some elementary cognits are innate (e.g., color perception, essential grammatical knowledge). The innate character of any form of knowledge, however, is not an essential premise of my argument. What is essential here is that cognits are made up of smaller structures of representation, some of which may be innate. Further, cognits are dynamic structures, subject to change with new experience. In cognitive development, the organism forms cognits of progressively greater magnitude and complexity by associations in space and time and by similarity. At the same time, by sensory discrimination and by reasoning—both inductive and deductive—the organism fragments cognits into cognitive categories of smaller magnitude or finer distinction between them. Learning takes place by the formation of new cognits from old ones, by composition and decomposition of preexistent cognits. This, incidentally, is also the essence of progress in science.

Cognits, the networks of knowledge that I postulate in the cortex, have immense variety in terms of their information content, their complexity, and the number and nature of their components. Their topography, that is, the architecture of the cortical networks that represent them, is just as variable. Their elemental sensory and motor components, however, are represented in relatively discrete locations of primary sensory and motor cortex that are mostly invariant from one individual to another. Because those elements of cognition are common to a large number of cognits, they are part of a large number of cortical networks. Those elements in primary cortex constitute the pillars at the base of a great many networks that fan out and upward into cortex of association. How those networks develop is a subject for the next chapter. In principle, the more complex a cognit is, and the more components it has, the wider is its cortical network. Further, as an item of knowledge becomes more specialized, personal, or idiosyncratic, the cortical network that represents it presumably differs more from one individual to the next, at least inasmuch as that same item has been acquired differently by different individuals.

It is a central tenet of this monograph that all cognitive functions consist in transactions of information within and between cognits. Thus, to the extent that cognits are represented in cortical networks, all cognitive operations are assumed to take place within and between cortical networks. Further, any cognit or cortical network can be the object of any cognitive operation. In other words, the same cortical networks can be used in perception, attention, memory, intellectual performance, and language. Different cognits have different and specific cortical distributions, but none of those different cognitive functions does. At any given time, a given cognitive function has the distribution of the active cognits on which the function is operating. It is the cognits and their networks that have topographic specificity, not the functions that use them. This, in my view, is a critical point.

This approach to neurocognition, of course, departs from the view that different cognitive functions reside in different brain locations. It is an approach more germane to the holistic notions of higher brain functions that I mentioned above in historical context. In cognitive neuroscience, it is beginning to be accepted that certain functions, such as memory and language, have wide cortical distributions, but it is still commonly held that these distributions are different for

different functions; in other words, that separate areas or regions of
the cortex are devoted to attention, to memory, to language, and so
on. Such notions, I believe, derive from faulty interpretation of facts.
For example, the results of stimulation or lesioning of certain cortical areas on a cognitive function, or the metabolic activation of those
areas during a behavioral task that depends on that function, are often
considered evidence for the cortical localization of the function. Instead, it may be evidence for the topography of the cognitive substrate
(i.e., the cognit, the cortical net) on which the function is active.

Thus, according to the point of view that has inspired this monograph, cognitive functions per se have no definite cortical topography.
Nonetheless, even if the five functions to be considered later in this
book share the same structural substrate, they will be discussed in separate chapters. The main reason for their separate discussion is the
compelling assumption of different neural mechanisms for each, even
though they are closely entwined with one another. To wit, perception
is part of the acquisition and retrieval of memory; memory stores information acquired by perception; language and memory depend on
each other; language and logical reasoning are special forms of cognitive action; attention serves all the other functions; intelligence is
served by all; and so on. In conclusion, for reasons of methodology,
temporal or spatial order needs to be analyzed separately for each
function. This is also true for the neural mechanisms that support
both the order and the function. Separate analyses and mechanisms
do not, however, imply separate neuroanatomical substrates. It should
be apparent in the ensuing chapters that any cognit or cortical network can serve several cognitive functions.

2

Neurobiology of Cortical Networks

*I*n this chapter I outline the present state of knowledge on the development of cortical networks, the postulated substrate of all cognitive functions. Separate sections are devoted to the ontogeny and phylogeny of the cortex, although the two are inextricably related. Much has been inferred about the evolution of the cortex from its development in the individual organism. Conversely, certain principles of natural selection at the core of evolution theory have been deftly applied to current reasoning on the development of neocortical structure and function. A persuasive line of reasoning is emerging on the interplay of genetic factors with neural activity and individual experience in the development of the neocortex. Nowhere is that line of reasoning more relevant to cognition than on the issue of cortical connectivity and its constituents, the synapses, axons, and dendrites that bind neocortical neurons into cognitive networks. This chapter deals successively with the evolution and ontogenetic development of the cortex, the principles of network formation, including the role of extracortical factors in that process, and the general structural characteristics of cognitive networks. Subsequent chapters will deal with their functional architecture and dynamics in each of the cognitive functions.

Phylogeny of the Cortex

Some 250 million years ago, in the early Mesozoic, a group of early reptiles (Therapsids) developed mammalian features. For a long time, scholars have considered them the earliest known mammals (for recent discussions, see Allman, 1984; Carroll, 1988; Jerison, 1990). One of those features was a new laminar neural structure in the dorsal aspect of the cerebrum or telencephalon, between the medially placed hippocampal pallium and the lateral—olfactory or piriform—pallium. That interposed *neopallium* (new mantle) was the structural precursor of the mammalian neocortex (Fig. 2.1). The precise evolutionary origin of this structure is a matter of unresolved debate (Northcutt and Kaas, 1995). Some argue that it derives, phylogenetically as well as ontogenetically, from the expansion of the other two

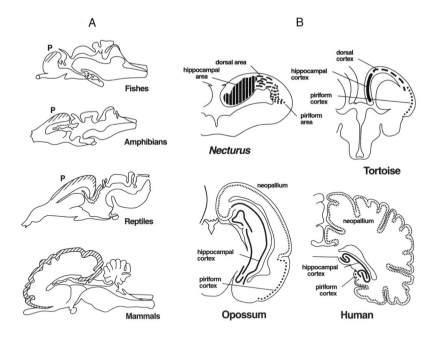

Figure 2.1. Diagrams of phylogenetic development of the cerebral cortex. *A:* Parasaggital sections of the brain in five classes of vertebrates; P, *pallium,* a generic evolutionary term for all cortex, paleocortex and neocortex. From Creutzfeldt (1993), after Edinger modified. *B:* Coronal sections of *Necturus,* a primitive amphibian, the box tortoise *(Cistudo),* the Virginia opossum *(Didelphis),* and the human. From Herrick (1956), modified.

mentioned telencephalic structures, one of them contributing to the new cortex a hippocampal germinal moiety and the other a lateral, olfactory, moiety (Sanides, 1970; Pandya et al., 1988). Others propose that the neocortex derives from a structure deeper in the telencephalon, the dorsal ventricular ridge (Karten, 1969; Butler, 1994), though this has been disputed (Aboitiz, 1999). There is no dispute, however, about the global homology of the neocortex in all mammals—though the homology of its individual areas is debatable. Nor is there dispute about the obvious retrospective evidence that the evolutionary development of neocortex has directly contributed to better adaptation to the environment, better communication with conspecifics, and longer life.

Comparative anatomy suggests that the cortex of those mammal-like reptiles, contemporaries of the early dinosaurs, was similar to that of certain amphibians now living, which consists essentially of one simple layer or zone of pyramidal cells with radially arranged apical dendrites (Herrick, 1956; Kemali and Braitenberg, 1969). Subsequent species in the mammalian lineage, however, are endowed with the characteristic layered structure of the neocortex, which, because of its uniformity throughout, has also been termed *isocortex*. Furthermore, comparative anatomy and the study of fossil records—such as that of cranial endocasts—substantiate the general conclusion that the neocortex has acquired mass as a function of evolution. In other words, as mammalian species evolve, their neocortex becomes larger and heavier (Stephan et al., 1981); this is the process of so-called neocorticalization (Jerison, 1990). In this process, which culminates in primates, the size of all brain structures maintains in all species a predictable relationship to brain size. That relationship, however, is nonlinear to varying degrees, depending on the structure (Finlay and Darlington, 1995). The deviation from linearity is maximal for the neocortices of primates (Fig. 2.2). In the 50 million years of primate evolution, as primate species evolve from prosimians to monkeys, to pongids, to the last hominid (*Homo sapiens,* first appearing about 250,000 years ago), the relative size of the neocortex accelerates; it grows disproportionately to such a degree that it seems legitimate to speak of a "neocortical explosion."

Since the cortex is a laminar structure, it is appropriate to ask whether its evolutionary enlargement takes place in thickness or in surface, or both. The answer is both, but disproportionately in favor

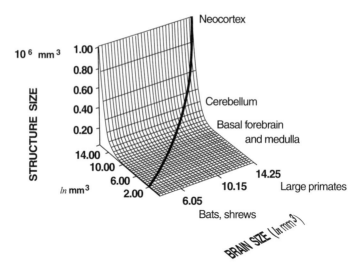

Figure 2.2. Marked increase in the volume of the neocortex (thick line) in the larger primates (human, chimpanzee, gorilla, and baboon). From Finlay and Darlington (1995), with permission.

of surface. With evolution, cortical thickness increases (Igarashi and Kamiya, 1972; Rockel et al., 1980), as can be inferred from measurements in assorted species of varying evolutionary age (Fig. 2.3). With thickening of the cortex, however, cell density tends to decrease (Jerison, 1973). In functional terms, more consequential than cortical thickening is the much greater evolutionary growth of the neocortex in surface. During evolution, the neocortex expands much more rapidly than the archicortex (hippocampal) and the paleocortex (olfactory), which flank it on either side. That expansion—about 1000-fold from mouse to man—is achieved by multiplication of the radial columnar units with relatively uniform cell numbers that, as we will see in the next section, constitute the basic elements of cortical ontogeny (Rakic, 1995). It is through the proliferation and apposition of those basic modules that new cortical areas are formed in the course of evolution (Northcutt and Kaas, 1995). Because the new areas develop out of simpler ones, they do not necessarily hold structural or functional homology from one species to another.

Changes in brain mass, however, do not provide more than a crude perspective of evolution in terms of neural function (Holloway,

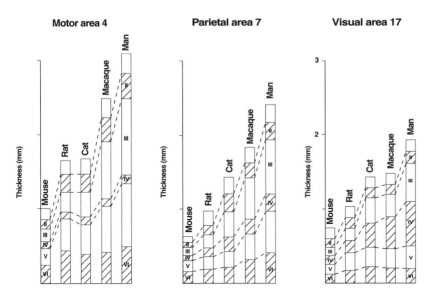

Figure 2.3. Thickness of the cortex of motor, parietal, and visual areas in several species. From Rockel et al. (1980), with permission.

1983). In the case of the neocortex, a better perspective is given by interspecies differences in cytoarchitecture, electrophysiology, and, above all, connectivity. Early mammals, at some stage after the ancestral Therapsids, already possessed the typical six-layer isocortex that is characteristic of present mammals. They did not have, however, the diversity of cytoarchitectonically and functionally distinct cortical areas of later species.

The comparative studies of living mammals by anatomical and physiological methods allow a degree of retrospective insight into the evolutionary development of the various cortical areas. Such studies are most instructive as they deal with sensory areas. The same five sensory modalities appear to be represented in the neocortex of innumerable species over a large phyletic range. Topographic cortical maps for vision and somesthesis are present in the earliest mammals (Northcutt and Kaas, 1995). What varies, and greatly, are the number of *specialized cortical areas* for each modality and the precision and range of their representational properties. In cortical evolution, parsimony and variability go hand in hand. An essential genome for the basic sensory and motor functions of the neocortex can cover the basic adaptive needs of all mammalian species, while slight modifications in that genome can generate enormous variability in behavior and cognitive ability (Krubitzer, 1995).

The biological process by which sensory cortical areas proliferate in the course of mammalian evolution is not yet known, though it is a subject of much research and discussion (see Deacon, 1990, for review). It has been suggested that the process may essentially consist in the duplication of areas by genetic mutation (Allman and Kaas, 1971; Fukuchi-Shimogori and Grove, 2001; Rakic, 2001). The concept appears plausible; for one thing, it is in accord with ontogenetic trends, especially in myelination. What appears untenable is the notion that, in primitive mammals, areas of undifferentiated cortex, which would correspond to what is now commonly understood by the term *association cortex,* somehow gave rise to the specialized sensory and motor areas. This hypothetical trend from nonspecificity to specificity is at odds with the evidence that some of those primitive organisms already had multiple and highly specialized cortical fields (Crewther et al., 1984; Krubitzer et al., 1995).

Most relevant to the phylogenesis of cognitive networks is the evolution of neocortical connectivity. Two categories of available data are especially revealing in this respect: one has to do with the dendrites of neocortical neurons, the other with the subcortical and callosal white matter. As noted above, the neocortex of mammals thickens with evolution, and this thickening is accompanied by a general diminution of neuronal density. This occurs even though both the lateral packing of neurons and their number per vertical column may stay roughly the same from the prosimian—and from the mouse— to man (Rockel et al., 1980). These changes occur together with the vertical *elongation of the dendritic processes* of pyramidal neurons. Such elongation is most conspicuous in the large pyramids of deeper cortical layers—V and VI—whose apical dendrites reach the superficial plexiform layer (I).

The elongation of dendrites has been documented by comparative and ontogenetic studies of the neocortex of several mammals by use of the Golgi staining method (Marín-Padilla, 1978, 1992). Such studies transpose to the phylogenetic domain the ontogenetic *sequence* that has now been established by other methods (see below, Rakic). The sequence consists of the following events: (*1*) formation of a primordial plexiform layer under the cortical surface, (2) formation, within it, of the cortical plate, which is the base for the layered adult neocortex and the destination of cells migrating—"inside out"— from the underlying ventricular zone, (3) outward migration of cells from that zone to the upper layer of the cortical plate, (4) relative descent of cell bodies to deeper cortex, and (5) proliferation of cortical layers—II to VI and their subdivisions—as descending cells settle at various distances from the surface. The first cells to migrate outward become situated in a deep layer as new generations of cells bypass the older ones (Rakic, 1974). The end result of these events is that, in the adult, cells are stacked up by order of antiquity, the older cells in deep layers and the younger in upper layers. Nonpyramidal cells, in their descent, lose their contact with the plexiform layer (I), while pyramidal cells retain it, and subsequently "hang" from that layer, so to speak, by their apical dendrite. As a consequence, pyramids generally lengthen their apical dendrites as a function of development. The older and larger pyramids in layers V and VI have the longest apical dendrites. Given that dendritic length correlates with spine numbers and synaptic contacts, the ontogenetic and phylogenetic prolongation of apical dendrites undoubtedly connotes a vast increase in the integrative and combinatorial, network-forming, power of neocortical pyramidal neurons.

The massive development of subcortical white matter (corpus callosum included) is another indication of the accelerating expansion of neocortical connectivity that takes place in the course of evolution (Fig. 2.4). In insectivores and primates, the volume of white matter under the neocortex (as measured relative to body size) increases even more rapidly than that of the neocortex itself (Frahm et al., 1982; Zhang and Sejnowski, 2000), which we have seen "exploding" in evolution. In a small insectivore *(Sorex minutus)*, the white matter constitutes volumetrically 6.7% of the aggregate neocortex–white matter, whereas in the human it reaches 41.9%.

In conclusion, the addition of neocortical areas and columns, the prolongation of apical dendrites, and the expansion of white matter reflect a phyletic increase, by several orders of magnitude, in the capacity of neocortical neurons to connect with one another and thus to form representational and operant networks. Logically from this perspective, those networks reach in the human brain their greatest complexity and ability to serve cognition.

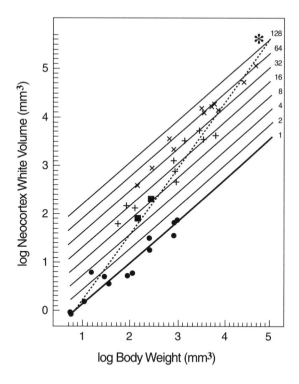

Figure 2.4. Volume of neocortical white matter plotted against body weight in double logarithmic scales. The thick reference line runs through averages from insectivores. (Thinner parallel lines, in multiples of 2, refer to size indices calculated from that reference.) The stippled line is the regression line for a total of 38 species: 13 insectivores (black circles), 2 tree shrews (black squares), 10 prosimians (+), 12 nonhuman simians (×), and man (asterisk). From Frahm et al. (1982), with permission.

Ontogeny of the Cortex

In ontogeny, as in evolution, the neocortex develops much more in size and volume than any other neuronal structure of the brain. Again this is especially true for the human, in whom the adult neocortex reaches maximum development—relative to brain and body size—in both thickness and spread (Fig. 2.5). Also in the human, from embryo to adult, the relative growth of the white matter underlying the cortex and associated with it—literally, its connective infrastructure—surpasses by far that of white matter elsewhere in the central nervous system.

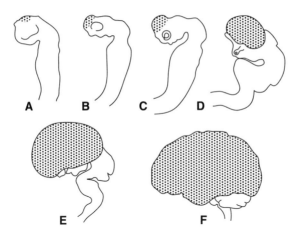

Figure 2.5. Sketches of human brain at various developmental stages to illustrate relative growth of cortex (stippled). *A* to *E,* prenatal: *A,* 2 weeks; *B,* 3 weeks; *C,* 4 weeks; *D,* 8 weeks; *E,* 6 months; *F,* adult. From Herrick (1956), with permission.

The neocortex emerges out of a germinal or proliferative layer of primordial cells lining the anterodorsal aspect of the neuroepithelium in the ventricular wall of the neural tube. Out of that germinal layer the neuroblasts proliferate that are to become cortical neurons (Rakic, 1988). In the course of embryogenesis, the newly formed neurons from the proliferative ventricular zone migrate in successive waves toward a stratum right under the surface of the potential cortex, the *cortical plate* (Fig. 2.6). The neurons migrate radially along glial fibers, apparently guided in accord with a contact-adhesion principle similar to that first postulated by Weiss (1939); in addition, the neurons migrate under some kind of attractive influence from developing thalamocortical and corticocortical axons (Rakic, 1981b). As they migrate, new cells overtake the older ones, which then descend in cortical depth as if pushed downward by the new arrivals. Consequently, as noted above with regard to pyramidal neurons in phylogeny, cells stack up in the cortical plate by order of antiquity, older cells in deeper cortex and newer ones above. As the process continues with successive neuron migrations and growth, the cortical plate thickens and the distance from proliferative zone to piamater, which in early embryogenesis is only $200-300$ μm, increases to the more than 2 mm of the fully developed cortex.

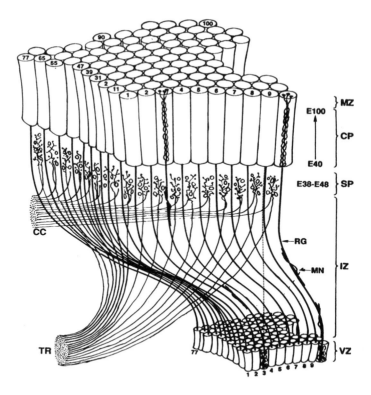

Figure 2.6. Migration of neurons, guided by glial fibers (RG), from the proliferative ventricular zone (VZ) to the cortical plate (CP) in the course of embryogenesis of the monkey. Throughout prenatal development, a topological relationship of neuronal migration is maintained between the columns of the proliferative zone and those of the expanding cortical plate. *Abbreviations:* CC, corticocortical connections; E, embryological age (in days); IZ, intermediate zone; MN, migrating neuron; MZ, marginal zone; SP, subplate; TR, thalamic radiation. From Rakic (1988), with permission.

Pasko Rakic, who has extensively investigated these processes in the human and the rhesus monkey (Sidman and Rakic, 1973; Rakic, 1981a, 1988, 1995), postulates that the ependymal cover of the embryonic ventricle—the proliferative layer—contains a genetically determined two-dimensional arrangement or matrix of proliferative cells. That arrangement would constitute a proto-map or *Bauplan,* a basic topological map of the future cortex. Cells proliferate and migrate within *radial columnar "units"* with their base in the germinal zone. At first, the radial units that guide neurons to their destination are almost virtual, barely outlined by glial fibers and terminal axons. Later in embryogenesis, the radial guiding units become the columnar modules of cytoarchitectonically mature cortex. Thus, through those radial units, morphological and potential functional specificity would gradually be transferred from the original primordial map to the fully developed neocortex. Although, as just outlined, the migration of cortical cells to their final destination takes place to a large extent radially, recent studies have shown that some cells—such as interneuron precursors—take long routes that are tangential to the cortical surface (Corbin et al., 2001). Based on the evidence of early plasticity, O'Leary (1989) argues that the cortex is initially entirely uniform and becomes differentiated exclusively by input (the *tabula rasa* model). This view is contradicted, however, by recent studies that demonstrate the interplay of genetic and environmental factors in all stages of cortical development. (For recent review of the relevant issues, especially the role of genetics, the reader is referred to the special issue of *Cerebral Cortex* introduced by Rubenstein and Rakic, 1999.)

In the human neocortex, by the end of the second trimester of gestation, neuron generation seems to have been completed. Afterward, however, cortical neurons continue to grow in size. Furthermore, by the time the infant is born, some neurons are still developing and migrating to their final location. As they grow, neurons develop their axons, which branch out and develop collaterals (Purpura, 1975; Mrzljak et al., 1990) (Fig. 2.7). Among these, already in the embryo, one can observe the incipient recurrent collaterals, which through neighboring cells can influence the cells that parent them (generally pyramids). In the pre- and postnatal periods, dendrites become longer and thicker, developing synaptic spines along their shafts (Fig. 2.8). Synaptogenesis begins with the third trimester of pregnancy and goes on at least until postnatal age 2 years. Later synapse formation in the human has not been demonstrated but cannot be ruled out.

In general, deeper layers of the cortex (IV, V, and VI) develop earlier and faster than upper layers (II and III) (Poliakov, 1961), the latter layers to accommodate much of the corticocortical integration of networks and functions. Concurrently with the neuronal developments outlined thus far, the glia and the capillary bed of the cortex also grow. The development of these structures accounts for further expansion of the neocortex in thickness and in depth. After it has acquired its full endowment of neurons, and most of them have

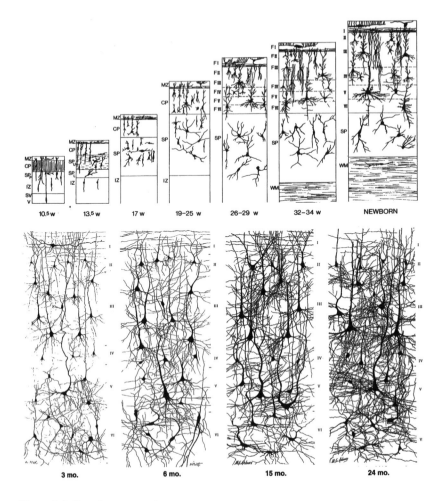

Figure 2.7. Development of neurons in the human cortex. *Top:* Prenatal period from 10.5 weeks to birth. From Mrzljak et al. (1990), with permission. *Bottom:* Postnatal period at 3, 6, 15, and 24 months. From Conel (1963), with permission.

reached their final destination, the neocortex grows further by in-folding and creating ridges, that is, by the formation of fissures, sulci, and convolutions (Fig. 2.9).

In the perinatal life of the human, as in all mammalian species, neurons, axons, dendrites, and synapses undergo periods of *exuberant growth* and overproduction followed by *attrition,* that is, by reduction in their size and number. Neuronal counts during these processes are difficult to establish morphometrically because of concomitant

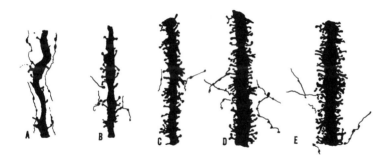

Figure 2.8. Developmental increase of spines on apical dendrites of pyramidal neurons of layer V in the human cortex at various ages: *A,* 5-month-old fetus; *B,* 7-month-old fetus; *C,* newborn; *D,* 2-month-old infant; *E,* 8-month-old infant. From Marín-Padilla (1970), modified.

changes in cell density. Thus, although the normal occurrence of cell death in the human cortex has been substantiated, its degree and timing are difficult to determine. Some axons, in any case, are known to retract in early postnatal stages. Others, coming into and leaving the cortex, grow to their final destination and then develop myelin sheaths over a period of months or years. Neocortical dendrites continue to grow after birth, mainly by elongation (Becker et al., 1984). In layer III, dendrites have been reported to nearly double in length between age 2 years and adulthood (Schadé and Van Groenigen, 1961). In some cortical regions, Broca's area for example, dendrites grow to considerable lengths postnatally (Scheibel, 1990). Along the shafts of dendrites existing at birth, synaptic spines increase in number until some time between the third and twelfth months of postnatal life, when they reach their maximum (Purpura, 1975; Michel and Garey, 1984; Huttenlocher, 1990); then they undergo a gradual decrease into adult life.

The significance and implications of the exuberant growth and attrition of neocortical elements are poorly understood. Undoubtedly these processes are to a large extent genetically determined, but there are indications that at certain times in postnatal life they are subject to a number of endogenous and exogenous factors that also contribute to their final outcome in the adult. Changeux and Danchin (1976) proposed an interesting hypothesis that not only explains exuberance and attrition but also makes these processes the biophysical foundation for the morphological and functional specificity of corti-

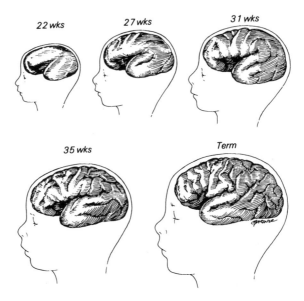

Figure 2.9. Schematic lateral view of the human cortex in gestation. From Barkovich (1995), with permission.

cal neurons, areas, and connections. The key element in their hypothesis is the synapse. They postulate an excessive number of connections originally specified between classes of cells—say, neurons in different cortical fields. Out of that original redundant overstock, epigenetic factors related to usage (experience, neuronal discharge, etc.) "select" the synapses that will interconnect the neurons of the definitive networks, while the rest of the overstock withers away. (This does not preclude some degree of prenatal selection.) The theory is eminently applicable to neocortical synaptology and has the merit of reconciling genetic determinacy with "nurture" and experience.

Among the epigenetic factors that foster or enable the development of the neocortex there is a host of neurochemical substances with varying degrees of trophic or growth-promoting influence upon neurons and connections. Because the mechanisms by which these substances regulate growth are not well understood, here I will refer only briefly to some of them that appear especially critical, beginning with a hormone, *thyroxine.* Mostly from the clinical consequences of deficit (hypothyroidism), especially within certain perinatal periods, it has long been known that the thyroid hormone plays an essential role in brain development, most particularly with regard to the neocortex (Eayrs, 1960). It can be reasonably assumed that thyroxine promotes and protects the normal development of the cerebral cortex.

In the past two decades, a category of related growth-promoting substances have been identified in the neocortex which are grouped under the generic name of *neurotrophins,* including the originally identified *nerve growth factor* (NGF). Neurotrophins (NTs) appear essential for normal cortical development and plasticity (Levi-Montalcini, 1987; Theonen, 1995). They are activity-dependent substances—that is, chemicals dependent on neuronal discharge—that are released chiefly from dendrites. Their role has been made especially evident in the visual cortex, whose function they protect from the consequences of visual deprivation during a critical postnatal period (Maffei et al., 1992). It would appear that experience (e.g., visual stimulation) promotes the genes that give rise to NT expression at dendritic terminals. It has been postulated that groups of synchronously activated neurons release NTs, and these enhance the formation of synapses and the efficacy of their transmitting properties (Katz and Shatz, 1996).

While the neocortex develops its cellular and connective architecture, it also develops its connections with other structures. Those two sectors of cortical development are in fact interdependent, though in ways that have not yet been fully clarified. As noted above, axon terminals from the thalamus and from the cortex contribute early to the guidance of neuronal migration. Anyway, the vast majority of connections developing in the neocortex are of local or distant cortical origin. Even in primary visual (striate) cortex, a sector of the neocortex that for its functions depends heavily on input from the thalamus (lateral geniculate body), at most 5% of its terminal axons is of thalamic origin; most of the other axons are of cortical origin (Peters and Payne, 1993). As we see later in this and the next chapter, there is an order to corticocortical connections. That order is laid out in functionally hierarchical steps above primary sensory and motor cortices. It also appears laid out along temporal maturational gradients, a subject of much controversy that here deserves some discussion.

The controversy began around the turn of the twentieth century, when Flechsig (1901) published his observations on the order of *myelination* of cortical fibers and, with it, proposed a new theory of neural association. He observed that, in human development, cortical areas myelinate in a certain chronological order (Fig. 2.10). For example, the motor cortex (Brodmann's area 4) and the primary sensory areas—with direct sensory afferents from the thalamus—show earlier myelination of their afferent and efferent axons than do the so-called areas of association interposed anatomically between them. Assuming that myelin makes axons more viable (we know now that at least it makes them faster transmitters), Flechsig (1920) concluded that the functions of the various cortical areas develop following the sequence of their myelination. Thus, primary sensory and motor areas would become functional before association areas, the latter to engage later in the most complex and experience-dependent functions of the cortex. The prefrontal cortex, for example, does not reach full myelination until puberty; thus, following that reasoning, this cortex would be destined to become involved in late-developing and com-

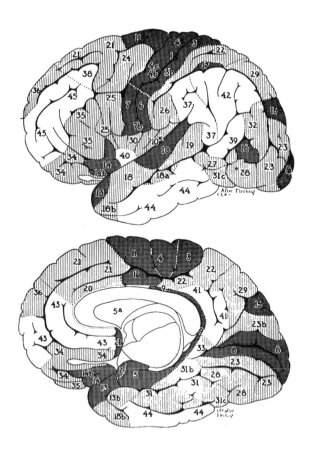

Figure 2.10. Order of myelination in the human cortex, according to Flechsig. From Bonin (1950), modified.

plex cognitive functions (e.g., language). We know that this is indeed the case, but the role of myelin in the process is far from obvious.

Despite a number of methodological problems, including the unreliability of certain fiber-staining methods, those early observations on the order of cortical myelination were confirmed by later investigators, albeit only in general terms, in the human (Conel, 1963; Brody et al., 1987) and the rhesus monkey (Gibson, 1991). Neuroimaging broadly substantiates the essentials of that histological order in the brain of the developing child (Salamon et al., 1990; Wolpert and Barnes, 1992; Barkovich, 1995). However, myelination is not an indispensable property of functional axons. Unmyelinated axons, in many neural structures of early development, can function perfectly well throughout the life of the individual. Furthermore, myelination is just one criterion of neural maturation. By other criteria, a chronological order of areal maturation fails to become apparent. One of those criteria is *synaptogenesis*. Detailed studies of synapsis formation and elimination in monkeys at various developmental stages do not show any asynchronies between areas (Rakic et al., 1986, 1994; Bourgeois et al., 1994). Synaptogenesis and subsequent synapse reduction seem to take place concurrently and at the same rates in all regions of the neocortex.

A more limited study in the human, however, has reported heterochronicity in synapse maturation between primary auditory cortex and association—prefrontal—cortex (Huttenlocher and Dabholkar, 1997). In this study, synaptic density in auditory cortex is claimed to increase to a peak at postnatal age 3 months, whereas in prefrontal cortex it does not reach a peak until age 15 months. Elimination of synapses occurs after those peaks, also with a time lag between the two areas. Thus, in the human, at variance with the monkey, synaptogenesis and synaptic regression appear to occur heterochronously in different cortical areas. The reason for the interspecies discrepancy is obscure and may be a product of methodological differences between studies; for one thing, the monkey studies are considerably more comprehensive than the human study. Further, the statistical comparison of the results between the monkey and human studies indicates that interspecies differences in synaptogenesis are not significant (Goldman-Rakic et al., 1997).

In any event, it is possible that in the human some synaptogenesis progresses from one cortical area to another pari passu with other phenomena of neural maturation, such as axonal growth and elimination, dendritic growth, and the myelination of subcortical white matter. In general, maturation appears to progress from primary sensory and motor areas to areas of association, without necessarily following the order stipulated by Flechsig. In some neocortical areas (e.g., prefrontal cortex), maturational changes seem to continue until puberty (Kaes, 1907; Yakovlev and Lecours, 1967; Mrzljak et al., 1990).

Along with axons, dendrites, and synapses, the cortex develops its substrate for *chemical transmission*. That too has a maturational timetable with periods of exuberance and recession, but these seem longer than those that apply to synaptic density. The timetable for the various cortical neurotransmitters varies somewhat between species. The development of monoamine neurotransmitters—norepinephrine (NE), dopamine (DA), and serotonin—has been extensively investigated in the prefrontal cortex of the rhesus monkey (Goldman-Rakic and Brown, 1982; Lidow and Rakic, 1992; Rosenberg and Lewis, 1995). At birth the monkey exhibits characteristic differences in monoamine distribution: NE and DA higher in frontal-lobe cortex and serotonin in posterior (postcentral) cortex. Postnatally, in all cortical areas, monoamine transmitters seem to increase to peak values around 2–3 years of age (early puberty in the monkey) and to decline gradually thereafter toward stabilization at adult levels. Especially noteworthy is the marked increase of DA in layer III, where it serves both excitatory and inhibitory synapses on pyramidal cells (Rosenberg and Lewis, 1995). Given that layer III is the source and termination of abundant corticocortical axons and recurrent axon collaterals on pyramidal neurons, it is reasonable to assume the importance of DA receptors in the development and functions of local as well as wideranging cortical networks.

In the human, our knowledge of the ontogenesis of connections between cortical areas is limited to a few broad inferences derived from the previously mentioned development of myelin and subcortical white matter. A little more is known in the nonhuman primate. The issue has been examined in the prefrontal cortex of developing monkeys by means of axon-tracing techniques (Goldman-Rakic, 1981). Early in fetal life, corticocortical fibers from the contralateral hemisphere have been observed to reach their prefrontal destination through the corpus callosum. At first, however, their distribution is coarse. Later in embryogenesis that distribution becomes topographically refined, in part by reduction of redundant axons and in part, it is believed, under the influence or guidance of preexisting structures, such as thalamocortical fibers. As a result of the final rearrangement, callosal fibers adopt a discontinuous pattern of distribution; the terminal arbor of each fiber innervates the cells in a vertical column or *module* of cortex. In cortical tissue sections, the terminal fields of callosal origin appear to alternate with others of ipsilateral cortical provenance. Two weeks before the monkey's birth, the mature segregated pattern of cortical axon termination has been attained.

In summary, then, there is clearly a genetic plan for the development of the entire observable structure of the neocortex. The plan covers all the macro- and microscopic features of that structure, including neurons and their connective appendices—dendrites, synapses, and axons. However, at every step of development the expression of that genetic plan, the structural phenotype of the neocortex, is subject to a wide variety of internal and external influences. These influences create the necessary and permissive conditions for the normal development of the neocortex and its neuronal networks. Among the essential factors is the interaction of the organism with its environment. Through sensory and motor interactions with that environment, the afferent, efferent, and association fibers of the neocortex will develop and form the networks that are to serve cognitive functions. The development of those networks involves most likely a process of selection of neural elements among those that in earlier stages have been overproduced (selective stabilization). A degree of competition for inputs among cells and terminals is probably part of that selective process. Thus the elements that succeed in the competition would thrive and survive the normal attrition; others would be eliminated. It is a kind of Darwinian process (Edelman, 1987) to which we will come back.

All the events of neocortical ontogeny have their timetable. Each has its *critical period,* a time window before or after birth during which a particular set of enabling factors is essential for normal development. It is also the time during which extraneous or injurious factors can most readily arrest or derail this development. The best-known critical periods, experimentally, are those that apply to the development of the visual cortex, especially in the cat (Wiesel, 1982). Kittens deprived of visual input during a certain postnatal period will develop abnormal axon terminals in the striate cortex. Correlated inputs from both eyes seem essential for the development of ocular dominance columns in that cortex (Löwel and Singer, 1992). On the other hand, lesions of peripheral sensory structures or cortical structures that are the normal targets of cortical connections can lead to the rerouting of cortical axons. This is especially the case if the lesions have been produced before or during a critical period (Goldman-Rakic, 1981; Frost and Metin, 1985; Sur et al., 1990). Axon rerouting has been adduced as evidence of cortical plasticity, in other words, as evidence of the potential of cortical structures to substitute for others that have been disabled. However, the clear proof of plasticity is the substitution of function. Auditory cortex cannot "see," even if visual inputs have been routed to it by experimental manipulation. This is not to deny the clinically well proven—but unexplained—evidence of functional recovery after massive cortical lesioning in early childhood. Nor is it to deny the evidence of functional plasticity in the sensory cortex of adult animals after the manipulation of peripheral sensory structures (Merzenich and Kaas, 1982; Pons et al., 1991). The latter evidence may be helpful in the forthcoming discussion to deal with the functional expansion of neocortical networks after their development has been essentially completed.

Cognitive Network Formation

So far we have discussed the development of the basic structure of the neocortex into its adult form. Here a few generalities about the "finished" structure are in order. Briefly, the fully developed neocortex contains a vast array of neurons grouped in columnar clusters or modules of varying dimensions—depending on the area—that are packed horizontally against one another. These clusters or modules fill the entire dorsal cortex of the cerebral hemispheres. This cortex is subdivided into a number of areas defined by cytoarchitecture, that is, by the size, shape, and vertical arrangement of their neurons. In certain areas, the neurons of each modular assembly are interconnected in certain ways to form a small local network, presumably representing a feature of the environment or of action upon the environment. Assemblies of neurons within an area are interconnected into larger networks supposedly to represent complex features. United neuronal assemblies from different areas form even larger networks that could represent even more complex features or sets of features. In that structural framework one can already discern the outline of a hierarchical organization of networks and representations (Chapter 3).

    After the developmental processes discussed in the previous section have taken place, the entire connective structure of the neocortex, including the corticocortical connections between areas, is virtually complete, at least as far as we can tell with present morphological methods. Functionally, however, the neocortex is incomplete. Life experience will continue to change it, especially at the synaptic level, and to increase the range of its functions. Thus experience will convert cortical networks into representations of the environment and of the subject's actions in that environment, in other words, into cognitive representations or cognits. Because the potential functional connections between neuronal assemblies and networks are practically infinite, there is no such thing as the complete cognitive development of the cortex. Networks and knowledge are open-ended. Never in the life of the individual do they cease to grow or to be otherwise modified. From that general fact derives the question now before us: How are the connective links within and between networks modified to form or expand cognitive networks and thus to represent the knowledge acquired by experience?

By merely asking that question we enter inevitably into the nurture versus nature debate. As it pertains to the cognitive development of the neocortex, the debate is basically between two camps of theoretical persuasion: selectionism and constructivism. *Selectionists* maintain that cortical representation is the result of the competitive selection of neural elements. Innate variation and adaptation play a role in both, the selection and the elimination of neural elements. The process in its totality has been compared to the sculpting of a statue out of marble. Exposure of the organism to the environment would cause competition—for sensory inputs, synapses, neuron groups, and so on—which would lead to the survival and specialization of certain sets of elements at the expense of others, which would disappear. In the connective aspects of that postulated selective process, axons play a more critical role than dendrites. Axons intervene actively in the "exploration" and selection of neurons for connection; axons are also easily subject to retraction if they fail to establish selective connection.

Constructivists emphasize the idea that cortical representation is the result of growth and combination of neural elements that develop in the cortical structure promoted by experience. Thus the emphasis is on the constructive work of experience, and for this reason constructivists have been called *latter-day empiricists*. In any event, it would appear that the debate between selectionists and constructivists is largely idle, like most debates concerning the nature–nurture issue. Both points of view are necessary to explain the making of cognitive representations in the cerebral cortex. The question then is not whether nurture or nature, but how much nurture and how much nature. In the cortex, it is a question still for the most part unresolved, and the answer may differ depending on the age of the organism, the cortical area, and the kind of network component we are dealing with, whether it is cell bodies, dendrites, axons, or synapses. Genetics and environment (internal environment included) interact with each other all the time. In the cortex, the works of genetics and experience co-occur throughout life. The precise time course of the two is not as important as the fact that they overlap. For the neurobiologist, that overlap is a necessary assumption in any attempt to comprehend by empirical means the development of cortical representation networks. In principle, then, the two conceptual frameworks, selectionism and constructivism, complement each other. Let us now briefly consider them separately.

Competitive selection is the essence of all selectionist views of the cortex, which are inspired by evolution and immunology. An eminently plausible selectionist model is at the center of the *neuronal group selection theory* proposed by Edelman (1987). This model accounts for the formation of representational networks out of preexisting neuronal populations through a selective process that takes place in close interaction with the environment. The original substrate is an epigenetically developed primary repertoire of cell groups (e.g., columnar neuron modules or assemblies) that respond more or less well to external stimuli. Some of these groups, which tend to discharge together and in a correlated manner in response to those stimuli, will be selected out by the strengthening of their synapses. Recurrence or reentry is an essential feature of some of the connections within and between the groups. It is also an essential feature of the functional architecture of computational models based on the theory (Tononi et al., 1992).

From that process of competitive selection in the primary repertoire of cell groups, which is a process fundamentally based on variability, correlation, and connective reentry, a secondary repertoire of neuronal groups will emerge. They will form a new representational map. The neuronal groups of this second repertoire, that is, of the newly formed map or network, will subsequently respond better to the individual stimuli that formed it. Further, the network as a whole will recognize those stimuli by responding to them categorically. Thus, by the selective process, the secondary network will have become a more effective representational and classifying device for perception, memory, and behavior than the original, primary repertoire of cell groups that became part of it. *Degeneracy*, a concept of immunological origin, is a critical property of that network. It refers to the network's capability to elicit the same response or lead to the same outcome when its separate structural components are stimulated. A degenerate response by the net is then tantamount to the categorization of the features that its structural components share in common. Those are the associated features that characterize the net, which is therefore the equivalent of our cognit. The concept of degeneracy, inasmuch as it coincides with that of categorization, is key to perception and to the understanding of perceptual constancy (Chapter 4).

Support for Edelman's model can be found in the results of certain studies demonstrating plasticity in the sensory cortex of adult monkeys after peripheral deafferentation. After the severing of nerves from the hand, extensive rearrangements can be observed in the receptive fields of the somatosensory cortex (Merzenich and Kaas, 1982; Kaas et al., 1983; Pons et al., 1991). Here the most relevant observation is the expansion of the receptive fields that represent nondenervated skin segments into areas formerly representing the denervated ones. That expansion of receptive fields at the expense of the deafferented fields indicates a remapping of the cortex as a result of imbalance in the normal competition of inputs. Inputs that have been eliminated yield their cortex to unaffected inputs. The experimental imbalance of inputs apparently recreates the selective competition that Edelman's theory postulates to have occurred in ontogeny with the passage from a primary to a secondary repertoire (map) of somatosensory neuronal groups. For a better appreciation of the reasoning and the evidence behind selectionism in the cortex, the reader is referred to the volume edited by Sporns and Tononi (1994).

The constructivist argument on the shaping of cortical representational networks is based to a considerable degree on the morphological evidence of cortical development as a function of *environmental influences*. Experience begins to play its structural, network-building role early in ontogeny, and that role persists throughout life. That is the essence of the constructivist approach (for reviews of various experimental aspects of constructivism the reader is referred to Black and Greenough, 1986; Purves, 1994; Elman et al., 1996; and Quartz and Sejnowski, 1997). In the previous section, I mentioned the apparent need of externally induced neuronal discharge for the development of thalamic axon terminals and for the epigenetic expression of certain growth-promoting substances such as the neurotrophins. Further, there is a long tradition of experimental work demonstrating a direct role of sensory experience in promoting the growth of the formal connective components of cortical networks, that is, synapses, dendrites, and axons. That evidence falls into two large categories: (*1*) stunted growth by sensory deprivation and (*2*) proliferation and expansion by sensory stimulation.

Sensory deprivation (e.g., rearing in the dark) leads to lower dendritic spine density and synaptic counts (Globus and Scheibel, 1967; Valverde, 1967; Cragg, 1975), shorter axons (Friedlander et al., 1991; McCasland et al., 1992), and shorter dendrites (Ruiz-Marcos and Valverde, 1970). Some of those effects are reversible upon restoration of normal sensory input (Valverde, 1971). Conversely, a rich sensory environment and increased *sensory stimulation* maintain the size and growth of dendrites and dendritic spines (Diamond et al., 1966; Globus et al., 1973) at the level presumably determined by genes. The stimulated animals become better performers of behavioral tasks (Rosenzweig, 1984; Diamond, 1988). However, the morphological effects of sensory deprivation or stimulation are not always as simple as stated here. For example, a lengthening of dendrites in an "environmentally enriched" animal may be accompanied by a lower number of *larger* synaptic spines (Møllgaard et al., 1971). There are reasons to suspect that, in general, the pruning of excess elements may actually be accompanied by the development of larger, probably more computationally effective synapses, axons, and dendrites. In any case, it can be reasonably argued that the so-called enriched environment of experimental studies simply provides the normal inputs that the brains of "control" animals do not have. In this light, sensory stimulation would restore the permissive conditions of normal genetic development.

If there is one thing on which all agree, selectionists and constructivists alike, it is the central role of the *synapse* (Fig. 2.11) in the making of cognitive networks. Everybody agrees that the neocortical representations of our internal and external environments, of our *internal milieu* and the world around us, are built by modulation of contacts between neurons. Not everybody, however, accepts the synapse as the only form of functional contact between neurons—probably it is not. Nonetheless, the fundamental role of synapses in the formation of representations, in the cortex as elsewhere, is commonly ac-

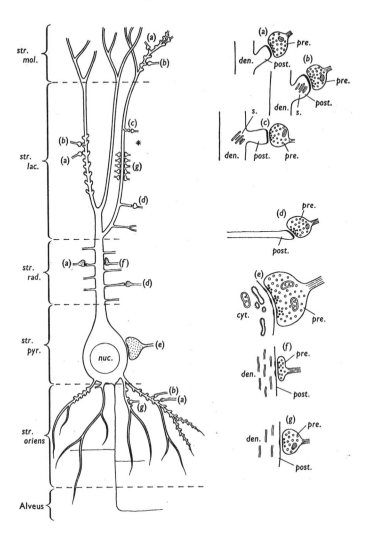

Figure 2.11. Diagram of a pyramidal neuron of the hippocampus and the various observable types of synaptic terminals on it. From Hamlyn (1962), modified.

cepted. That idea, first proposed by Tanzi (1893) and Cajal (1894), has now taken solid hold, and the evidence for it is impressive, especially in invertebrates and in the mammalian hippocampus.

Nonetheless, the mechanism is not yet known by which a synapse or an *ephaptic* contact becomes a link, or part of a link, in a net of neocortical neurons representing a feature of the environment or a memory of it. The best current conjecture is that the linkage takes place according to the principles proposed by Hebb (1949). His famous rule, which is the best known of those principles, postulates that whenever one cell (A) repeatedly takes part in the firing of another (B), "some growth process or metabolic change takes place in one or both cells" such that the efficiency of the first cell in firing the second is increased. In invertebrates (e.g. mollusks), the temporal coincidence of pre- and postsynaptic firing has been shown to enhance the efficacy of preexisting synapses and thus contribute to learning (Kandel, 1976; Krasne, 1978).

In the mammalian hippocampus, which is phylogenetically ancient cortex, the phenomenon of long-term potentiation (LTP) is considered another example of the operation of Hebb's rule—that is, the increase in the strength of synapses by transmission of impulses through them. The tetanic electrical stimulation of the perforant path, a major entry of neocortical input to the hippocampus, induces an enhancement of the excitability of the synapses of dentate granule cells, upon which that path terminates (Bliss and Lømo, 1973). That enhancement can persist for hours, days, or even weeks after cessation of the electrical stimulus (Swanson et al., 1982; Teyler et al., 1989). Many efforts have been made to substantiate the molecular and electrochemical basis of LTP and to apply the hebbian rule to it (Lynch and Baudry, 1984; Brown et al., 1990). The issue is yet to be resolved.

In addition to the temporal coincidence or correlation of pre- and postsynaptic firing, there is another condition (Hebb's second rule) leading to synaptic facilitation (Fig. 2.12); this condition is the *temporal coincidence* of presynaptic inputs arriving to the same cell or to different cells of the same assembly. Hebb also envisioned the importance of this condition for memory network formation. He wrote, "any two cells or systems of cells that are repeatedly active at the same time will tend to become 'associated,' so that activity in one facilitates activity in the other. . . . [Here] I am proposing . . . a possible basis of association of two afferent fibers of the same order—in principle, a sensori-sensory association" (Hebb, 1949, p. 70). He did not precisely define, however, the hypothetical circuitry of the "two cells or systems." In any case, he admitted the possibility that "the two afferent fibers" acted on the same cell, perhaps on the same synaptic "boutons," whereby synaptic facilitation would be caused by temporal summation.

Marr (1969) and Stent (1973) provided substantial theoretical support for the application of Hebb's second rule—also called the

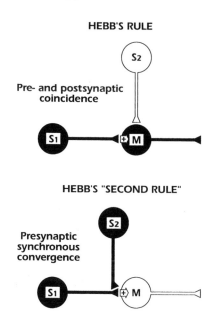

HEBB'S RULE

Pre- and postsynaptic
coincidence

HEBB'S "SECOND RULE"

Presynaptic
synchronous
convergence

Figure 2.12. Hebb's basic principles. *Top:* Synaptic facilitation occurs between cell S_1 and cell M when the first repeatedly causes the second to fire. *Bottom:* Synaptic facilitation occurs between cells S_1 and M, as between S_2 and M, when signals from S_1 and S_2 arrive at M at the same time.

principle of synchronous convergence (Fuster, 1995). Stent, in particular, based on the synchronicity of binocular inputs on the striate cortex (Wiesel and Hubel, 1965), provides an exceptionally cogent argument for the enhancement of synaptic efficacy by synchronous inputs. The second hebbian postulate has also received empirical support from invertebrate studies (Carew et al., 1984; Buonomano and Byrne, 1990) and from the discovery of associative LTP in the hippocampus (McNaughton et al., 1978; White et al., 1990) and in the cortex (Iriki et al., 1989).

Given certain assumptions of neural circuitry and excitability, the second rule can be reduced to a special case of the first. Further, Hebb's principles do not exhaust the possible explanations for synaptic, use-dependent facilitation or for the linkage of neocortical neurons in network representations. Some use-dependent links may consist of nonsynaptic contacts (Bach-y-Rita, 1993). Nevertheless, those principles are compatible with a large body of neurobiological data and continue to be useful working hypotheses. In any endeavor to model cortical networks, Hebb's rules cannot be ignored, for they have two features that are essential to any plausible neural model of cognitive representation: (*1*) the association by temporal coincidence (correlation) and (*2*) the linkage of inputs in cerebral structure. Note, however, that hebbian rules presuppose the existence of synapses. Thus, in hebbian terms, no synaptic plasticity can result from environmental influences before the synaptic infrastructure has been genetically established. Those influences can thereafter modulate synapses but not make them.

In any event, important qualifications must be made to hebbian rules to make them applicable to the building of cortical networks. The first qualification is on the issue of synchronicity. Clearly, absolute temporal coincidence, down to the millisecond, cannot be a valid constraint to Hebb's second rule (synchronous convergence). Neurons have excitatory cycles, their membrane is not always in the best ionic environment for reception, inputs from sensory signals have different durations and different time constants at peripheral receptors, and so on. With a strict simultaneity constraint, two brief stimuli could never be associated centrally if they arrive more than a few milliseconds apart from each other. Yet we know that separate stimuli need not overlap in time to be associated at the cognitive level.

There are several possible mechanisms by which the central effects of temporally separate, nonoverlapping stimuli upon a cell could coincide in time. One plausible mechanism would be the reentry of excitation through recurrent circuits. For example, earlier stimuli would be maintained in neural circuits by cyclic reentry (reverberation) until the arrival of later stimuli to the net. Then output from those circuits would act together with input of the later stimuli to facilitate synaptic transmission to an associative postsynaptic cell or set of cells. Hebb did suggest a reverberation mechanism for short-term memory. In Chapter 6, I will attempt to show empirically the plausibility of that mechanism for so-called working memory, which I construe as a form of attention.

A second qualification to the synchronicity rule is that the presynaptically converging inputs need not be external (sensory). Some of the inputs that facilitate synapses by synchronous convergence may be internal, generated in other parts of the cortex. Thus, the coinciding inputs that build connections that build a cortical network may come from other networks. These other networks may be activated by recognition of an external object, for example. Then the sensory input from the object coincides with the internal input that its recognition elicits. The provision for internal inputs has, of course, important implications for cognitive network formation and operations. If correct, that provision essentially frees cognitive networks from the outer world.

The average pyramidal cell has some 10,000 synapses and is embedded in a mesh of connectivity of enormous complexity. Thus, for the building of a representational network, what happens in individual synapses and cells is inconsequential, unless it also happens at the same time in many other synapses and cells, and unless those cells share connections with other cells. Under those conditions the outcome of an association of inputs is cooperative, and Hebb's second rule becomes the *principle of cooperativity* of Miller (1991). We have transcended cell A and cell B and pulled cell groups A and B together to obey that principle. We have, in other words, transcended cell dynamics and entered population dynamics. It is this critical step that allows selectionists to theorize in population terms while still adhering to hebbian principles (Edelman, 1987).

Extracortical Factors

Network formation in the neocortex depends to a large extent on the modulating influences from other brain structures and from neurotransmitter systems of subcortical origin. These extracortical influences have global potentiating roles and do not per se confer representational specificity on neocortical networks. That specificity derives from the specificity of thalamic projections and the organization of corticocortical connections. Nonetheless, it is appropriate to consider here, however briefly, the permissive and mediating role that limbic and subcortical structures play in the formation of neocortical connections.

Largely by inference from the results of damage in humans and animals, the *hippocampus,* which is phylogenetically old cortex, has been supposed to play a crucial role in the acquisition and consolidation of memory and thus in the construction of neocortical representations. In humans, the bilateral lesion of the hippocampus—especially region CA1—causes severe anterograde amnesia (Scoville and Milner, 1957; Cohen and Squire, 1980). The deficit affects conspicuously the capacity to remember declarative memory, that is, memory of events and facts, while not affecting other kinds of memory (reviews in Squire, 1986, and Cohen and Eichenbaum, 1993). In monkeys, hippocampal lesions also induce deficits in performance of certain memory tasks (Mishkin, 1978; Zola-Morgan and Squire, 1985). Such lesions impair the capacity to consolidate new representations (Zola-Morgan and Squire, 1990); they do not impair representations over 4 weeks old, which presumably have already been consolidated in the neocortex.

The hippocampus exerts its memory-making role over the neocortex probably through the connections that reciprocally link the two structures; these connections course through the parahippocampal gyrus (Fig. 2.13). In the rhesus monkey they possess two general features with important implications for the formation of neocortical representations. First, the neocortical connectivity of the hippocampus is limited to areas of association; no hippocampal fibers seem to terminate or originate in primary sensory or motor cortex. Second, the hippocampal connectivity not only reaches into large sectors of the posterior cortex of association, behind the central sulcus, but also extends to associative areas of the frontal lobe, that is, to the prefrontal cortex.

The first implication of those anatomical facts is that only the associative areas of the neocortex need the input from the hippocampus for the formation of new representations. Primary sensory and motor cortices do not. This may have to do with the innate characteristics of sensory and motor representations in primary cortices. At birth, these cortices contain those representations of the environment and of organismic action already built into their structure. They do not seem to need hippocampal inputs for the formation of elementary sensory and motor representations, whereas the cortex of association does need those inputs in order to accommodate the new memories of the individual and presumably to retrieve them.

A significant implication of the hippocampus-prefrontal connections is that the hippocampus participates in the making not only of perceptual memory (declarative) but also of motor memory (*procedural* or *executive*). As we shall see in the next chapter, the cortex of the frontal lobe, as a whole, is implicated in action. The primary motor and premotor cortices are involved in skeletal motor actions and speech, whereas the prefrontal cortex is involved in the formulation of action plans, that is, in the highest and most idiosyncratic forms of executive representation (Fuster, 1997). Thus, a reasonable inference from anatomical connectivity is that the hippocampus, in

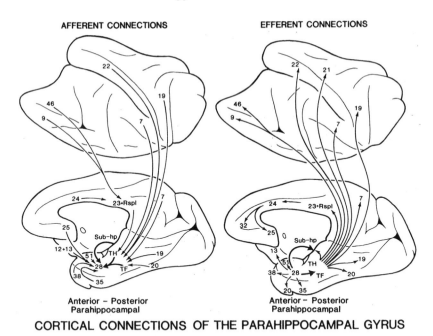

CORTICAL CONNECTIONS OF THE PARAHIPPOCAMPAL GYRUS

Figure 2.13. Bidirectional connectivity between the hippocampus and the neo-cortex through the parahippocampal cortex in the monkey. Area 28 (Brod-mann's) is a major node of connections linking the hippocampus with associative areas of the neocortex. From Van Hoesen (1982), with permission.

addition to its role in memory formation, contributes to the forma-tion of the neocortical representations of the most complex actions of the individual.

The hippocampus is not the only temporal-lobe structure impli-cated in the formation of cognitive networks. Lesions of the entorhi-nal and perirhinal cortex (areas 28, 35, and 36) also produce deficits in monkeys' performance of memory tasks (Zola-Morgan et al., 1989). One reasonable deduction from these results is that those lesions in-terrupt the connectivity between the hippocampus and the neocortex, which is funneled in both directions through those areas. Further-more, lesions of the amygdala, the most important nuclear complex of the limbic system, also cause memory deficits (Mishkin, 1978). In view of its well-known role in the attribution of emotional significance to external stimuli (Gloor, 1960; LeDoux, 1993), the *amygdala* may impart to the neocortex the affective and motivational inputs that play such an important role in the registration of memories. The con-

nections between the amygdala and the neocortex are both direct
and indirect, through the thalamus.

The building of network representations in the neocortex is also
subject to *neurochemical modulation* of subcortical origin. The neocortex is the recipient of several neurotransmitter systems originating in
the brainstem. These systems are critically involved in general state
functions, such as sleep, wakefulness, and alertness, which bear heavily on the capacity of the neocortex to form new representations.
Monoamine transmitters undoubtedly play a critical role in the formation of cortical networks. In the simpler neuronal circuitry of the
mollusk *Aplysia,* the neurotransmitter serotonin, a monoamine, intervenes crucially in the mechanism of synaptic facilitation at the root
of learning (Kandel, 1991).

Gamma-aminobutyric acid (GABA) is the most abundant inhibitory neurotransmitter in the cortex, especially in synaptic terminals of nonpyramidal interneurons. Neural inhibition is an important
mechanism in cognition, notably in attention processes, and probably also plays a role, through collateral and feedback connections,
in the making of representational networks. The cholinergic system
(acetylcholine), with its origin in the nuclear complex of Meynert,
also appears necessary for learning and memory. This can be inferred
from the pathology of that system in certain forms of dementia, notably Alzheimer's disease, which are characterized by severe memory
deficits (Whitehouse et al., 1982).

The precise modes of operation of these neurotransmitter systems in the formation of cognitive cortical networks are not known.
Experiments in animal learning with local or systemic injection of ag-
onist or antagonist substances indicate that some of the transmitters
interact with each other at many levels of neural function (review by
Decker and McGaugh, 1991). Some of the interactions appear to
occur within the amygdala, which most probably intervenes in neocortical memory formation by virtue of its presumed role in emotion.

Glutamate is the most abundant excitatory neurotransmitter in
the central nervous system (Westbrook and Jahr, 1989). Among the
glutamate synaptic receptors, N-methyl-D-aspartate (NMDA) stands
out as a putative mediator of neocortical associations in network representations. It has properties that make it exceptionally suitable for
that role, such as the capacity to induce long synaptic currents, which
facilitate the temporal integration of not precisely synchronous inputs (see the previous section). Furthermore, hippocampal NMDA

appears to participate directly in the induction of LTP (Nicoll et al., 1988). In both hippocampus and cortex, glutamate, through NMDA receptors, may activate second messengers in postsynaptic cells, and thus induce protein changes that sustain LTP as well as other lasting phenomena of network formation (Schuman and Madison, 1994). Finally, in the neocortex, NMDA receptors are most common in layers II and III (Cotman et al., 1987), which are the preferred terminations of corticocortical axons, and thus the potential site for corticocortical network links.

Basic Structure of Cognitive Networks

The development of representations in the neocortex is the continuation of a process that began with cortical evolution in ancestral mammalian species. The phylogenetically oldest representations are those of the simplest physical features of the world and of motor adaptation to it. They are present at birth in the structure of the primary sensory and motor cortex. That structure by itself could be considered a form of memory. It contains information—about the world and the organism in it—that has been "stored" in evolution and that can be "retrieved" as needed by the organism for adaptation to its surrounding. That memory seems to need rehearsal at the beginning of life in order to be able to render faithful "recognition." This is a teleological but plausible interpretation of the physiological significance of critical periods for sensory and motor functions. During such periods, sensory and motor areas need to be stimulated, or else their structure deteriorates or develops abnormally; they lose their capacity to function well or at all (Blakemore et al., 1978; Wiesel, 1982). Those critical periods are periods of greatest vulnerability for the structure of sensory and motor systems. They are also periods in which plasticity, namely, the surrogate or competitive development of alternate structures, is most likely to occur (Frost and Metin, 1985; Sur et al., 1990). As already mentioned, thalamic terminals are essential for the proper ontogenetic development of sensory cortex, and those in turn need sensory input for their development. The developmental role of the connections of the motor cortex with subcortical structures (e.g., basal ganglia) is still unclear.

To repeat an important generality, the formation of neocortical networks in the developing individual is the continuation of processes that took place during phylogeny and early ontogeny in primary areas, and that in subsequent life extend into areas of association. Thus, neocortical network formation would be part of a continuum extending from phylogeny into the life of the individual, all perhaps following a discrete number of fundamental neurobiological principles within certain structural constraints. These structural constraints would include the connectivity of cortical columnar modules and the areas that contain them. In the next chapter we will deal in more detail with areal connectivity, which is the structural essence of cognitive networks. Here I will briefly sketch that connectivity and note that, to some degree, it follows the maturational gradients of neocortical development.

Beginning in primary sensory and motor areas, a series of cortico-cortical paths toward higher associative areas can be traced anatomically. These paths are reciprocal throughout, composed of ascending as well as descending fibers. Every step in those paths between cortical areas is made up of both *diverging and converging fibers.* The relationship between connectivity and maturity cannot yet be precisely determined, however. In both the monkey and the human, it is only possible to discern a very general correspondence between the trend of cortical connectivity and the trend of cortical maturation.

The neocortical networks for cognitive representation develop in the same direction as cortical connectivity, presumably gaining in width of distribution with every step as they fan out into more and higher areas, where they intersect other networks of different origin. That intersection of networks would support in those areas, among other things, the cross-modal representation of objects—that is, the representation across sensory modalities. In network formation, there is not only convergence (synchronous) but also divergence. Divergent connections facilitate the synchronous convergence of inputs of different origin in widely dispersed areas. Both convergence and divergence have been well demonstrated anatomically in the patterns of fibers that flow from the occipital visual—striate—cortex into other areas of the cortex, reaching as far as the frontal lobe (Van Essen, 1985).

Cognitive networks are largely self-organized by *auto-association.* They are formed by inputs arriving simultaneously, in temporal correlation, to cell groups of existing networks of association cortex, where those inputs establish new associations. Thus the new associations are simply expansions of preexisting nets. That is basically a bottom-up process. However, as we will see in the chapters dealing

with attention and memory, some sensory stimuli are favored or selected by top-down influences that flow from higher levels, that is,
from higher associative cortex. In general, as networks expand into
higher levels of the neocortical hierarchy (Chapter 3) and away from
primary areas, the process of network formation becomes freer from
the outer world and more top-down. Thus, as networks expand, progressively more of the network-forming inputs are internal.

In the next chapter, I shall discuss network architecture in greater
detail. Here, however, I close this chapter by recapping some general
features of that architecture and its dynamics in the building of cognitive networks. Figure 2.14 illustrates the most elementary modes of
neuronal connectivity to which I have made reference in this chapter.
In this figure they are schematized at the level of single neurons; but
in cortical networks, as already mentioned, the same modes of connectivity can link cell groups and populations. Figure 2.15 schema-
tizes the formation of a cortical memory network associating two visual stimuli with each other and a visual stimulus with a tactile one.

Cortical networks are to some extent *layered networks,* like some
of the conventional computational network models of neural representation and processing. Like them, cortical networks have input
layers, output layers, and processing layers between them. They also
contain three processing features, to which I have repeatedly referred, that are central to the most plausible network models of the
brain: convergence, divergence, and recurrence. However, the layer-
ing of cortical networks, as well as the processing in them, have cer-

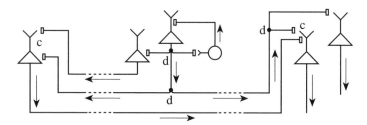

Figure 2.14. Elementary modes of connection between cortical neurons. Pyramidal cell bodies are symbolized by triangles, a recurrent interneuron by a circle;
arrows indicate the direction of axonal flow, and dashed lines indicate interareal
corticocortical axons. *Abbreviations:* c, convergence of axons on a cell; d, point of
axonal divergence.

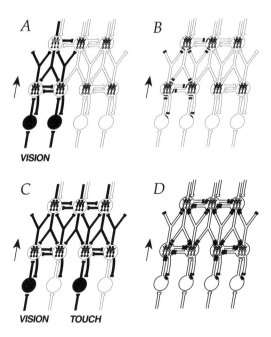

Figure 2.15. Four schematic diagrams of a cortical network extending through three stages of a sensory processing hierarchy (*arrows* indicate the direction of processing). The network contains 11 neuronal groups—4 in the two lower stages and 3 in the upper one—interconnected in the basic modes illustrated in Figure 2.14: collateral, convergent, divergent, and recurrent. *A:* The network associating two coincident visual stimuli. *B:* Memory of the associated visual stimuli represented by a pattern of facilitated synapses *(in black). C:* The network associating a visual stimulus with a tactile stimulus—as from an object perceived simultaneously by sight and palpation. *D:* Synaptic enhancements representing the associative visual-tactile memory.

tain peculiarities that distinguish them from those models and that in fact complicate the attempts to model computationally the real cortical networks.

　　One of the structural peculiarities of cortical networks is that they are mostly layered horizontally, tangential to the surface of the cortex. Another peculiarity is that the connective structure within and between networks allows parallel as well as serial processing. As we shall see, in the act of perception, for example, a cognitive cortical network can process large amounts of information in parallel, all at the same time; the same network, in attention, can process limited amounts of information in series, one bit at a time. Finally, a functional characteristic of cortical networks is their *emergent property*. This property is the one most obscurely related to structure and, therefore, the most difficult to define and to model. At low levels of the hierarchy of cortical networks, the representations they sustain are largely determined by associations between external inputs and by the constraints of connectivity in or near primary areas. There, network building is mostly bottom-up. The periphery governs, and the content of the networks is potentially reducible to their components and the applicable psychophysical algorithms. However, as networks fan out and upward in associative neocortex, they become capable of generating novel representations that are not reducible to their inputs or to their individual neuronal components. Those representations are the product of complex, nonlinear, and near-chaotic interactions between innumerable elements of high-level networks far removed from sensory receptors or motor effectors. Then, top-down network building predominates. Imagination, creativity, and intuition are some of the cognitive attributes of those emergent high-level representations.

3

Functional Architecture of the Cognit

Current debate on the neural foundation of cognition is often mired in fruitless attempts to defend or refute one of two apparently opposite, but reconcilable, ideas. The contentious alternatives abound: innate versus learned, hierarchical versus heterarchical, parallel versus serial, module versus network, convergence versus divergence, and so on. At some time, somewhere in the cerebral cortex, each of those alternatives is true. While so much evidence is still missing, it is unproductive to take a stance for an alternative and to advocate its generality at the expense of the other, or others. Here again, eclecticism is the reasonable position, not only out of ignorance, but also because solid neural data weigh on the side of any of the prevalent theses or their antitheses. If there is one distinction that the cognitive neuroscientist should attempt to keep sharp, it is the distinction between the *representation* and the *processing* of knowledge. This is not always easy; to study the cortical anatomy of a memory, we must test the processing of it, and to study the latter we must often tamper with the former—or observe what happens when disease or trauma does it. How do we know for sure that our data reflect a loss of structure and not of function, or vice versa? Failures to resolve this issue have left a trail of confusion in the literature on every cognitive function. In this book I take the position that all five cognitive functions share the same representational substrate of cells and connections. What differs, depending on the function and the circumstances, is the portion of that substrate that is in use at any given time and, of course, the processing within it. No cognitive function has a fully dedicated cortical area or network. Conversely, a cortical representation or network is at the disposition of any and all functions. In this chapter I consider the structural characteristics of cognits, that is, the morphological features of the cognitive networks of the cerebral cortex. In following chapters I will consider how these networks serve the various cognitive functions.

Structure of Knowledge in Connectionist Models

Knowledge about oneself and the environment is the subject matter of cognitive science and the matter of all cognitive functions—perception, attention, memory, intelligence, and language. For more than a century, neurologists and experimental psychologists have endeavored to assign one or another aspect of cognition, beginning historically with language, to one or another sector of the cerebral cortex. The study of the effects of brain lesions has been by far the leading methodology, and the only one for a long time. In recent times, electrophysiologists and experts in neuroimaging have joined the effort. As we saw in Chapter 1, that long endeavor led to the postulate of the distributed nature of knowledge and cognitive functions. From this idea and from a better understanding of cortical physiology, in particular the properties of cortical neurons, the connectionist models of cognition arose. These models attempt to explain how nerve cells *might* function in cognition. They do not lead to a neural topology of knowledge. They do possess, however, certain distinctive properties that can be reasonably attributed to the cortical substrate of knowledge and that can be tested in the living brain.

Largely because it derives from neural inferences, connectionism has become the most plausible model of the organization of knowledge in the cerebral cortex (McClelland and Rumelhart, 1986; Rumelhart and McClelland, 1986; Müller et al., 1995; McLeod et al., 1998). There are several variants of that model, which differ in their architecture and their computational algorithms, but all have common properties, which here I attempt to summarize. To begin with, all connectionist and neural network models assume the *distribution* of knowledge in assemblies of *units, neurons,* or *nodes* that constitute and represent the component elements of knowledge. In sensory systems, those elements would be sensory features; in semantic systems, words. The nodes are interconnected in various ways. The connections or *synapses* of the neural network are used not only to pull the nodes structurally together but also to transmit activation between them. The networks are *layered,* such that the information from one layer can be processed and transmitted to the next. Some of the connections between layers are reciprocal, and thus information can be processed and transmitted forward as well as backward. Feedback *reentry,* in some cases skipping several layers, is an essential feature of most connectionist models.

The flow of feedforward as well as of feedback connections between layers has three major characteristics. To wit, some connections are segregated in separate parallel channels; others originate in several nodes and converge onto one; and still others diverge from one node into several. These three configurations of connectivity allow, respectively, *parallel processing, integration,* and *distribution* of information. Thus, along separate channels, nodes can pass information to other nodes in subsequent layers on such variables as, for example, the levels of input to the network. Nodes can also integrate information from a previous layer and can make certain decisions, such as whether or not a certain threshold of activity has been reached. Figure 3.1 depicts a schematic connectionist model simulating the representation and processing of information along the visual pathway, together with the computational transformation performed by a unit in the model.

Neural networks *learn.* By virtue of their architecture and processing algorithms, they can be taught to acquire and store new information. In some models, the learning is *supervised,* that is, guided by certain algorithms in their design (e.g., backpropagation) that impose certain quantitative relationships between input and output. In other models (self-organizing), the learning is *unsupervised,* in that the model is allowed to determine those relationships by itself. In either case, the learning takes place by the change or adjustment of *weights* (transmitting capability) in the connections or synapses between nodes. This process, of course, is analogous to that assumed to take place in the nervous system in accord with hebbian principles (Chapter 2). The self-adjustment of weights in self-organized associative networks (Kohonen, 1984) constitutes the most plausible simulation of cognitive associations at higher cortical levels, and thus of the acquisition of new knowledge. Its most attractive feature is the facili-

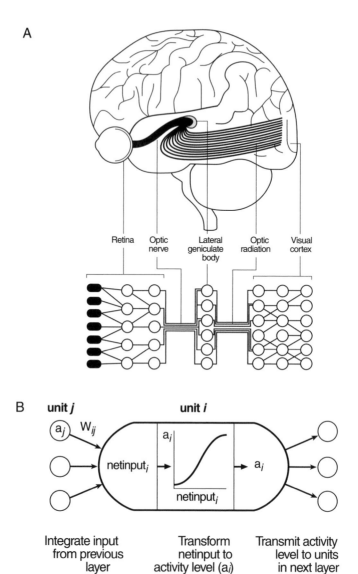

Figure 3.1. A: Information processing in the visual system construed in the form of a layered connectionist network. B: Computations performed by a unit (*i*) in a connectionist network model. From McLeod et al. (1998), with permission.

tation of synapses by the temporal coincidence (*synchronous convergence*) of sensory inputs upon units of the same level or *layer*—in connectionist terms.

Trained network models exhibit the most remarkable properties, some of which are extraordinarily reminiscent of those that the brain exhibits. Here I will enumerate only a few, without elaborating on the architecture and algorithms that support them. For example, associative networks that have been trained to recognize patterns, that is, to reproduce an output pattern present at the input, will do so despite the presence of internal or external noise. A network avoids error under these circumstances by "cleaning up" the representation of the pattern. In the presence of internal perturbations, the networks' performance declines only gradually, displaying what has been termed *graceful degradation*. Further, their output can reproduce the entire object or pattern in the presence of only one part of it at the input. This is one of the reasons why these networks are called *associative,* as they simulate the brain's associative retrieval of memory by completion of partial objects or patterns. Of course, their properties of *regenerative representation* and *completion* in the presence of noise or internal disturbance are very much akin to the restorative capacity of associative cortex after injury.

Because of their layered structure and the disposition of their connections, neural networks are architecturally suited to integrate information in progressive stages between input and output. Thus they are broadly suited to categorize and to generalize information, to abstract the essential features of input stimuli. They are hypothetically suited to recognize stimulus constancy despite variance, as well as relations of topology and isomorphism. To some degree, connectionist networks can perform some of these operations, though only imperfectly, in no way near the versatile manner in which the brain does.

Categories of Knowledge

The categorization of knowledge, which the brain does so much better than computer models, is the essence of all cognitive functions. Perception is the classing of the world into categories. Discrimination is the reclassing and decomposition of sensory information. Attention is the focusing on a class or subclass of sensory or motor information. All our memories are categorized by content, by time, by place, and so on. Reasoning and intelligence are closely dependent on the proper categorization of phenomena, external and internal. And the use and comprehension of language depend on the classing of words and sentences by meaning, despite enormous variations in phonetics, pitch, loudness, and the size or style of print.

Knowledge about the world can be categorized according to a practically infinite number of criteria and parameters. Living organisms do it according to the criteria and parameters that they and their species have found adaptive. Scientists do it to discover order and causality in the universe. The brain does it with all the information that it receives from the senses or sends to the muscles. In behavior, reasoning, and language, categories of perception lead to categories of action. Probably nobody has described the processes of cognitive categorization better than Hayek (1952).

To understand how the brain categorizes cognitive information and how it stores it, which is our task in ensuing sections, it is helpful to focus briefly on perceptual knowledge, as has been done before by many, from empiricist philosophers to Gestalt psychologists to psychophysicists. Here we attempt to do it with the aim of defining or at least sketching an order that may well match a comparable order in the neocortex. To be sure, many concepts in current cognitive science, including those discussed below, are based on neural facts, however fragmentary or inadequately understood. Thus, in this chapter, I cannot disclaim a degree of tautology.

The most obvious characteristic of perceptual categories is *their hierarchical organization*. They are organized in cognitive hierarchies of progressive integration and generality, with sensory percepts in low levels and abstract or symbolic percepts in higher ones. At the bottom of the hierarchy are the sensory qualia of each modality. Here it is immaterial whether those elementary sensations are the irreducible building blocks of sensory perception, as Mach (1885) first proposed, or are themselves the product of prior evolutionary association, in other words, of *phyletic memory* or memory of the species (Chapter 2). Above that basal level, sensory qualia are grouped or *bound* to form higher classes or categories, in other words, percepts of greater generality. These in turn form classes of classes in higher levels of cognition, and so on. At any level, a class component can be a member of more than one category. Its contribution to the category is determined by context, that is, by the other components. For example, the contribution of an ambiguous character to a word is determined by neighboring characters (Fig. 3.2).

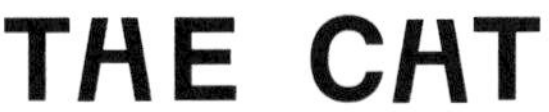

THE CHT

Figure 3.2. The importance of context. We perceive the same stimulus as a different letter, depending on the context. From Selfridge (1955), modified.

Each class is thus defined by its members and the relationships between them, and not by their sum. Consequently, the categorization of perceptual knowledge does not necessarily imply a proliferation of basic features in every higher category, for the categorization is often accompanied by a degree of generalization, abstraction, and symbolization. Features that have commonly been perceived together are unified to form broader categories, where some basic features stand for others as labels for the entire class. Perception, in sum, consists in the classing of objects by the *binding* of characteristics that have co-occurred in the past and thus have been associated by prior experience (Chapter 4). That binding is what segregates each object from its background. There is, however, a form of perceptual categorization that is not based on co-occurring sensory stimuli, but rather on sequences of them. That categorization may be viewed as a process of multiple classification over time or as the binding of temporally separate percepts (temporal integration). Temporal binding is extremely important in language. As we shall see, it is one of the essential functions of the cortex of the frontal lobe.

Finally, the hierarchical organization of perceptual categories does not imply that all learning (categorizing) occurs from the bottom up. Many associations, probably most, occur between hierarchical levels, between higher or abstract categories and lower ones, or horizontally within higher levels. In adult life these kinds of *heterarchical* categorization of percepts are probably not the exception but the rule. This does not negate, however, the general principle of a hierarchical organization of knowledge and a cognitive framework for it that has been laid out before, by early experience and education.

Paralleling a hierarchy of perceptual knowledge, there is a *hierarchy of action knowledge,* a hierarchy of the modes of response to surrounding events and to the percepts they evoke. Motor or executive knowledge, memory, and categories are all part of that hierarchy. As is the case with percepts, all the actions of the organism can be categorized, from the bottom up, and stacked in a hierarchy of motor cognits. At the bottom reside the elements of action that are defined

by discrete movements and muscle groups. Above them are the categories of action defined by goal and trajectory; and higher yet are the
programs and plans. Again the categorization *in time* is paramount,
especially with regard to language. Here, small temporally dispersed
categories (e.g., phonemes) are temporally integrated into larger categories (e.g., words), and these in turn into yet larger ones (e.g., sentences), and so on up the hierarchy. And here again, the temporally
integrative role of frontal cortex will become essential.

Cortical Modularity

One of the most striking characteristics of the mammalian neocortex
is the uniformity of its internal structure—hence the alternate desig-
nation *isocortex*. It consists in its entirety of six layers, each with its
characteristic content and architecture of cells and fibers. Every layer
has within it certain predominant types of cells with their own predominant connections (Fig. 3.3). In brief, layer IV receives thalamic
projections, while pyramids of layer II project principally to ipsilateral
cortical areas, pyramids of layer III to contralateral areas, and pyramids of layers V and VI to numerous subcortical structures, including
the thalamus, basal ganglia, midbrain, and spinal cord (Jones, 1984).
In addition, cells in all layers, including pyramids, project locally to
other cells in the same or a different layer.

     Without deviating from the six-layer template, cortical areas dif-
fer considerably in cytoarchitecture and in extrinsic connectivity—
that is, in the sources and targets of their connections. These structural differences are certainly the basis for the special functions of all
cortical areas, even though those functions are not yet fully understood. Indeed, the function of every area or subarea of the cortex is
defined by its afferent and efferent connections with other structures,
as well as by its intrinsic processes.

     Almost overshadowed by the stratified architecture of the neo-
cortex is the iterative vertical structure of its cells and fibers. As can
be best noted in microscopic sections, the apical dendrites, cell bodies, and axons of pyramids are arranged vertically, and apical dendrites are bundled up in vertical arrays. The entire cortex appears
parceled out in vertical *columns* of cells and fibers that span the width
of the cortex and are separated by regular intervals of sparse connectivity and low cell density. The width of those columns varies from
area to area, generally within the range of 30–50 μm. Columns orig-

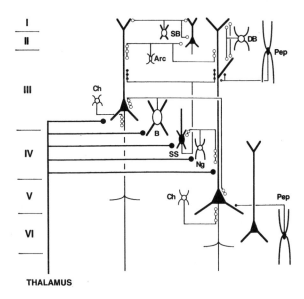

Figure 3.3. Schematic diagram of cortical neuron types and their connections. Cell types: Arc, arcade; B, large basket; Ch, chandelier; DB, double bouquet; Ng, neurogliaform; Pep, peptide cells; SS, spiny stellate; SB, small basket. *Solid dots*, excitatory contacts; *open circles*, inhibitory contacts; *solid cells*, excitatory; *open cells*, inhibitory. From Mountcastle (1998), adapted from Jones (1991), with permission.

inate in the primordial matrix of the proliferative layer (Chapter 2), each column resulting from the upward migration and superposition of about 100 neurons—more in visual cortex. Mountcastle (1998) considers this aggregate of closely interconnected cells, which he calls a *minicolumn,* the smallest processing unit of the neocortex.

Early electrophysiological studies revealed that cells of similar function in primary somatic cortex (Mountcastle, 1957), visual cortex (Hubel and Wiesel, 1968), and motor cortex (Asanuma, 1975) are grouped in ensembles that take the form of vertical bands or slabs across the thickness of the cortex. The unifying functional parameter for the cells of one such *module* varies considerably, depending on the modality. In somesthesis, it may be the receptive field for touch on a sector of the skin; in vision, the stimulation of a retinal field or a certain stimulus orientation; in audition, a sound frequency range; in motility, a muscle or muscle group. The dimensions of those functionally homogeneous cellular aggregates or modules vary also, depending on the species, cortical region, and modality. Their width generally ranges between 50 and 500 μm. Because in most instances that width exceeds the width of the minicolumn, especially outside of somatic cortex, it has been postulated that columnar modules are made up of coalesced minicolumns. In any event, the functionally defined column is broader than the anatomically and developmentally defined minicolumn. Nonetheless, connectivity is a defining factor in both. The cells of a column, like those of a minicolumn, are unified by a common set of extrinsic connections, afferent and efferent, with another cortical or extracortical structure. Undoubtedly connectivity and function go hand in hand in both kinds of modules.

Outside of primary sensory and motor cortices, functional modularity seems to loosen up or disappear. Anatomically, vertical arrangements of cells and fibers can still be discerned in cortex of association. Moreover, interarea connections have been noted to terminate in vertical patches of 200- to 500-μm width, with maximal density in supragranular layers (Jacobson and Trojanowski, 1977; Schwartz and Goldman-Rakic, 1984). Functional modularity, however, has not been conclusively demonstrated in cortex of association. Arguably, the "right parameters" to stimulate that cortex have not yet been found. At any event, in cortex of association, sensory, behavioral, or psychological variables have failed to elicit common responses in cellular aggregates that might thus be construed as functional modules. There is one notable exception, in inferotemporal cortex (Fujita et al., 1992; Tanaka, 1993). It is an exception that confirms the rule, however, for the modularity there is considerably looser than in sensory cortex, at least in terms of sensory tuning. Most importantly, relatively large modules of inferotemporal cells seem to encode *associated* features of the visual world (Fig. 3.4).

The findings just cited—from Tanaka and collaborators—are indicative of an expanding trend, in the substrate of cortical representation, toward progressively higher stages of the hierarchy of sensory processing areas. Both anatomical and physiological evidence makes it clear that the inferotemporal cortex is unimodal association cortex, an important stage in the hierarchy of cortical regions dedicated to the processing of visual information. In this sense it is a transitional or intermediate step between primary visual cortex and the higher areas of polymodal convergence. Inferotemporal neurons are characterized by broad visual tuning, large receptive fields, and specific reactivity to complex visual stimuli—some with behavioral sig-

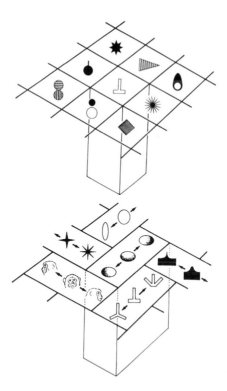

Figure 3.4. Vertical modules of cells attuned to various complex visual stimuli in the inferotemporal cortex of the monkey. Adjacent neurons in horizontally elongated slabs or conglomerates of columnar modules react to different but physically related stimuli. From Mountcastle (1998), adapted from Tanaka (1993), with permission.

nificance (Desimone et al., 1984). These general traits of inferotemporal cells, together with the finding that they associate visual features, provide strong suggestive evidence for the upward expansion of representation in the cortical hierarchy of visual processing areas.

The chemical senses, taste and olfaction, have their first cortical areas of representation in the paralimbic cortex at the base of the frontal lobe (orbitofrontal cortex)—immediately rostral to the junction between the temporal and frontal lobes. Taste cortex lies lateral and adjacent to olfactory cortex. A modular structure for either cortex has not been discovered. If there is one, it cannot be easily revealed, among other reasons probably because of the nontopological nature of chemical senses. Beyond primary cortex, the pathways for

processing and categorization of chemical-sense information have
not been clearly identified.

The primary motor cortex occupies a functionally symmetrical
position with regard to primary sensory cortices. With regard to somatosensory cortex, its position is not only functionally but also
anatomically symmetrical, for the two cortices face and mirror each
other across the central (rolandic) sulcus. Like somatosensory cortex,
motor cortex is somatotopically organized, in that the various sectors
of motility are topologically mapped onto it. The motor cortex lies at
the base of the cortical hierarchy of motor representations, much as
sensory cortices lie at the base of the hierarchies of sensory representations. It is subdivided into vertical modules of cells dedicated to discrete aspects of motility. Recent studies, however, emphasize the population dynamics of motor cortex. Cells are unified in ensembles
dedicated to the performance of synergistic movements by groups of
muscles (Georgopoulos et al., 1986; Sato and Tanji, 1989). Therefore,
modules of yet unclear geometry would seem to serve movements of
specific trajectory.

To recap, discrete neuronal modules of specific function have
been identified only in primary sensory and motor cortex. From their
functions we can deduce the elementary features of the sensorium
and of motility that they *represent*. They seem to represent the simplest
components of cognition, the elementary "memory" that the species
has acquired in the course of evolution in its perennial striving to
adapt. We can say, figuratively, that phylogeny delivers to ontogeny
those primary modules as items of old knowledge (*phyletic memory*), so
that the new organism will be capable of adapting to new situations
and of acquiring new knowledge about itself and the world. Each primary sensation, each elementary motor action, is an act of *re-cognition*
of sorts, a reactivation of the knowledge of the species that is deposited
in the structure of the modules of primary sensory or motor cortex.

Beyond primary cortices, the search for cortical modularity may
be futile. This presumption is based on the mounting evidence, from
a variety of methodologies, that all connective trends away from primary areas lead into areas that process and represent acquired complex knowledge, in other words, complex individual experience or
memory. Because that memory is fundamentally based on the association and integration of information within and across modalities,
across space, and across time, it is unlikely that it can be encoded in
discrete domains of cortex. Instead, what is more likely is that the new

knowledge will be distributed in large-scale networks of association cortex. Each junction or node in those networks will not represent a specific item of personal experience but instead mediate the association between several items that make up the experience. It is well to keep in mind, however, that each of those items is originally based on the modules of primary cortex that represent the common memory of the species, that is, the elementary sensations and the simple acts.

Cortical Hierarchy of Perceptual Networks

Pyramidal neurons of each primary sensory area—V1 for vision, A1 for audition, S1 for somesthesis—send axonal connections onto adjacent or nearby areas of somewhat different cytoarchitecture that constitute further processing steps for analysis within that modality. In the visual cortical pathway, for example, beyond V1 (area 17), some of these areas specialize in the analysis of such visual features as motion, shape, and color (Felleman and Van Essen, 1991). These areas send fiber projections to other areas of occipital, temporal, or parietal cortex that specialize in the processing of more complex information of the same modality. All areas in the three cortical pathways dedicated to the processing of modality-specific information beyond primary cortices have been characterized as cortex of *unimodal association*. Pandya and colleagues (Pandya and Yeterian, 1985), in the monkey, group them into three successive cortical regions for each modality— first-, second-, and third-order association cortex (Fig. 3.5).

All connections in the sequence of cortical areas that constitute a unimodal processing and association pathway are reciprocal, in that successive areas in it are linked by fibers flowing forward, away from the primary area, and by fibers flowing in the opposite direction (Fig. 3.6). Further, the interarea linkages in both directions include topologically organized parallel connections, convergent connections, and divergent connections. Thus the neural wiring is available for parallel processing, as well as for integration and distribution of information in both directions, that is, bottom-up and top-down.

Each unimodal pathway, at various stages, sends long-distance projections to three broad cortical regions: frontal lobe cortex, paralimbic cortex, and areas of multimodal convergence in parietal and temporal cortex. The connections to frontal cortex serve sensory–motor associations, those to paralimbic cortex (gateway to the amygdala and hippocampus) serve emotional associations and memory,

Cortex and Mind

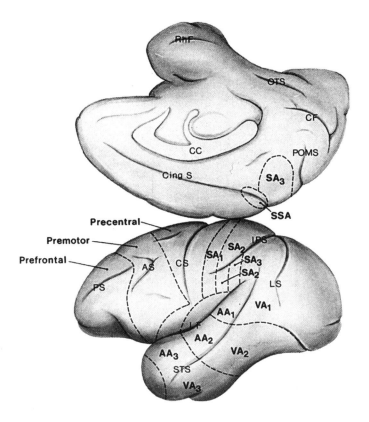

Figure 3.5. Schematic map of the unimodal association areas of the monkey's cortex: visual (VA), auditory (AA), and somatic (SA) areas of first, second, and third order (respectively marked by subscripts 1, 2, and 3). *Abbreviations:* AS, arcuate sulcus; CC, corpus callosum; CF, calcarine fissure; Cing S, cingulate sulcus; CS, central sulcus; IPS, intraparietal sulcus; LS, lunate sulcus; OTS, occipitotemporal sulcus; POMS, parieto-occipitomedial sulcus; PS, principal sulcus; RhF, rhinal fissure; SSA, supplementary somatic area; STS, superior temporal sulcus. From Pandya and Yeterian (1985), with permission.

and those to multimodal areas serve cross-modal associations. These three sets of long cortico-cortical connections are reciprocal. The temporal and parietal areas of multimodal convergence, presumably serving intermodal association, have been termed *transmodal areas* by Mesulam (1998), who has applied to the human some well-reasoned inferences from the cortical connectivity of the monkey (Fig. 3.7). In the human, transmodal areas include large sectors of the midtemporal cortex, Wernicke's area at the junction of temporal and parietal

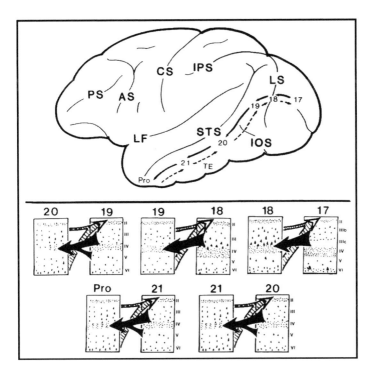

Figure 3.6. Interconnected areas in the cortical visual pathway departing from area 17 (V1). All connections between successive areas are reciprocal: some are sensory-fugal (*continuous arrows*) and others sensory-petal (*broken arrows*). Arrows in the lower part of the diagram mark the cortical layers of predominant origin and termination of connective axons. *Abbreviations:* AS, arcuate sulcus; CS, central sulcus; IOS, inferior occipital cortex; IPS, intraparietal sulcus; LF, lateral fissure; LS, lunate sulcus; STS, superior temporal sulcus; Pro, proisocortex; PS, principal sulcus; TE, inferotemporal area. From Pandya and Yeterian (1985), with permission.

cortices, and limbic cortex (entorhinal, parahippocampal, and hippo-campal).

In the monkey as in the human, the streams of connectivity from primary sensory to transmodal areas mark not only trails of sensory processing but also an ascending ladder in a hierarchy of representations of perceptual knowledge. A massive literature of cognitive neuroscience substantiates this hierarchy. Essentially, the supporting evidence is of two kinds: (*1*) lesions in progressively higher connective stages lead to deficits in the availability of progressively higher cate-

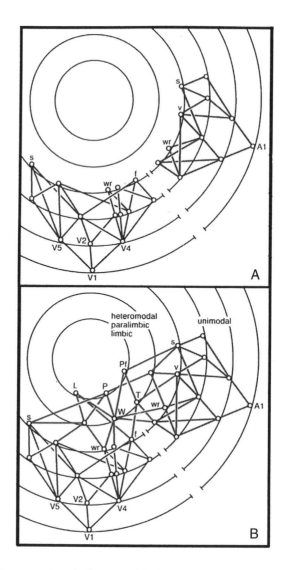

Figure 3.7. Patterns of cortical connectivity in the human, as inferred by Mesulam from those verified in the monkey. *Concentric circles* denote hierarchical levels of representation and processing. *Small circles* denote anatomical cortical areas or network nodes. *Unidentified circles* denote intermediate or nonlocalized areas. In *A*, the visual and auditory pathways are depicted. In *B*, transmodal pathways are added. *Abbreviations for visual areas:* V1, primary visual cortex; V2, V4, V5, additional visual areas; s, area specialized for encoding spatial location (visual); wr, area specialized for encoding word forms (visual); f, area specialized for face encoding. *Abbreviations for auditory areas:* A1, primary auditory cortex; wr, area specialized for encoding word forms (auditory); v, area specialized for identifying voice patterns; s, area specialized for encoding spatial location (auditory). *Abbreviations for transmodal areas:* L, limbic and paralimbic cortices; P, heteromodal posterior parietal cortex; W, Wenicke's area; T, heteromodal lateral temporal cortex; Pf, lateral prefrontal cortex. From Mesulam (1998), with permission.

gories of knowledge and (2) neurons in progressively higher stages fire in correlation with sensory stimuli that activate—thus make available—progressively higher categories of knowledge. By *higher categories of knowledge* I mean knowledge of greater abstraction or generality, including, in the highest stages, cross-modal semantic and symbolic knowledge. Since the evidence of deficit or neuronal correlation has been obtained by testing sensory discrimination or memory performance, some of that evidence will be cited in relation to the cortical dynamics of perception (Chapter 4) and memory (Chapter 5). Here my objective is to outline the principles of organization of knowledge that derive from cortical neurobiology and connectivity, and that are supported by cognitive neuroscience. How is that ladder of perceptual knowledge formed? What is the anatomical structure of that knowledge? We will address these questions at the three broad hierarchical levels discussed above with regard to the connectivity between them: primary sensory cortex, unimodal association cortex, and transmodal association cortex.

The module of *sensory cortex* is the smallest and hierarchically lowest perceptual network. It is the circuitry dedicated to the representation of an elementary sensory feature. In addition to potentially active cells and synapses, that circuitry contains the essentials of memory networks, including recurrent connections, to maintain a representation active while present in the environment and even afterward, for a few moments (iconic memory). As we proceed upward to *unimodal association* areas, we find sensory representation slightly more dispersed in brain space. Modules are larger, and the information they represent is more complex than that in primary cortex. Cells are more broadly tuned to stimulus parameters and less demanding with regard to those parameters. Receptive fields are larger, and cells respond to stimuli despite wide variations of stimulus parameters. Thus the cells at these higher levels appear to respect stimulus constancy to some degree, a crucial requisite for perception and its categorizing function. In sum, the cells of unimodal association areas are part of representational networks that encode more complex and multidimensional stimuli than the cells of primary cortex. Some of the dimensions to which those cells respond extend beyond the sensorium and the associations of a given modality within it. Those extrasensory dimensions include the behavioral significance and motor responses that the stimuli are supposed to elicit.

Because the cells of unimodal association respond to stimuli that are more complex and spread over wider sectors of cortex than those of primary cortex, it is reasonable to conclude that they are part of networks representing those complex stimuli. Those networks, we can further infer, bind together the features that constitute the percepts they represent. Thus those networks would be formed by integration of the stimulus features that have been individually analyzed in sensory cortex. Not all the features of a stimulus might be integrated and represented by the network, but only those that categorize that stimulus as a perceptual cognit. On the other hand, any of a network's components can be part of many other networks. In Chapter 4 we will deal with the electrophysiology of perceptual binding.

Thus, what we call a cognit in unimodal association cortex is a network of cells that are interconnected to represent associated features of a complex stimulus or group of stimuli of the corresponding modality. The network has been formed by prior repeated co-occurrence of those constituent features. The strength of the binding, and thus the robustness of the cognit, are functions of several factors. Notable among these factors are (1) temporal contiguity, (2) spatial contiguity, (3) repetition, and (4) emotional or motivational connotations. There is considerable trade-off between these factors but, in general, the greater any or all of them are, the more solid is the cognit, the easier it is to retrieve it in cognitive operations, and the more resistant it is to cortical damage.

Compound representations that are formed by simultaneous and spatially contiguous features of a given modality tend to coalesce in relatively discrete portions of unimodal association cortex. A notable example is that of individual *faces,* which are represented in discrete areas, presumably by small networks, of visual association cortex (Desimone, 1991; Young and Yamane, 1992; Tanaka, 1993). Faces as a category of objects of more generality, however, have a wider, more distributed representation, with network nodes in temporal, fusiform, and prepiriform cortex. Some of these nodes or netlets of face representation reside in paralimbic areas, which may have to do with the encoding of the emotional connotations of faces. Emotional or motivational association is one of the reasons why the networks of unimodal association cortex extend into other areas; it is also a reason why the perceptual cognits of one modality are distributed beyond the region of representation for that modality. Another reason is the associations of those cognits with behavioral action. These sensory–motor associations are mediated by the long reciprocal fibers, already mentioned, between unimodal cortex of the posterior regions of the hemisphere and areas of the frontal lobe.

Imaging studies indicate that separate areas of unimodal association cortex are activated by the semantic retrieval of categories of animate and inanimate entities, such as animals and tools (Damasio et al., 1996; Martin et al., 1996). Moreover, clinical studies implicate certain areas of unimodal visual and auditory association cortex in the representation of, respectively, word forms and word sounds (Mesulam, 1998).

In the upper reaches of their respective hierarchies, the cortical pathways of unimodal association converge on areas of *multimodal* or transmodal association of posterior cortex. In the monkey, several such areas can be identified in the banks and depths of the superior temporal and intraparietal sulci. In the human, one large convergence region, apparently comprising several multimodal areas, occupies the junction of the occipital, temporal, and parietal lobes. That region includes the cortex of the angular gyrus and the superior half of the superior temporal gyrus, Wernicke's area. Clinical evidence and imaging studies implicate both of these cortical areas in the representation of the meaning of words and sentences (Chapter 7). Lesions of these areas often result in agraphia and semantic aphasia (Penfield and Roberts, 1966; Geschwind, 1970; Luria, 1970).

Nonetheless, the role of transmodal areas in cognitive representation is poorly understood and probably transcends language. Lesions within them can cause agnosias that extend to nonverbal material encoded in more than one sensory modality (Walsh, 1978). Those areas, therefore, seem to contain representations of cross-modal information. At the same time, they may constitute the nodes of wide networks encroaching on many areas of unimodal and cross-modal association. These wider networks would represent abstractions and concepts by tying together the common nodes of many cognits represented in more concrete constituent networks at lower hierarchical levels. Later we will deal further with this issue.

The progressive expansion of knowledge categories with the upward progression of the perceptual hierarchy explains the different degrees of vulnerability to damage at different levels of that hierarchy, as well as the different consequences of damage. At the lower level, in sensory cortex, representation is highly concrete and localized, and thus highly vulnerable. Local damage leads to well-delimited sensory deficit. In unimodal association cortex, representation is more cate-

gorical and more distributed, in networks that span relatively large
sectors of that cortex. With the possible exception of areas representing certain categories of sounds, objects, and faces, resistance to
local lesions is greater than in sensory cortex. Lesions must be larger
than in sensory cortex for deficit to ensue.

As noted, in transmodal areas representation is even more widely
distributed. The content is more general, for it is based on multimodal networks. It consists of categories of knowledge that have been
acquired through multiple experiences and through several senses.
Because that knowledge is widely distributed, damage does not so
much obliterate it as disjoint its components, breaking large networks
and the associations between those components. Lesions thus produce the *disconnection syndromes* of Geschwind (1965b) in the form of
aphasias, agraphias, and agnosias of various sorts. Only large lesions
affecting several of those transmodal areas lead to the deterioration
of conceptual cognits and thus to what Goldstein (1959) calls the loss
of the *abstract attitude.*

Cortical Hierarchy of Executive Networks

Earlier I alluded to long connections from posterior cortical areas to
areas of the frontal lobe. These connections constitute the functional
linkage between the two cortical hierarchies, one for perception in
posterior cortex and the other for action in frontal cortex. The lowest stages of both hierarchies are the cortical processing areas at the
interface between the cortex and the environment: sensory cortex at
the input interface and motor cortex at the output interface. In the
course of behavior, the two hierarchies are engaged in a cybernetic
cycle of dynamic interactions with the environment that I have termed
the *perception-action cycle* (Chapter 4).

Above the motor cortex of area 4, or M1, the next level up in the
motor hierarchy, is the premotor cortex of area 6. All three unimodal
association cortices (visual, auditory, and somatic) send projections
to premotor cortex. In addition, they send some to the next frontal
level up, which is the prefrontal cortex (areas 8, 9, 10, and 46). All
these projections are topologically organized (frontal-lobe connectivity reviewed in more detail in Fuster, 1997). The frontal lobe reciprocates, with projections of its own, all the projections it receives
from posterior areas (Fig. 3.8). The reciprocal, backward projections
are also topologically organized. As outlined below, motor represen-

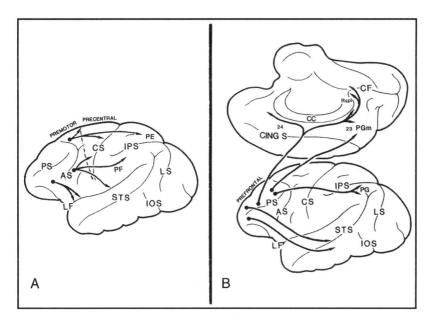

Figure 3.8. Fiber projections from the frontal lobe to areas of posterior cortex. From Pandya and Yeterian (1985), with permission.

tations are hierarchically arranged by ascending order of generality and temporal dimension in the three frontal stages: motor, premotor, and prefrontal. This order parallels the sensory order in posterior cortex. In very general terms, long connections link corresponding levels of the two hierarchies. Thus, the unimodal association areas are reciprocally interconnected with premotor areas, whereas the multimodal areas of posterior cortex are interconnected with multimodal areas of the lateral prefrontal convexity.

In addition, the prefrontal cortex has reciprocal connections with limbic structures. Its dorsolateral areas are connected with the cingulate, hippocampus, and parahippocampal cortex. These connections have probably much to do with the formation of motor memory and its representations in the frontal cortex. On the other hand, the orbital prefrontal cortex, either directly or through anterior thalamic nuclei, is connected with the amygdala, which plays a role in the evaluation of the motivational significance of external stimuli. Influences from the amygdala may also play a role in the acquisition of motor memory, inasmuch as those stimuli are essential to the configuration of motor behavior.

As noted in Chapter 2, the formation of cognits of action may be subject to the same basic mechanisms as the formation of perceptual memory. Hebbian principles probably apply here too, and synaptic connections in motor networks may be facilitated by synchronous convergence in the same manner as in perceptual networks. Motor networks may thus be formed by coincident motor inputs (e.g., efferent copies of movement through recurrent fibers from the pyramidal system) and sensory inputs (proprioceptive and other) from posterior cortex. In the upward progression of the action hierarchy, from motor cortex to prefrontal cortex, networks would come to represent progressively higher categories of cognits of action.

In the *frontal lobe* the connectivity within the motor or action-related hierarchy generally courses from the top down. As in the sensory hierarchy, three connective patterns prevail: parallel, convergent, and divergent. In the execution of motor actions, parallel processing down the cortical hierarchy, through subcortical loops (basal ganglia, cerebellum, lateral thalamus), seems at least as important as serial processing (Alexander et al., 1992). Here too, integration via convergent fibers and distribution via divergent fibers seem to play complementary roles.

At the top of the executive hierarchy is the prefrontal cortex, which in the monkey as in the human seems to contain neuronal networks that represent programs or plans of action. The next level underneath in the cortical connective chain is the premotor cortex, where actions are represented in more concrete form, defined by trajectory and goal. At the bottom is the primary motor cortex, which represents specific movements defined by groups of muscles working in synergy and genetically preassigned to the cell populations or motor modules of area M1. In premotor and prefrontal cortex, a modular organization has not been conclusively demonstrated. Behavioral electrophysiology provides evidence of cell clusters encoding stimuli that the animal uses as cues in memory tasks (e.g., delay tasks), but such clusters are large and widely scattered. Further, their cells seem to respond to the stimuli mostly or only inasmuch as these are components of temporally organized actions.

At the level of the *motor cortex* (M1), cell populations similar in dimension to modules of sensory cortex encode specific movements (Asanuma, 1975). As already noted, their activation leads to muscular movements that are defined in terms of direction (Georgopoulos et al., 1986; Sato and Tanji, 1989). Muscles are grouped and represented by their *desired effect.* That means that in M1 the representations are not strictly organized somatotopically, but rather by intended action. When those representations are activated and the action is implemented, the activation of M1 cells precedes the movement by a fraction of a second.

Judging from electrophysiological and lesion data, the representations of movement in *premotor cortex* (area 6) are more global and more distributed than in M1. Several areas, however, can be distinguished within that cortex, each with somewhat different characteristics with respect to the actions it represents. In the band of cortex that constitutes premotor cortex proper (area 6b), immediately in front of motor cortex, cells are attuned to the kinematic properties of movement, especially trajectory (Weinrich and Wise, 1982; Crutcher and Alexander, 1990). Their activation by a sensory stimulus may precede the movement by as much as a few seconds, and therefore those cells seem to intervene in movement preparation. Some premotor cortex cells are involved not only in the representation of movements defined in body-centered coordinates, but also in that of movements at a somewhat more abstract level. Such cells, for example, will be activated by the observation of specific movements performed by a human subject (Di Pellegrino et al., 1992). Because these units seem to reflect the other subject's action, they have been termed *mirror units.*

Units at an apparently higher level hierarchically, in the upper and more medial premotor cortex (area 6a), which has been called the supplementary motor area (SMA), are activated before and during the execution of specific *sequences of movements* (Mushiake et al., 1991). Cells are not tuned to any of the component movements of a sequence but to the sequence itself. Note that we have entered a higher level of abstraction, executive *abstraction in the time domain.* The representations are no longer defined solely by spatial coordinates but also by the temporal coordinate. Imaging studies corroborate the cellular evidence on a regional scale (Colebatch et al., 1991; Grafton et al., 1992).

Furthermore, some neurons in premotor cortex proper, as in the SMA, are subject to influences that must be characterized not only in kinematic terms, but also in such terms as interest, biological significance, and goal. These factors will enhance the activation of premotor cells in the preparation and execution of movements. Their role is epitomized by units of the SMA that are activated not only by sensory stimuli that call for specific movements or sequences of movements, but also by an internal decision in anticipation of *self-initiated* movement (Mushiake et al., 1991). The readiness potential (Kornhuber and Deecke, 1965), a slow surface negative potential just before a self-initiated motor action, seems to originate in the SMA. Furthermore, lesions of the SMA in the human impair the ability to initiate movements (Halsband et al., 1993). Evidence of this kind has led some authors to conclude that the SMA is the source of voluntary movement (Eccles, 1982).

The evidence that premotor neurons take part in the preparation and execution of biologically motivated actions, and the evidence that the role of those neurons is enhanced by interest and self-initiation, point to influences from limbic structures upon those neurons. Further, the available evidence argues for the participation of limbic connections in the representation of actions, not just in their execution. Whether these connections are direct or mediated by neurons in the prefrontal cortex, which lies above premotor cortex in the motor hierarchy and receives profuse limbic inputs, cannot yet be ascertained.

The temporal dimension of action representation is paramount in *lateral prefrontal cortex*. In animals and humans, lesions of this cortex lead to deficits in the learning and performing of tasks that depend on the temporal integration of sensory and motor information. Such deficits can be observed best in delay tasks (e.g., delayed response, delayed matching), where the animal must integrate a sensory cue (the position or color of an object, for example) with a later stimulus in order to perform an appropriate action. In the human, the deficit is observable not only in delay tasks but also in other integrated sequences of cognitive acts. One of the most characteristic symptoms of lateral prefrontal damage is the impairment of the capacity to formulate and carry out *plans of action*. The difficulty of integration in the temporal domain is also manifest, of course, in the spoken language (Chapter 7). If the lesion is in the lower convexity of the left frontal lobe (Broca's area), the deficit affects the most elementary aspects of syntax (Geschwind, 1970). If the lesion is in the dorsolateral convexity, the language deficit may be more subtle and may affect only the construction of novel and elaborate speech (Luria, 1970). In either case the patient has difficulties integrating language in time. Behind those difficulties there is probably a deficit in the representation of linguistic sequences. Neuroimaging shows prefrontal activations by the internal representation of plans of action and speech (Ingvar, 1983; Roland, 1985; Frith et al., 1991).

During the execution of delay tasks, cells in prefrontal cortex show sustained and cue-specific activations in the delay interval between the cue and the later sensory stimulus with which the cue has to be integrated (Fuster, 1997). That form of discharge has been widely interpreted as a manifestation of working memory (of the cue), which is one of the executive functions of the frontal lobe (Chapter 6). It is probably also a manifestation of the activation of a widely distributed representation of a structure of behavior (the delay-task trial) of which the cue is only a part. Other parts of that structure are the expected cues and consequent movements in preparation. Therefore, it is not surprising that in the dorsolateral prefrontal cortex the *working-memory* cells are accompanied by *motor-set* cells (Quintana and Fuster, 1999). Nor is it surprising that the sustained activation of massive numbers of both types of cells results in a slow surface negative potential between cue and response, the *contingent negative variation*. All are manifestations of the activation of a large, widely distributed executive cognit and its temporally separate components, sensory and motor.

Finally, there is evidence from lesion and imaging studies that cortical executive representations are not permanent, especially those in prefrontal cortex. Animals with lesions of this cortex have difficulty learning to perform certain tasks, such as delayed-response tasks. After extensive training, however, they do learn them. This is evidence that other motor structures at lower hierarchical level (e.g., premotor cortex, basal ganglia) can play a surrogate role and accommodate the executive memory of a delay task after the frontal lesion occurs. Human subjects with frontal lesions can perform automatic movements but have lost their ability to perform them on command or voluntarily. Further, the activation of prefrontal cortex during the learning of skilled sequential movements disappears after the movements have become routine, while that of basal ganglia increases (Grafton et al., 1992; Jenkins et al., 1994). These observations suggest that the prefrontal cortex represents mainly or only the new and complex executive cognits. As they become automatic, the old and well-established cognits migrate or are relegated to lower structures of the executive hierarchy. The perception-action cycle continues to operate, but mainly at subcortical levels.

Summarizing, at the lowest cortical level of the executive hierarchy, in M1, skeletal movements are represented in discrete neuronal networks that may be characterized as motor modules. In the level above, the premotor cortex, motor networks and their representations are more ample and defined by goal and trajectory; in one premotor area, the SMA, some of the cognits represented consist of movement sequences. In prefrontal cortex, the highest executive level, the representations of action are made up of more extensive networks that encode novel, temporally extended schemas, plans, and programs of action, including linguistic sequences.

Heterarchical Representation in Association Cortex

In the previous two sections, I have described two parallel and complementary hierarchies of cortical networks: one in posterior cortex for the representation of perceptual cognits and the other in frontal cortex for the representation of cognits of action. For heuristic reasons, I have outlined two tiers of stacked cognits of increasing breadth as we ascend in either hierarchy. This picture, although correct in general terms, may be misleading. It conveys the idea that every representation is formed and retained at a certain hierarchical level, sensory or motor, and that all memories of the world and the self are neatly compartmentalized by level. Most memories, however, are probably represented in networks that span two or more levels. They are *heterarchical* (I hesitate to use this term because it implies dissimilar organization, instead of dissimilar ranking of network components, but the term has been condoned by usage as the opposite of *hierarchical;* certainly *anarchical* wouldn't do!).

As noted in Chapter 2, inputs that meet at the same time to facilitate a set of synapses and thus to build a network need not be of external origin (sensory). They may originate internally by activation of previously formed networks of whatever hierarchical rank. Thus, for example, an incoming sensory input activates an old network of associative memory by virtue of the fact that some of that input is a component of that network, as it was one of its originally associated constituents, or closely related to one. The new input then becomes associated with the old reactivated network, expanding and updating the latter. Of course, the old memory may have a very different ranking in the cortex than the new information, and consequently the new memory will be heterarchical. For example, the sight of a good deed by the good Samaritan will elicit and become associated with the concept of charity, a cognit of high ranking that is probably widely distributed in the cortex and based on—that is, abstracted from—previous experiences of the same kind.

That admixture of networks of different hierarchical rank is inherent in perception, inasmuch as perception is a top-down interpretation of the world in the light of prior experience (Boring, 1933). Hayek (1952, p. 143) expresses it this way:

> All we can perceive of external events are therefore only such properties of these events as they possess as members of classes which have been formed by past "linkages". The qualities which we attribute to the experienced objects are strictly speaking not properties [of those objects] at all, but a set of relations by which our nervous system classifies them or, to put it differently, *all* we know about the world is of the nature of theories and all "experience" can do is to change these theories.

Those "theories," by definition, have a higher rank as categories of knowledge than the new experience, which they help to categorize. A sensory event cannot be converted into a new cognit unless it is related in some manner to concomitant or past events. The integration of that event with others can only occur at a higher level than the primary sensory cortex—despite, for example, the apparent integrative properties of some *hypercomplex* cells of visual cortex. Further integration with other cognits of higher category, in terms of abstraction or generality, must involve higher levels of associative cortex. The integration with information of other modalities must involve areas of transmodal association cortex. Finally, the integration with prospective action must involve the cortex of the frontal lobe, the prefrontal cortex in particular.

Given that one cortical hemisphere can learn what the other is being taught, integration of new cognits can also take place across *interhemispheric* commissures. At any level of associative cortex, information can be sent across the corpus callosum and become associated with material in the other hemisphere. Thus, callosal fibers can become part of heterarchical networks representing perceptual or executive cognits. In sum, because cognits can be formed within and between hierarchical levels, information from many sources, internal as well as external, can contribute to the formation of a cognit of any category, that is, of any level of abstraction or generality, even across hemispheres.

However, the upward abstraction and generalization of cognits that appear to take place with progressively higher integrative operations conjure another misconception: the notion of pyramiding networks toward a *grandmother network* that will represent a concept or general fact somewhere in upper cortex. This simplistic notion is contradicted by overwhelming neuropsychological evidence from lesion studies. The process of upward abstraction and generalization is probably quite the opposite of pyramiding. Networks tend to spread through their divergent connections and to occupy wider cortical space as they penetrate higher hierarchical levels. Therefore, it is reasonable to suppose that, at those higher levels, cognitive networks of lower and separate origin will be more likely to intersect, to interact, and to be integrated than at the lower levels. Multiple high-level interactions and integration are the most plausible mechanisms behind the merging of lower-category cognits into higher, more abstract and general ones. Thus a high-level cognit (e.g., an abstract concept) would be represented in a wide network of association cortex that has contacts with multiple lower-category networks with which it is associated—and which have contributed to its formation. In that sense, cortical high-level cognits are both degenerate and complex (Edelman and Gally, 2001). This view is not incompatible, however, with a degree of semantic or abstract convergence in certain domains of cortex.

Further, the misconception of the cognit as a discrete and isolated cortical network is contradicted by evidence that cognits change with and without additional experience. We know they can be elicited or retrieved in modified form by changing circumstances and experiences, apparently as a result of changes in other remotely associated cognits—by reasons of similarity, contrast, and other factors. Therefore, a cognit cannot be a discrete and isolated network, uninfluenced by changes in other networks. A more appropriate view is that of a network with relatively firm connections at the core, made of repeatedly enhanced synaptic contacts, as well as weakly enhanced and *noncommitted* contacts "around the edges." It is difficult to determine with present methods what are the boundaries of the core and of the more plastic or labile periphery. In any case, strength of connection is at the root of cognit formation, cognit boundary, and cognit loss. Contiguity, repetition, and emotional load seem to be the most decisive strengtheners of synaptic contacts in the making of a cognitive network. Aging, disease, and trauma, on the other hand, undo connections and the cells that keep them.

4

Perception

*I*n the previous chapter, I outlined the principles of organization of the cortical networks that make up perceptual cognits, which are the units of knowledge acquired through the senses and chiefly distributed in posterior cortex. On the basis of developmental and connective gradients, as well as some functional evidence, I proposed that those networks and the knowledge they represent are hierarchically organized in layers by order of complexity or generality of cognitive content. These layers correspond to cortical stages for the processing and representation of sensory information. Further, the perceptual networks are amply interconnected within and between layers, as well as with the motor networks or cognits of frontal regions. One of my goals in this chapter is to assemble evidence of an order in the cortical processing of sensory information that corresponds isomorphically to the mental or *phenomenal* order of perception. The first two sections of the chapter deal with psychological aspects of perception; the last three deal with the mechanisms by which networks of posterior and frontal cortex process sensory information in perception.

Perceptual Categorization

To philosophers and psychologists of all times, from Heraclitos (fifth century BC) to contemporary psychophysicists, perception is the representation of the world entering the mind through the senses. At various times, some have argued for a major role of ideas, knowledge, or reason in the perceptual experience, but hardly anyone has ever denied the fundamentally sensory foundation of this experience. To some, in fact, *perception* and *sensation* are different terms for the same mental faculty. In modern neuroscience, perception is widely assumed to be reducible to the effects of sensory stimuli upon dedicated receptors, pathways, and nerve cells—essentially a late version of Müller's old principle of the *specific energy of nerves* (Boring, 1942), now extended into the brain.

Any definition of perception, however, that is based solely on the sensory analysis of physical attributes is inadequate, as it ignores an essential trait of perception, namely, its historical or autobiographical character. Bishop Berkeley (1709/1963) first, and two centuries later Helmholtz (1925), adduced with powerful arguments that our perceptions of the world are under the influences of the past, inasmuch as they are molded by previous memories and guided by selective attention, which, like memory, is anchored in past experience. Contemporary neuroscience acknowledges these influences, but treats them collectively as some kind of *top-down control* of sensory input from higher centers by mechanisms that are still obscure. Yet perception is not only under the influence of memory but is itself memory or, more precisely, the updating of memory. We perceive what we remember as well as remember what we perceive. Every percept is a historical event, a categorization of current sensory impressions that is entirely determined by previously established memory. This view becomes more plausible if we accept that all sensation, even the most elementary, is the retrieval of a form of ancestral memory— phyletic memory or memory of the species (Chapter 2).

Thus, every percept has two components intertwined, the sensory-induced *re-cognition* of a category of cognitive information in memory and the categorization of new sensory impressions in the light of that retrieved memory. Perception can thus be viewed as the interpretation of new experiences based on assumptions from prior experience—in other words, the continuous testing by the senses of educated hypotheses about the world around us (Hayek, 1952). Hence the essentially active character of perception, a concept far removed from the passive, receptive view of that faculty that Locke (1690/1894) held, echoing the Stoics of ancient Greece (*tabula rasa*). To this day, however, psychophysics and cognitive science tend to dismiss this active character of perception. The former does it because of its emphasis on the sensory analysis of physical features; the latter because of its emphasis on the symbolic nature of cognitive operations, which are admitted to be released by sensory input but are considered independent of it. Both psychophysics and cognitive science also tend to ignore the basic fact that the bulk of perceptual processing is executed in parallel and unconsciously.

Indeed, in much of the perceptual categorizing of sensory information, consciousness is *optional* (Barsalou, 1999). We are unaware of massive amounts of that information while our brain is engaged in processing it. Outside of consciousness, we test and verify myriad hypotheses about the world. Most of that testing and verifying takes place in parallel, concurrently along several channels of one or more sensory modalities. One part of it, however, is conscious and largely executed in series, that is, in successive steps. That is the part of perceptual processing that is guided by selective *attention,* a top-down cognitive function that, like memory, determines the course of categorization (Chapter 6). Attention can be aroused by unexpected percepts, in other words, by sensory inputs that falsify hypotheses—so to speak—about the surround and alert us to novelty, danger, or the need to take unanticipated adaptive action. Attention can also arise from preconceived plans or searches, as in the creative or scientific endeavor. In any case, the outcome of the role of attention on a percept or series of percepts is usually, at some level, a new discrimination of the environment, a reclassification or recategorization of that environment. In sum, attention is an aid to the categorizing function of perception. As we scan the world in search of meaning and of new categories of reality, or new ways to discriminate them, we orient our senses to the aspects of the environment where we know from experience that those can be most readily found. Our search is driven not only by salient changes in the physical dimensions of sensory stimulation, but also by educated, memory-based expectations of significance or of relevant difference at the source of that stimulation. Furthermore, discrete aspects of perception are selectively modulated from experience, that is, enhanced or gated to maximize the yield from the processing of sensory information that experience tells us is most relevant at a given place and time.

The limited capacity of sensory systems to process sensory information is the primary reason why selective attention serves the categorizing in one particular sector of perception at the expense of all others. Hence the two major components of selective attention: inclusion and exclusion. The inclusive component is what is widely understood by focus of attention, namely, the selection of a limited sector of sensorium for the intensive analysis of the information within it. The exclusionary component, conversely, consists in the attenuation or suppression of information from other sectors that may interfere with the analysis of what is in focus at the time. Both components of selective attention, inclusive and exclusionary, will be further discussed in Chapter 6.

Finally, the categorizing function of perception is subject to *affect* and *value*. Both influence perception through attention. Our mood determines to a large extent the scope of the perception of the world around us. Depression is commonly accompanied by anhedonia and by lack of interest, both of which limit the breadth of attention, though in some instances adverse events may intensely attract attention. Further, when low mood prevails, events are often misperceived adversely. Trivial somatic sensations may lead to hypochondriacal interpretations. On the other hand, heightened mood of whatever origin (e.g., pathological hypomania) tends to sharpen attention, though it also makes it temporally inconsistent and abnormally vulnerable to distraction. Both depression and elation can induce mood-congruent perceptual imagery that may well serve the creative artist.

Personal values will also color perception and steer through attention the categorization of sensory information. The motivational significance of sensory stimuli with regard to those values is a powerful attractor of attention. Emotional connotations are an important factor in the perceptual categorization of sensory information, whether that categorization takes place consciously or unconsciously. In states of apprehension or anxiety, perceptual ambiguities are resolved on the side of danger or threat. Emotional tone in the spoken language may lead to misunderstanding of its cognitive content. These facts are so well known as to border on the trite. Here I mention them simply to highlight the variety of influences from our organism that intervene in the perceptual processing and categorization of the information that reaches our senses.

In our daily lives we perceive, consciously or unconsciously, a staggering amount of information. We spend most of our day in a continuous classifying of sensory impressions from the environment—including the internal environment. As already noted, perception constitutes to a large extent a projective, *centrifugal* process from memory, a continuous *doing* guided by our past. Most of it takes place outside of awareness. Only a minuscule part of that massive active process leads to further cognitive or behavioral action. That is the sector of activated perceptual cognits that are linked to executive cognits and, through them, to action. As we shall see, this translation of perception into action involves the extension of posterior cortical networks into the frontal lobe.

To conclude these psychological considerations, the categorizing from memory that forms the percept is essentially a *matching act* guided by attention, affect, and value. Presumably, the matching takes place between a set of sensory impressions and a preestablished cognit, that is, the activated cortical network that represents it. For the matching to occur, the sensory impressions must be organized in a manner similar to that of the cognit (i.e., its network). If the match is inadequate, the organism will modify that cognit accordingly or will project other cognits on present reality in search of a better match. In any event, the essence of perceptual categorization is the matching of sensory organization to mnemonic organization.

Gestalt

Sensory information and cognits are organized by specific sets of spatial and temporal relations between elementary parts or features—the latter possibly in modules of sensory cortex. It is those specific relations of elements that define sensory and cognitive items as configurations or structured units of sensation and knowledge, respectively. At the beginning of the twentieth century, the Gestalt school of psychology made those configurations the center of its epistemology of perception (Koffka, 1935). Based on the study of the human vision of forms and patterns, Gestaltists created an eminently logical, self-contained, and testable theory of perception that explained how we identify objects and regularities in the world we sense. Some members of that school even theorized about the way in which the brain apprehends those objects and regularities. They postulated certain cortical *fields* of electrical activity that would represent the apprehended Gestalten (in English commonly termed *gestalts*), which is the name they created for their relational configurations or articulated wholes.

Gestalt psychologists maintained, further, that the meaning of a gestalt was inherent in the phenomenon of experiencing it, a meaning that was innate and immediate. This concept cast a cloud of nativism over the entire movement, somewhat contributing to its discredit. Yet Gestalt psychology remains to date probably the most plausible approach to the investigation of the isomorphism between perception and brain function. Stripped of its unsustainable nativism (there can never be a satisfactory theory based on the a priori), Gestalt psychology is clearly of current relevance to cognitive neuroscience. Though generally unacknowledged, it has been eminently successful in shaping much of contemporary sensory physiology and psychophysics, which have adopted several of its principles. Most of the methodology of Gestalt psychology developed around visual perception and its spatial dimensions. The basic question it attempted to clarify is how we perceive objects as individual entities, how we segregate them from others around them—and from the background—and thus identify them. A related question is how that identity is preserved despite discontinuities, distortions, or partial occlusions from sight (Fig. 4.1).

To explain these phenomena, particularly the segmentation of objects in visual scenes, Gestalt psychology developed a number of *principles of organization*. At least at first, those principles were mainly intended to explain the separation of figure from ground. Among the most important are the principles of proximity, similarity, continuation, and closure (Fig. 4.2). All of them explain the grouping of elements in a gestalt and its contour. All are based on regularities in the spatial relationships between the constituent elements of that gestalt. All principles contribute to the tenet that the whole is more than the sum of its parts. Because regularities are crucial for the segmentation of that whole from the background, regularities are also crucial for identifying the gestalt as a separate entity. Here Gestalt theory intersects with information theory, which defines a highly identifiable figure as one with high internal redundancy (Attneave, 1954).

Because of their power to explain a great variety of configurations in human cognition, the laws of Gestalt psychology have been

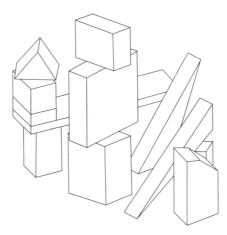

Figure 4.1. A complex set of lines, some of them broken, evokes the perception of solid objects. From Anderson (1995), adapted from Winston (1970), with permission.

generalized to several cognitive functions, including learning and thinking. The essence of the value of those laws in these domains, as in perception, is that they help define all manner of cognitive structures by relationship. Here, their usefulness to us lies in the structural parallels between a gestalt and a cognit, both of which are defined by *relationships*. In the case of the cognit, those relationships consist of neural associations, that is, the associations of the network supporting that cognit. If the same laws that apply to gestalts apply to cognits and networks, we would be able to establish the isomorphism between perceptual structure and neural structure.

To be useful to our study, however, the principles of Gestalt psychology must apply to organization not only in the spatial domain but in the temporal domain as well, to other sensory modalities in addition to vision, and to multiple levels of hierarchical organization in terms of complexity and abstraction. Curiously, *temporal gestalts* were one of the prime topics of Wertheimer (1967), a pioneer of the Gestalt movement. But the interest in spatial gestalts quickly overtook the field, in part because temporal structure is harder to investigate than spatial structure. Likewise, the consideration of auditory or tactile gestalts, for example, was largely overshadowed by visual topics. Where Gestalt psychology has been clearly deficient, but could be most useful in the present context, is on the issue of its applicability

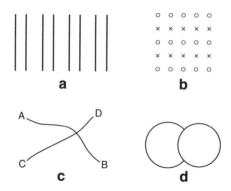

Figure 4.2. Four examples of gestalt principles of organization: (*a*) proximity, (*b*) similarity, (*c*) good continuation, and (*d*) closure. From Anderson (1995), with permission.

to multiple levels of perceptual categorization and its neural corre-lates. This extension of its field should help us resolve two major problems in the cerebral cortex: *perceptual constancy* and *symbolization*.

The problem of perceptual constancy has puzzled generations of psychologists and neuroscientists. How is it that, despite enormous variations in size, shape, and color, among other things, we are able to identify an object as one and the same or as one of the same class as others? How is it that a melody retains its identity despite changes in tempo, key, or the musical instrument with which it is played? At the phenomenal level, the solution to those problems, at least in prin-ciple, lies clearly in Gestalt theory. What defines a gestalt or the per-cept of an object is the relationships between its elements (and be-tween them and the background), not the absolute values of those elements in terms of frequency, length, pitch, hue, or what not. For the cognitive neuroscientist, however, the problem of perceptual con-stancy still looms large and unresolved. Some form of neural hologra-phy has been proposed as the solution. Holographic models (Gabor, 1968; Willshaw, 1981) are based on the reduplication of informa-tion—and relationships—in multiple locations. Such models remain plausible but unverified. A more attractive solution seems to lie in se-lectionist principles (see the next section).

Neither Gestalt psychology nor neuroscience has yet solved the equally vexing problem of symbolization. How is it that sensory cog-nits are abstracted into symbols? How are symbols represented in the cortex? How do they become surrogates for sensory representations in cognitive operations? In the next two sections, I attempt to show how these questions may be answered by applying relational connectionist principles to the cortical substrate of perception. This approach, I believe, leads to plausible as well as testable conclusions.

Cortical Dynamics of Perception

Perception is the activation through the senses of a posterior cortical network, a perceptual cognit, that represents in its associative structure a pattern of relationships (a gestalt) present in the environment. Following upon our previous discussion, this definition applies to an infinite variety of cognits at several hierarchical levels, as well as to an infinite variety of external gestalts. The definition transcends any given sensory modality and applies to polysensory networks; it transcends gestalts of spatial relations and applies to those of temporal relations as well. Our definition of perception spans the entire hierarchy of cognitive representation: from the physically concrete of a simple shape or tune to the conceptually abstract of a semantic memory, from a twig in the wind to the concept of movement, from the color of the ink to the pattern of symbols on the written page, and to their meaning.

In the act of perception, sensory impulses come to a perceptual apparatus that is ready-made for them, much as in the immune system a pattern of antibodies is ready-made for a wide array of antigens (Edelman, 1987). This apparatus, as we have seen, consists of a highly complex, hierarchically organized system of cortical networks, that is, perceptual cognits, that represent established knowledge. Such a system will recognize and process the arriving information. Essentially, as noted in the initial section, the perceptual processing will be one of categorizing that information in accord with prior experience, by matching the new to the old and by modifying the old with the new. The modification will consist of synaptic changes that will expand or in some other way alter the associative structure of a cognitive network (Chapter 2). In perceptual categorization, sensory stimuli are recognized (matched) by a given network because those stimuli, or others similar to them, at an earlier time participated in the formation of that network by association and hebbian principles. Upon their recurrence, the arriving stimuli gain access to the same network by rapid— serial and parallel—processing through cortical paths. As they arrive at the network and are recognized by it, they activate the network *d'emblé*, the entire cognit at once. The rapid ignition of a distributed cortical network is the essence of the rapid categorization of objects that is at the root of the dynamics of perception (Lamberts, 2000).

The recognition of sensory stimuli or gestalts as cognits in storage does not require a perfect match. It is sufficient that the stimuli or the gestalts contain certain relationships or regularities within them that qualify them as members of the same class, the same cognit. *Degeneracy*, as meant by Edelman (1987), is here a useful term. In the present context, degeneracy implies an approximate or highly probable fit between the structure of the network, in connective terms, and the structure of the external gestalt in relational terms. Because of the factors of approximation and probability, and because several cognits share common features, an incoming gestalt or part thereof can activate several networks before the best match and categorization occur.

The perceptual process of matching and categorizing takes place simultaneously on many aspects of the environment. That environment is ordinarily complex, constantly changing in many dimensions as the organism moves within it, changing the orientation and exposure of its sensory receptors. Consequently, perception must proceed along many channels at once within a given sensory modality. The parallel processing of environmental information is especially necessary in vision, as the visual scene changes rapidly in many diverse aspects simultaneously. In audition and touch, serial processing dominates, as changes in these modalities occur mainly in the time axis.

Which networks or cognits will be activated by sensory inputs at any given moment, and at which hierarchical level, will depend on the nature of those inputs and on a series of internal factors enumerated in the first section of this chapter. In a complex environment, several gestalts will reach perceptual systems at the same time. If a given gestalt contains relationships between its elements that match relationships in an existing cognit, it will activate it. Because of associations of similarity, several networks can be activated simultaneously in a parallel process of successive match and rematch of gestalts to cognits. Familiar gestalts will quickly find their match in higher areas of association, at the semantic or symbolic level. New complex gestalts will undergo a more elaborate process of analysis, segmentation, and successive matchings at lower levels before their categorization at a higher level (Lamberts, 2000). Temporal gestalts will be integrated in the time axis before they are categorized. Some of these processes will be guided—top-down—by attention and may occur consciously. The vast majority, however, will occur unconsciously in rapid succession.

Because the perceptual categorization of sensory gestalts depends on the structure of the categorizing networks, it is appropriate to briefly review the cortical structure of the perceptual apparatus discussed in Chapter 3. At the lowest, most peripheral stages of cortical sensory systems, perceptual cognits are purely sensory, and are thus fit to categorize information defined by physical parameters only. Those cognits are made up of local networks in sensory cortex, enabled by certain processes during perinatal ontogeny to represent the basic sensory features of the world (Chapter 2). Sensory networks are thereby ready to represent and analyze those features when they appear in the environment in new configurations. The perceptual representation in those networks—truly a primitive form of *recognition*—will be immediate and faithful to that environment. The early-life formation of sensory networks in sensory cortex does not mean, however, that those networks are thereafter fixed and invariable. We know that they retain a degree of plasticity throughout adult life (Gilbert, 1998). They can "learn" and be modified by perceptual usage at any age. They can also be used in imagery, which is internally generated perception.

Out of sensory cortex, parallel streams of cortical connectivity flow to higher sensory areas, which are dedicated to the representation and analysis of sensory information of the same modality as that of the cortex from which it comes. The connectivity within each stream consists of collateral, convergent, divergent, and recurrent fibers. It has been extensively investigated in the visual and somato-sensory systems, especially the former (Felleman and Van Essen, 1991). Those higher areas, some of which retain retinotopy or soma-totopy (their neurons have discrete receptive fields in the retina or skin), specialize in the processing of certain sensory features, such as color, orientation, motion, pressure, and pitch. In some of these secondary sensory areas, such as area V2, cells exhibit the ability to detect illusory contours, thus obeying at least one Gestalt principle. We can reasonably infer that their cognitive networks represent discrete sensory features and possibly have some capacity to integrate them within a limited sector of sensorium. Networks in those lower uni-modal sensory areas are fit to categorize relatively simple percepts of the corresponding modality.

In higher areas of unimodal association, for example the inferotemporal cortex for vision, the representation and hence the processing specialize in more complex features. There, as we saw in the previous chapter, neurons have broad receptive fields and respond to the presentation of complex forms, such as faces and patterns. Cognitive networks in those areas seem to represent categories of objects—for example, faces—defined by universal and highly consistent spatial relationships between their components. The specific identity and other associations of a particular face, for example, involve extensions of those networks into other associative areas at the same or other level(s). Thus, the perception of a face activates not only the visual components of a network but also those components of other modalities that encode other attributes of the person. If the face carries an emotional expression, the activated network will probably extend into limbic cortex or the amygdala.

Beyond unimodal association cortices, the processing streams flow into large expanses of heteromodal and limbic or paralimbic cortex, collectively termed *transmodal cortex* by Mesulam (1998). Lesions of this cortex, depending to some degree on the particular area affected, lead to agnosias or deficits in the recognition of categories of objects, words, or lexical structures; they may also lead to semantic aphasias. The cognitive networks in this cortex appear therefore to encode considerably broader categories of cognition than do the networks in lower cortical stages. We have entered the substrate for the perception of symbols, which are highly abstract cognits.

Symbols are derivative gestalts. They are formed in the perceptual apparatus of the cortex by repeated experience with variants of the gestalt they represent or with other symbols (e.g., words) that represent those variants. Symbols abstract the essential features of an object across practically infinite variations of the same. A boat, a symphony, a table, a cry of distress, a cloud—all can vary widely, but each has certain essential sensory characteristics that define it. That set of special characteristics forms the symbol, which is still a gestalt defined by a specific set of relationships, albeit of a more general nature than that of its individual instantiations. As such, a symbol, which may consist of a verbal expression, is a high-ranking perceptual cognit resulting from profuse convergence of information from below (Fig. 4.3). Because of the multiplicity of individual forms they represent, that cognit and its network can be characterized as highly *degenerate,* in Edelman's sense. Although generally treated as *amodal* by cognitive

Public Transport

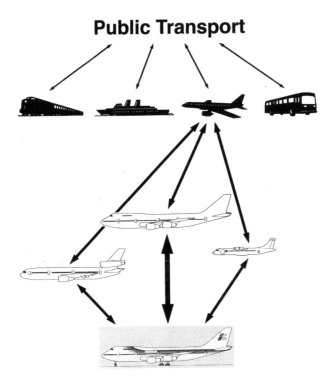

Figure 4.3. Hierarchical categorization of visual cognits of vehicles for public transportation: at the *bottom,* one particular airplane; in the *middle,* several types of airliners; at the *top,* several general kinds of vehicles in quasi-symbolic form. *Arrows* represent the connectivity between layers of representation. Alternate classifications can be made by carrier company, passenger capacity, power source, supporting medium (aerial, terrestrial, maritime), and so on.

science, symbols are solidly based in perception by virtue of their perceptual origin and the nature of their perceptual retrieval (Barsalou, 1999). Some are formed or retrieved only through one modality, others through several.

The patterns of connectivity within and between hierarchical levels that have been observed in lower cortical stages of sensory systems—convergent, divergent, collateral, and recurrent—can also be found at higher levels (Chapter 2). This allows for the versatile binding of associated properties that characterize a cognit at any level, as well as that of heterarchical cognits that span several levels—binding sensations with symbols, for example. The same connectivity serves

the activation of networks in perception as it serves the cognitive processing within and between them. Upward convergence assists the
binding of properties into higher categories, while upward divergence assists the distribution of common properties to different categories. Collateral connectivity serves the binding of categories at the
same level. Recurrent connectivity serves reentry in heterarchical
binding and top-down processing.

The patterns of connectivity within and between hierarchical
levels have several important general implications for the representation and processing of percepts. These implications can be stated as
follows: (*1*) A cognit can be defined by a net that connects dispersed
attributes in associative cortex; (*2*) a high-level cognit can pool attributes from widely dispersed cognits of lower levels, thus forming a
more general category of perception; (*3*) at no level is there a need
for convergence into sharply localized cognits; (*4*) on the contrary,
specific attributes may be dispersed upward to higher categories that
possess those attributes in common. Accordingly, the upward progression of cognits and categories may be accompanied by gradually
more widely dispersed representation.

In the human, language and arithmetic add collateral hierarchies of symbolic representation to the perceptual hierarchy derived
from sensory categorization (Chapter 7). In the course of development and by education, words become symbolic representations of
cognits that, like them, become hierarchically organized. The word
chair, for example, has a higher ranking than *armchair* and *rocking chair*,
and these in turn have higher rankings than the semantic character-
izations of individual specimens of them. Like the percepts and concepts they represent, words and linguistic structures are encoded in
distributed neuronal networks of posterior associative cortex.

What then is the neural structure of symbols? There is no conclusive evidence to answer this question. Nevertheless, by extending
our previous reasoning to the higher cortices of association, it seems
appropriate to construe the neural structure of a symbol as a neuronal network representing in its connectivity the pattern of general
relationships that defines it. At higher associative levels, this pattern
would be formed by convergence of specific patterns of relationships
residing in lower and collateral areas of associative cortex. Note that
by postulating an upward translation of relationships, we avoid the
absurdity of the convergence toward a *grandmother cell*. At the same
time, however, we leave open the possibility that higher gestalts are

relatively localized in the form of network-like *nodes* of connectivity. Here the concept of *zone of convergence* (Damasio, 1989a) seems applicable. Symbolic networks, integrating information from lower levels, would be narrowly distributed within zones of convergence of posterior association cortex.

Indeed, a large body of neuropsychological evidence indicates that those hypothetical nodes of categorical information, the higher cognits that we call symbols, are distributed within regions of higher association cortex. Included among these cortical regions is the cortex of the inferior, medial, and superior regions of the temporal lobe, Wernicke's area, and the posterior parietal lobe. That evidence is somewhat confounded, however, by considerable variability across studies. Some of that variability is inherent in their methods, derived mainly from the heterogeneity of the cortical lesions investigated. Some of the variability, however, may reflect real intersubject variance. It is reasonable to suppose that in the ascent toward higher cortical areas, the relative constancy of distribution and localization of networks that prevails at lower—sensory—levels is gradually lost. The precise distribution of higher cognits in higher cortex is probably idiosyncratic and varies considerably between individuals.

Let us summarize the tentative principles of perceptual categorization in posterior cortex that have emerged thus far from our discussion. In the lowest stages of the cortical hierarchy, external gestalts are analyzed, mapped, and integrated by their sensory features. Objects may be segmented at a rudimentary level by spatial contrast. Illusory contours may be completed and blind spots filled (blind sight). The individual features of new sensory configurations are analyzed and passed on to higher unimodal levels. New temporal structures of different modalities are serially analyzed in their respective unimodal cortices and passed on to higher levels, where they are integrated. In unimodal association cortices, objects are not only segmented but also integrated into categories within the corresponding sense modality. Highly familiar visual configurations, such as faces, are categorized in certain areas of visual association cortex. Networks representing visual symbols for objects probably retain topological relations with the objects they represent, and are thus able to categorize the objects across retinal translations in terms of magnitude or location. In cross-modal and transmodal association cortex, sensory gestalts are categorized as perceptual symbols across several sensory and nonsensory dimensions. Network connections with limbic structures mediate the categorization of sensory information in biological, affective, and emotional dimensions.

It is not possible to ascertain with present knowledge the neural basis for *perceptual constancy,* that is, for the categorization of a gestalt or pattern of sensation despite potentially infinite variations in its sensory components. The physiological and neuropsychological evidence indicates that constancy increases with ascending level in the hierarchy at which categorization takes place (thus with degeneracy). Constancy is low in sensory cortices and high in transmodal cortex. It appears that, in the upward hierarchical progression of the visual system, constancy for objects across visual dimensions and location begins to occur in inferotemporal cortex (Tanaka, 1993). Constancy for highly variable graphic symbols, such as letters and words, does not seem to occur before the cortex of Wernicke's area and surrounding areas. It is reasonable to suppose that constancy goes hand in hand with the abstraction of the essential characteristics that define a class by relationships between them. The fewer those characteristics, and the more symbolic the abstraction, the greater the perceptual constancy. The increased constancy probably results from the topological mapping of the essential traits of a class into networks made up of progressively fewer but more firmly established nodes. This, incidentally, would contribute to the greater resistance of higher perceptual categories to cortical injuries, and thus the greater resistance to categorical amnesia from those injuries (Chapter 5). To sum up, perceptual constancy seems to increase upward in the hierarchy of perceptual areas, together with increased abstraction of the information perceived.

If a perceptual act results in selective attention or working memory, the activation of the categorizing network will be maintained by reentry of excitation. At the same time, other networks will be reciprocally inhibited, especially those that represent elements of context or background that are excluded from attention. If that were not the case, a discrete sensory stimulus would lead to a cascade of activation through innumerable associative links of context and past experience. In other words, the stimulus would lead to an excitatory explosion and to the submersion of the cognitive gestalt that it evokes in a morass of associative noise.

The above discussion outlines our present understanding of the principles of organization and dynamics of perception in the cerebral cortex. Most of the knowledge we have used thus far to infer these principles comes from anatomical and neuropsychological studies in humans and nonhuman primates. Now we will examine further the relevant functional evidence of recent years, especially from micro-electrode and neuroimaging studies, in an attempt to further substantiate those principles.

Perceptual Binding

Perceptual binding is the term used by psychologists to characterize the unification of the associated sensory features of an object in the perception of that object as an identifiable (segmented) entity or gestalt. To us here, perceptual binding is the activation of the neural network or cognit that represents that object in its associative neuronal structure. That is the same network that, as we have seen, not only represents but also categorizes the object and initiates whatever cognitive or behavioral operations the organism will perform with it. Thus, following our reasoning thus far, perceptual binding is the joint activation of all of the network's neurons, whether it is induced by the presence of the entire object or by one of its associated parts. By *joint activation* we mean the *synchronous* or nearly synchronous increase in the firing frequency of the neurons that constitute the network.

Berger (1929), the discoverer of the EEG, claimed that rapidly oscillating brain waves—in the upper beta range, about 20 cycles per second or higher—could be recorded from the scalp of subjects performing mental operations, such as arithmetic. High-frequency (HF) neuroelectrical oscillations—20–60 Hz or higher—were subsequently recorded in several animals, including monkeys, from a variety of brain structures, cortex included. Such oscillations can be recorded by the use of field-potential electrodes (EEG), microelectrodes, and magnetoencephalography (MEG). They can be observed in several behaviorally or psychologically defined states and cognitive functions such as arousal, attention, emotional excitation, active short-term or working memory, and perception.

The biophysics and physiological significance of *HF activity* are matters of continuing debate. Some take the position that HF activity is an inherent tendency of neurons to oscillate in certain brain structures, notably the thalamus, and that cortical HF activity can be a manifestation of reverberation in corticothalamic loops (Llinás and Ribary, 1993; Steriade, 1993). Others take the position that HF activity in the cortex is generated in corticocortical circuits and has en-

coding properties—in the form of a spike-interval code—to serve a
number of cognitive functions, notably perception (Singer, 2000). As
I will discuss further in Chapter 6 with regard to working memory and
our research of it, our view is that HF activity reflects cortical encoding, but indirectly. HF activity does not encode a cognit in a time
code, but is a manifestation of the activation of the network that encodes the cognit in cortical space—that is, in the connectivity of the
network. Thus, HF activity reflects the functional architecture of that
network and the reentrant activity within it.

Freeman (1975) was the first to attribute perceptual binding
properties to HF activity—in olfaction. According to him and to others who have observed similar activity in several animal species, oscillatory HF activity is an expression of the coherence of the percept, of
the unification of all its components and of the relationships between
them (Von der Malsburg, 1985; Bressler, 1990; Singer and Gray, 1995).
There seems to be general agreement that the phenomenon is the
manifestation of synchronous HF firing of nerve cells in the act of
perception. What is unclear, however, is how that electrical phenomenon can register a mental phenomenon that occurs so fast and
seems to antecede any record of oscillatory HF activity. With a focus
on vision, it has been argued (Von der Malsburg, 1985) that the oscillatory HF activity must be preceded by a rapid wave of correlated
discharge that ignites the entire network by virtue of its tight inter-
connections. Its neurons thereby would act as *coincidence detectors,*
highly sensitive to correlated inputs (Abeles, 1982).

Singer and Gray (1995) adduce that the correlation persists beyond the arrival of the signal, which is encoded by that correlation in
a well-delimited though widely distributed network (assembly) of cortical neurons. The coherence of the encoded gestalt, according to
them, is ensured by the synchrony of the neurons, which treat that gestalt as a unit in accord with Gestalt principles, such as those of proximity and continuity. That the assembly is held together by corticocortical connections is strongly suggested by evidence that lesions of
the white matter or of the interhemispheric commissures attenuate
or obliterate the synchrony (Engel at al., 1991).

Whether the gestalt is encoded by a temporal code of neuron firing or rather, as I maintain, by a network whose activation entails the
synchronized firing of its neurons, cortical neurons tend to drift in
and out of certain frequencies and temporal patterns (Bodner et al.,
1998). We view these frequencies and patterns as *fixed-point attractors,*

that is, states that are defined by the functional architecture of the net and to which its cells gravitate. Some of the patterns, in the monkey's association cortex, are oscillatory in the HF range. The critical question is whether, in the act of perception, a cognitive network resonates with synchronous attractors to the gestalt that the network recognizes and thereby categorizes. That question has been addressed in the human by analysis of field potentials recorded through the skull.

To that end, Tallon-Baudry and her colleagues (1995) utilized visual stimuli designed by Kanizsa, a Gestalt psychologist. Subjects were presented with three images, each of them with three Pacmen or incomplete black circles (Fig. 4.4, left). The first enclosed the line figure of a triangle, the second enclosed an illusory triangle, and the third, where the Pacmen did not face one another, did not enclose any figure, real or illusory. The gestalt of the triangle was thus maximally coherent in the first figure, illusory in the second, and incoherent in the third (a *pseudogestalt*). The analysis of the power spectrum of the EEG immediately after figure presentations showed an orderly distribution of frequencies as a function of the coherence of the image of the triangle (Fig. 4.4, right). At 100 ms after stimulus onset, frequencies in the 28- to 42-Hz range showed a peak that was maximal at 28 Hz for the fully coherent figure. At 300 ms after stimulus onset, the spectrum clearly and significantly differentiated the three figures: a peak at 30 Hz was highest for the fully coherent figure and lowest for the incoherent figure, with the illusory figure in between. These results indicate that, at 300-ms latency, the perception of a coherent image induces cortical synchronization at high frequencies, whereas the perception of an incoherent image does not. In another study (Joliot et al., 1994), HF oscillatory activity (40 Hz) — recorded by MEG—was associated with coherence in the temporal domain; here coherence was experimentally manipulated by changing the time interval between successive clicks.

Other studies, by EEG (Lutzenberger et al., 1994; Pulvermüller et al., 1997) or MEG (Eulitz et al., 1996), lead to comparable results with the use of symbolic gestalts: words, either written or spoken. These studies show a greater incidence of HF oscillations (30–60 Hz) after real words than after pseudowords or false fonts, whether the verbal configurations are perceived through the visual or the auditory modality. Here, therefore, we have HF correlates of coherence at the symbolic level. Perceived coherence is again accompanied by a higher incidence of HF oscillations of field potentials over widespread cortical

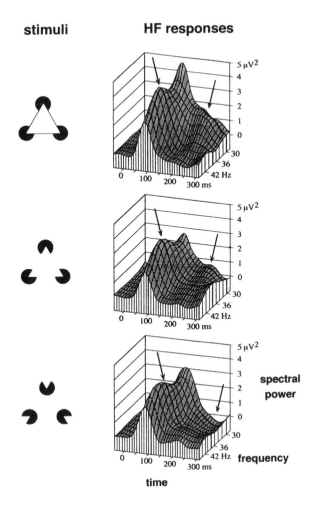

Figure 4.4. EEG spectral responses to presentation of a complete triangle, an il-lusory triangle, and a pseudotriangle. Coherent stimuli (*top* and *middle*) induce a response greater than 30 Hz (*right arrow*). From Tallon-Baudry et al. (1995), mod-ified, with permission.

regions. In most studies the coherence-induced differences have been observed in posterior cortical regions, that is, occipital, temporal, and parietal. The prevalent frequency with coherence is usually around 30 Hz, and it occurs within 300 ms of stimulus onset.

In summary, field-potential studies in the human support the oc-currence of HF *attractor frequencies* in cortical networks. These fre-quencies appear to relate to the degree of *coherence* that a perceived sensory stimulus carries, whether as a physical gestalt or as a gestalt with meaning. It is reasonable to assume that an attractor frequency is related to the encoding of the cognit that a network represents, and that the neuronal elements of that network *resonate* to the gestalt by firing synchronously at a given frequency. Each network may have its signature frequency, and in this sense that frequency could be construed as the temporal encoding of the information that the gestalt carries and that the synchronized neurons of the network reproduce (Singer, 2000). It seems more likely, however, that the information is encoded in the connective architecture of the network—of the cognit, that is—and the frequency of oscillation is a by-product of the activation of that architecture by reentrant loops. According to this view, the encoding is defined topologically by connectivity, rather than temporally, and the frequency is determined by the activated architecture of the particular network that carries the code. We should be able to substantiate this topological view of perception by the imaging of activated networks in perceptual acts.

The neuroimaging of the human brain has become a powerful tool for exploring the activation of neural networks. PET and fMRI are now widely used in the study of the cortical dynamics of cognitive functions. These methods, however, still have a number of shortcomings that hamper the topographical definition of activated cognitive networks. Among these shortcomings are the limitations in spatial and temporal resolution of the image, the uncertainties surrounding the relationship between neural activity and blood flow (which those methods measure), and the difficulty of establishing statistical criteria of neural activation. The last problem is aggravated by the use of the subtractive method to contrast cortical activation under a given cognitive function against activation under control conditions. This method makes the activation from that function difficult to assess. Nevertheless, careful studies can at least yield reliable estimates of the location of maximal cortical activation in various cognitive states. Those estimates are inadequate to describe an active network but are probably adequate to locate the heavily activated nodes of that network, or *epicenters* of its excitatory neuronal activity, as a function of a condition or cognitive variable under study.

Cabeza and Nyberg (2000) conducted an extensive and thorough review of the published literature on the imaging of cognitive functions. Their review—of 275 studies—can be characterized as a *meta-analysis,* inasmuch as conclusions are drawn from it that transcend any particular study. In light of the problems enumerated in the previous paragraph, that review is exceptionally valuable, especially because of its expert evaluation of methodologies. The majority of the studies of perception deal with vision. Figure 4.5 illustrates the location, by published stereometric coordinates, of the peaks of activation by perception described in the various studies and coded in the figure by the characteristics of the testing stimuli utilized. As expected, all those peaks are in posterior cortex, with the exception of two olfactory peaks in the orbital prefrontal cortex near the frontal operculum, where the primary areas for the chemical senses are located. Also, as expected, there is an apparent dichotomy of distribution for visual percepts of objects (in lower cortex) and percepts of space/motion (in upper cortex). Nonetheless, in light of the previous discussion, we cannot avoid the impression that in the graphic results of the meta-analysis, we are looking at the "tip of an iceberg." Thus, the peaks of activation portrayed in the figure convey a modular image of perceptual recognition and categorization that deviates considerably from our network concept of those processes.

By contrast, another recent review of neuroimaging data, by Mar-

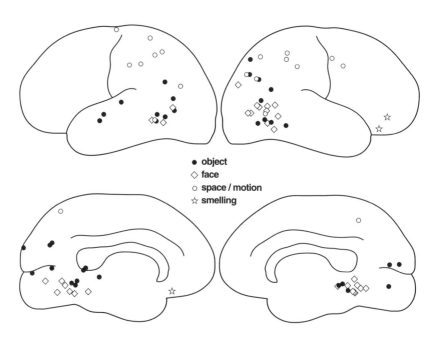

Figure 4.5. Location of cortical activation maxima induced by four kinds of stimuli, from neuroimaging studies reviewed by Cabeza and Nyberg (2000), modified, with permission.

tin et al. (2000), is guided by the network concept, and its results are interpreted in that light. The authors, after reviewing their own studies and those of others, produce convincing evidence that semantic object representations are based on the activation of cortical networks that associate the sensory features of the objects that those representations categorize. No semantic category appears localized anywhere, but its representation is the product of the activation of the *prelexic semantic primitives* that define it. The authors support their argument with data indicating that the presentation of objects or words for objects with a salient physical attribute, such as color or motion, activates areas in the vicinity of sensory areas that specialize in the analysis of that attribute (Fig. 4.6). The network representing and categorizing the object as a semantic entity would be made up of neuronal assemblies in parasensory areas representing those attributes. Here again, however, the graphic display of activation maxima exaggerates localization. A category is inferred to be localized in the area of maximal activation induced by its salient feature (e.g., color). A

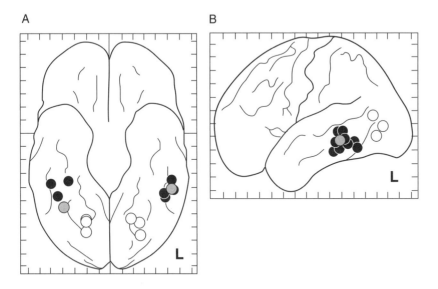

Figure 4.6. Location of cortical activation maxima in studies reviewed by Martin et al. (2000). A: *White circles,* activation in color perception; *black circles,* activation by color words; *gray circles,* activation by color imagery. B: *White circles,* activation in motion perception; *black circles,* activation by action words; *gray circle,* activation in verb generation. From Martin et al. (2000), with permission.

truer picture of the category would be provided by the activation of all its components, including the lesser features, that together define the cognit, the network, and the category. Such a picture would also be more congruent with the point of view presented in this chapter.

My view of widely distributed cognits, however, is not incompatible with the notion previously stated in this chapter that certain object categories—for example, animals, faces, and tools—are relatively well localized in certain cortical areas. This notion has been espoused by several investigators (for example, Caramazza and Shelton, 1998) and is supported by a large body of neuropsychological evidence from lesions. It is also supported by incipient evidence from microelectrode recording in medial temporal areas of the human (Kreiman et al., 2000). Nonetheless, the overriding idea in this chapter should be that an object is represented at several hierarchical levels, from the sensory to the symbolic. The perception of the object can activate its representation at any of those levels. Under most circumstances, it will activate a heterarchical cognitive network that represents sensory as well as symbolic—that is, semantic—aspects of the object. It is conceivable, however, that the cognitive networks for common objects with salient sensory features have associative nodes of heavy representation in unimodal association cortex. This does not rule out, however, the possibility that the same network represents the semantic aspects of an object in more or less discrete areas of higher cortex of association. In any case, a given parasensory area can be activated by several objects that share the sensory feature that the area represents. On the perception of one of the objects, that feature will draw activation from a wide network of higher cortex toward the area of unimodal association representing that feature. Parasensory areas, however, are not the only ones to be activated top-down by sensory associations. Internal imagery can activate sensory areas as far down in the hierarchy as the primary sensory cortex (Kosslyn and Thompson, 2000).

Perception-Action Cycle

Perception may lead to other acts of cognition (attention, working memory, retrieval of long-term memory, or further perception) or it may lead to behavioral action. The conditions under which this will occur, and the nature of the cognitive or behavioral action resulting from a percept, will depend on a number of factors that can be grouped into two major categories. The first is the internal conditions of the organism, including the drives and motives prevailing at the time; the second is the behavioral, cognitive, and emotional associations of the percept.

At all levels of the central nervous system, the translation of perception to action is mediated through connections between sensory and motor structures. Both sensory and motor structures are hierarchically organized along the entire length of the nerve axis, the two tiers interconnected by reciprocal polysynaptic pathways that form a sort of ladder of connections between the sensory moiety and the motor moiety of the nervous system. Sensory structures constitute the dorsal or posterior tier and motor structures the ventral or anterior one. In the spinal cord, the connections run through interneurons and link the posterior (sensory) with the anterior (motor) neuronal aggregates. In the telencephalon, the two moieties of the cerebral cortex, posterior and frontal, that respectively represent perceptual and executive networks or cognits, constitute the highest stages of the anatomical substrate for sensory–motor integration. As we have seen in Chapter 3, profuse fiber connections run from posterior to frontal cortex. All of them are reciprocated; thus projections from posterior neurons to frontal neurons are reciprocated by projections in the opposite direction.

That connectivity between posterior and frontal cortex is topologically and hierarchically organized. In general, areas of posterior cortex are interconnected with areas of comparable hierarchical rank in frontal cortex. Thus, the two hierarchies of cortical cognits, perceptual and executive, appear interlinked at all stages. Networks in a given stage of perceptual representation and processing are reciprocally connected with networks in a corresponding stage of executive representation and processing. The correspondence is not complete, however, and there is considerable heterarchical connectivity between the two hierarchies. Interhemispheric sensory–motor connections can also be heterarchical.

The cognitive interactions of a primate with the surrounding world are governed by what I have named the *perception-action cycle* (Fuster, 1995). This interactive cycle is the extension to cortical processes of a basic principle of biology that characterizes the dynamic adaptation of an organism to its environment. It was first proposed by the biologist Uexküll (1926), who deduced it from behavioral observations in a large number of animal species. Essentially, it

can be stated as follows. An animal's behavior consists of a succession
of adaptive motor reactions to changes in its external and internal environments. These motor reactions produce changes in those environments, which in turn are detected by sensory or internal receptors
and generate or modulate subsequent actions. Thus, behavioral
adaptation is based on the continuous operation of a universal mechanism of circular processing through the central nervous system: sensory or internal signals lead to actions that generate feedback that
regulates further actions, and so on.

    Instinctual, reflexive, and well-learned sensory–motor integra-
tions take place in circular loops of neuronal connectivity at lower
levels of the neural hierarchies (spinal cord, basal ganglia, hypothalamus, etc.). At higher levels, however, the circular processing of information in behavior, speech, and reasoning engages the perceptual
and executive regions of the cerebral cortex. There perception is integrated into action through loops of corticocortical connectivity that
mediate the feedforward as well as the feedback components of the
perception-action cycle. Figure 4.7 illustrates schematically the flow
of functional connectivity between cortical structures that supports
the operations of that high-level cybernetic cycle.

    On the sensory side of the cortical substrate of the perception-
action cycle is the hierarchy of posterior areas for the representation
and processing of perception; on the motor side is the hierarchy of
executive areas. As mentioned, the two hierarchies are reciprocally
connected at every level. Goal-directed behavior depends on the
continuous operation of the cycle at several cortical levels simultaneously. The more automatic and routine behaviors will be integrated
at lower levels, mainly with the participation of primary sensory and
motor cortices. More complex and novel behaviors will bring in the
cortical areas of association. In the progression toward a goal, posterior and frontal cortices will engage each other in the continuous and
circular processing of mutually dependent signals and acts. What I
am essentially proposing, therefore, is the orderly and timely interplay of perceptual and executive cognits, across the central fissure
and the interhemispheric commissures, in the pursuit of behavioral
and cognitive goals.

    One of the functions of the perception-action cycle is to bridge
time. The sensory and motor components of a behavioral—or linguistic—structure toward a goal are commonly separated by time.
Time separates sensory signals that guide behavior, it separates sig-

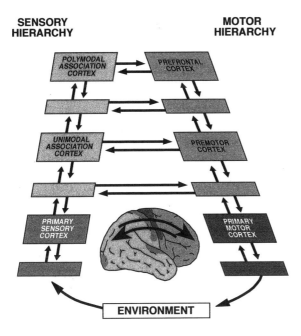

Figure 4.7. Schematic structure of the cortical perception-action cycle around a diagram of the human brain. Blank quadrangles are meant to represent intermediate areas or subareas of adjacent—labeled—regions. For example, blank quadrangles between sensory association cortices and between the top two frontal cortices are supposed to allow for the fact that some unimodal association areas are interconnected with some prefrontal areas. All connections (*arrows*) between cortical areas or regions have been substantiated in the rhesus monkey.

nals from consequent actions, and it separates sensory feedback from further action. This implies that the organization of any complex structure of behavior necessitates the integration across time of percepts with other percepts, actions with other actions, and percepts with actions. Integration across time is a basic function of the prefrontal cortex and the basis of its cardinal role in the temporal organization of behavior.

The *prefrontal cortex* sits on top of the executive hierarchy of cortices in the frontal lobe and thus constitutes the highest executive structure in the perception-action cycle. In Chapter 3 we attributed to it the *representation* of the highest motor and executive cognits, the schemas of behavioral, cognitive, or linguistic action. Here we have to consider the prefrontal cortex as the functional substrate for the *exe-*

cution of those schemas or temporal gestalts of behavior. We have to consider how the representational networks of the frontal lobe become operational.

The role of the prefrontal cortex in the execution of a structure of behavior is initiated and maintained, in large part, by inputs from posterior cortex. Such inputs are the result of the activation of perceptual cognits by sensory signals and are also the result of the processing of those signals by the networks that support those cognits. In the act of perception, a sensory stimulus can gain access to a perceptual network and activate it by association. If, by previous associations with specific action, the activated network has established connections with an executive network of the frontal lobe, it will then activate that executive network through posterior-anterior connections to it. That will lead to the initiation of motor action. Motor action will lead to sensory feedback, which will be processed in posterior cortex and provide new input to frontal cortex. The perception-action cycle will have been set in motion.

Thus, in its role of temporal integration, the prefrontal cortex works in close coordination with posterior cortices. These provide the prefrontal cortex with a steady stream of sensory and perceptual inputs that allow it to perform its integrative role. The prefrontal cortex, in turn, closes the cycle at the top by providing posterior cortex with integrative signals to sensory systems, notably in the processes of attention and working memory that support a behavioral or cognitive sequence (Chapter 6). Together with those integrative signals, the prefrontal cortex sends inhibitory feedback to posterior cortex that ensures the suppression of extraneous perceptual inputs into the cycle. This *inhibitory feedback* serves the exclusionary aspects of current attention, while the latter is focused on the essential cognitive components of the sequence. In sum, the temporal organization of behavior, especially if the behavior is novel and complex, requires the serial, successive, and alternating engagement of frontal and posterior cortices in the perception-action cycle. The prefrontal cortex contributes temporal integration as well as inhibitory control to the smooth and goal-directed operation of the cycle.

5

Memory

Memory is the capacity to retain information about oneself and one's environment. In everyday parlance, we understand as memory the ability to remember the mental traces of experience, of past events and learned facts. This common view of memory is essentially based on the conscious acquisition and recall of information. Cognitive science and neuropsychology, however, have now made it imperative to broaden that definition. Certainly the definition of memory must include all the knowledge that we acquire, retrieve, and utilize without conscious awareness. It must include motor skills as well as perceptual knowledge, most of which is utilized unconsciously (Chapter 4). In sum, the definition of memory must include an enormous fund of experience that the organism has stored throughout life in its nervous system to adapt to its milieu, whether at any time it is consciously aware of it or not. All that has been said in previous chapters about the formation and organization of knowledge applies also to memory, for memory is made up of knowledge and knowledge of memory. In this chapter we will discuss the cortical substrate and mechanisms of memory. Thus we will revisit the making, the organization, and the retrieval of cognits, now as items of memory.

Formation of Memory

The difference between knowledge and memory is a subtle one. Phenomenologically, knowledge is the memory of facts and relationships between facts, which like all memory is acquired by experience. One distinction between autobiographical memory and knowledge lies simply in the presence or absence of time constraints: the contents of memory have such constraints; those of knowledge do not. New memories have a date and undergo a temporal process of consolidation before they are permanently stored or become knowledge. Established knowledge is timeless, even though its acquisition and content may be dated.

Despite those temporal qualifiers, the subtlety, or rather artificiality, of the distinction between memory and knowledge becomes obvious by considering the functional interactions between the two in both the cognitive and neural spheres. The first consideration is that there is no such thing as a totally new memory. Any new memory is no more than the expansion of old knowledge. As noted in the previous chapter, all perception involves remembering in that it is an interpretation of the world according to prior knowledge. In that process of interpretation, sensory percepts are instantly classified in the light of old experience. Thus, a new percept leads to a new memory by building upon old memory. Without prior knowledge, a new percept is uninterpretable and thus unencodable as a new memory. It goes without saying that the interaction between perception and memory also takes place in the reverse direction. After becoming old knowledge, a memory will shape new memories with new percepts.

Undoubtedly the reader has already recognized in the foregoing comments the conceptual thread of this book. What I wish to restate here, to follow that thread, is that, from the point of view of neurobiology, knowledge, memory, and perception share the same neural substrate: an immense array of cortical networks or cognits that contain in their structural mesh the informational content of all three. Later in this book, we will add other cognitive functions to that same structural framework.

Stored memories, like cognits, *are* cortical networks. Their formation takes place by the same mechanisms, and obeys the same principles, as the formation of cognits. Both principles and mechanisms were discussed in Chapter 2. Here they will be briefly recapitulated with a different emphasis. Some of the new emphasis will be on the temporal aspects of network formation, where a somewhat defensible but tenuous distinction may be made between memory and knowledge. That distinction, nonetheless, supported by questionable evidence, has led to the unjustified inference of two separate neural systems, one for short-term memory and the other for long-term memory.

First, let us emphasize a general point, which is that memory is fundamentally an *associative* function. All memory is associative in one way or another and for one reason or another. The basic biophysical process at the root of memory formation is the modulation of transmission of information across synapses, the neural elements anatomically associating cells with one another (Hebb, 1949; Kandel, 1991). That process is to a large extent the result of the temporal association of inputs upon cells (synchronous convergence). It can be argued that even so-called phyletic memory, that is, the structure of sensory and motor cortices has been formed in the course of evolution by associative principles. The bulk of individual memory is formed and stored in neuronal networks of cortex of association, so named because its areas connect sensory and motor systems within and between themselves. Cortical memory networks, as we have seen, are formed in and between neuronal populations or nets (cognits) by a self-organizing associative process (Kohonen, 1984; Edelman, 1987). Finally, the retrieval of memory—recall, recognition, remembering—is essentially, as we shall see below, an associative process. It is therefore unwarranted to identify any particular type of memory as associative and others not.

By mechanisms that were discussed at some length in Chapter 2, the formation of the associations between cortical cell populations that make up memory networks takes place under the functional control of limbic structures, especially the *hippocampus* (Fig. 5.1). This is a reasonable inference from the long-established fact that human subjects with lesions of those structures are unable to form new memories. The landmark observations in this regard (Scoville and Milner, 1957) were made on H.M., a patient with epilepsy who, for the treatment of his condition, underwent bilateral surgical ablation of medial temporal-lobe structures. After the operation, the patient preserved his long-term autobiographical memory but was unable to form new memories. He was unable to remember recent events or to recognize persons he had met a few minutes before. Repeated encounters did not help. Subsequent studies with similar cases have

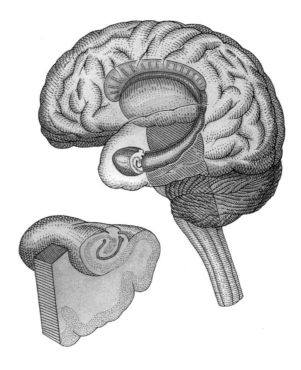

Figure 5.1. Cross section of the hippocampus and adjacent midtemporal cortex in the human brain. From Squire and Kandel (1999), modified, with permission.

confirmed that, indeed, midtemporal structures, the hippocampus in particular, intervene in the deposition of new memory, supposedly in neocortex (Squire and Kandel, 1999).

One particular inference from hippocampal studies, however, appears to me unreasonable and unsupported. It is the inference that the hippocampus, together with neighboring cortex, constitutes the depository—however temporary—for a special kind of memory, the so-called declarative memory. This form of memory is supposed to comprise all mnemonic traces that the subject can verbalize, whether they are semantic or episodic. That inference is based not only on the clinical evidence noted above, but also on two yet unproven assumptions. One is that the subject without hippocampus is deprived of the store for new declarative memories. The other is that the subject is perfectly capable of forming new memories of other kinds—for example, nondeclarative, implicit, and procedural. The first assumption ignores the distinction between the store (neocortex) and the

means to store (hippocampus and possibly other subcortical structures—e.g., thalamus). Midtemporal ablations in monkeys performing delayed-matching tasks do not resolve the issue, because the use
of such tasks as models of declarative memory is questionable. The
second assumption is based on evidence that patients like H.M. can
learn and perform certain motor and perceptual skills, such as pencil-
tracing figures and reading words through a mirror. A problem here
is that the standards of performance of those skills by normal subjects
may not have been well established. Furthermore, the effort and difficulty of forming declarative memory may not be equal to those of
forming procedural skills. Thus, the inference of specificity of midtemporal structures for declarative memory may be another instance,
common in neuropsychology, of an unjustified conclusion derived
from relative differences in performance.

Attention, rehearsal, repetition, and practice are cognitive operations that work synergistically in the making or strengthening of the
synapses that form the memory networks of the cortex. The *consolidation* of a memory consists essentially of synaptic modulation under
the assistance of those cognitive operations. It is a process that in the
cognitive field is known as the *encoding* of memory, although some
prefer to use this term only for the initial stage of memory acquisition. As noted, the hippocampus plays an important role in this process—though there is some evidence that, for any new item, this role
is time-limited (Kim and Fanselow, 1992). The *amygdala,* which is the
evaluator of the affective and motivational value of stimuli, probably
also plays a role here, though the possible mechanisms underlying
this role are still obscure.

Undoubtedly the synaptic modulation of cortical synapses that
underpins the consolidation of memory includes *inhibition* as well as
excitation. Like any other neural function, the making of a memory
network probably involves a degree of excitation of some neuronal
groups together with the reciprocal inhibition of others. With regard
to attention, the issue is discussed in the next chapter. Nowhere in the
central nervous system is there effective excitatory integration without some reciprocal inhibition. Inhibition enhances contrast. It is
reasonable therefore to suspect that, in the cortex, with regard to
memory, the formation of new associations, new discriminations, and
new relationships of context is accompanied by a degree of inhibition
of the opposite or the obsolescent.

Several *neurotransmitters* probably participate in the formation of a memory network in the cerebral cortex. In recent years, NMDA has emerged as a very likely candidate, particularly in view of the calcium dependence and voltage dependence of its receptors, as well as the long time course of the NMDA-induced synaptic changes (Nicoll et al., 1988). Further, NMDA receptors, which are common in the cortex (Cotman et al., 1987), are implicated in the generation of LTP, a presumptive mechanism of memory formation. Perhaps not coincidentally, the strength of experimentally induced LTP seems to decrease as a power function of time (Barnes, 1979), just as memory does.

In the formation of a mnemonic or cognitive network, synaptic modulation takes place along many cortical pathways and at several layers of the cortical hierarchies. To a large degree, this occurs autonomously and simultaneously in different locations, by self-organization and according to *hebbian principles,* especially synchronous convergence. To some degree the process is guided top-down from higher cortical areas, as are many attentive processes (Chapter 6). The temporally coincident inputs that construct new memory can come from many sources, some external and some internal. Among the external inputs, sensory stimuli and outputs from sensory processing areas are the most important. Internal inputs include those from the organism's internal milieu, which through the limbic brain carry to the neocortex information on the visceral and affective connotations of sensory stimuli. Other internal inputs are those from preexisting cognitive cortical networks, also activated associatively by sensory stimuli in the act of perception (Chapter 4).

The coinciding inputs to form the new network need not come from areas of the same hierarchical rank (sensory, motor, unimodal association, transmodal association, etc.). Some originate in small nets (*netlets*) of specific sensory or motor cortex, others in large-scale poly-associative cognits of higher cortex; thus, some carry specific-feature information and some symbolic information encoded in higher levels and triggered or activated by current peripheral stimulation. The point I wish to make here is that, in the formation of memory, *heterarchy of inputs* is the rule and not the exception.

Here another point, which is a direct corollary of the postulated architecture of cognits, is worth repeating (Chapter 3). Because the informational content of a cognit or memory is defined by relations, and not by the sum of its components, *any neuron or group of neurons anywhere in a cognitive hierarchy can become part of many memories.* The multiple intersections and overlaps of memory networks account for considerable redundancy of representation, or degeneracy—that is, the capacity of different structures to yield the same outcome. They also account for the potential for recovery after injury, in addition to such phenomena as false memory. The intersection and overlap of memory networks are, I believe, the key to understanding the robustness of memory and the apparent nonspecificity of certain amnesias after lesions occur, especially in higher cortex.

For the consolidation of memory into cortical long-term nets, there must be mechanisms of synaptic modulation that outlast the sensory impressions or internal inputs that form a memory. We have mentioned LTP as one such putative mechanism at the local level. Another, at the network level, seems very likely in view of the pervasive connective recurrence in cortical circuitry: the *reverberation* of impulses through recurrent circuits. Hebb (1949) was the first to postulate reverberation as a mechanism of memory retention; this mechanism is as plausible now as it was when he proposed it. Another plausible mechanism is the reactivation of the modulating inputs by repetition or rehearsal of sensory impressions. This is especially true for perceptual memory; practice would do the same for executive memory. For the reinforcement of a memory, the reinduced inputs need not be identical to those that generated it. Associations of similarity, perceptual or motor constancy, and symbolic representation can recreate effective inputs to enhance a memory network. By any or all of these potential mechanisms, the associated components of a network remain active for consolidation during their "stay" in what has been called short-term memory.

Short-Term Memory

Experimenting on himself, Ebbinghaus (1885), the pioneer researcher of human memory, made a singular discovery. By testing his ability to retain lists of nonsense syllables at various intervals after learning them, and by plotting the results of his tests, he produced graphs with an inflected curve. In the first 24 hours, his forgetting was precipitous; by the end of that time he was capable of remembering only 40% of the material. By the third day, retention was down to 30%. Thereafter, however, it descended very slowly to 20% at about 30 days. Clearly, he and many others thereafter reasoned, something happened in the first 3 days that stabilized memory or at least drastically diminished the rate of forgetting. That was the origin of the concept of a transition from short-term to long-term memory. Indeed, the argument was compelling. The memory that remained after 1 month, even in the absence of interim rehearsal, seemed to have passed to a more stable store. That change appeared to have allowed the memory to withstand further loss. What had been lost, it was thought, was short-term memory; what stayed was long-term memory. Subsequent research established seemingly beyond reasonable doubt the existence of *two forms or stages of memory*. The first, short-term memory, was characterized by limited storage capacity—which someone eventually estimated to be for a maximum of seven items—and relatively rapid decay. The second, long-term memory, had unlimited capacity and little or no decay. Both benefited from repetition and rehearsal.

With the "cognitive revolution" of the 1960s, memory researchers began to postulate the existence of two separate storage compartments for the two forms of memory, suggesting two dedicated brain structures. Atkinson and Shiffrin (1968) proposed a model, simplified in Figure 5.2, that became immensely popular and spearheaded a great deal of research on human memory. The model was supported by the evidence that subjects performing certain memory tasks were able to recall items with different degrees of proficiency, depending on the time that had elapsed between presentation and recall. A subject presented with a list of words, and required afterward to repeat the words regardless of order (free recall), can usually recall well the first words in the list (primacy effect) and the last words (recency effect), but not so well the words in the middle. The insertion of distracting stimuli, or of tasks between word presentation and recall, interferes with the recency effect, not with primacy. It has been argued, in support of the two-system model of memory, that at the time of recall the first words have already passed to long-term memory and resist interference, while the last words are still in short-term memory and vulnerable to interference.

The neuropsychology of the hippocampus also weighed on the side of the two-system linear model of memory. Since some hippocampally injured patients could remember very recent events but could not form long-term memories (anterograde amnesia), it was argued that short-term memory is stored somewhere else, though the hippocampus is necessary for its transfer to a permanent store. Further, some amnesic patients seemed to have lost the primacy effect of free recall while retaining the recency effect. The dual-storage model was challenged, however, by cases such as that of K.F. (Warrington

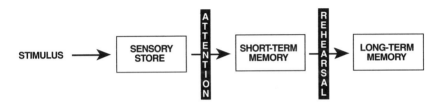

Figure 5.2. The model of human memory by Atkinson and Shiffrin.

and Shallice, 1969), in which the reverse was observed: good primacy and poor recency. Thus, the neuropsychology of memory favored but did not conclusively support the linear two-store model.

The distinction between short- and long-term memories, even as discrete stages if not stores of memory, began to falter when it was shown by appropriate analysis that the curve of forgetting was not inflected, as had been widely believed, but monotonically gradual (Wickelgren, 1975). When plotted on double-log graphs, data such as those of Ebbinghaus became straight lines. More precisely, they conformed to a power function. In logarithmically plotted curves of retention as a function of time, the inflection was no longer present (Fig. 5.3). Forgetting appeared to be simply subject to negative acceleration with time. There was no need to postulate the asymptotic stabilization of memory. Furthermore, numerous studies demonstrated what had been known or suspected all along, namely, that the forgetting and the slope of its curve are greatly dependent on the number and complexity of items in so-called short-term memory. The greater their number and complexity, the harder the remembering and the faster the forgetting. In any event, remembering is reinforced by rehearsal and impeded by distraction. Forgetting is naturally subject to the converse effects of rehearsal and distraction.

While human psychology was debating the two "systems" of memory, animal experiments produced evidence for the gradual consolidation of memory in a single store along a temporal continuum. The first such evidence was the observation that certain procedures, such as an electric shock to the head, obliterated recent memories or conditioned behaviors, and they did so as a function of time after learning (Glickman, 1961; McGaugh and Herz, 1972). Thus, the more remote a memory, the more resistant it was to electroshock. The retroactive interference with memory deposition induced by such procedures, together with the temporal characteristics of the effect, indicated that

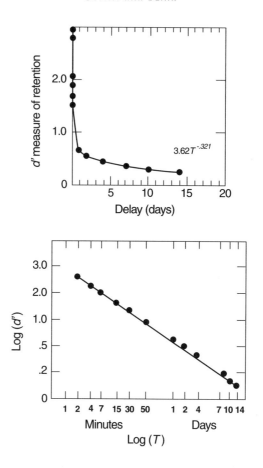

Figure 5.3. Ability to recognize words (measured by retention index *d*') as a function of time (delay) after presentation. The data in the upper graph are replotted on logarithmic scales in the lower graph. From Andersen (1995), adapted from Wickelgren (1975), with permission.

somewhere in the nervous system memory underwent a period of consolidation, as discussed in the previous section. Interference with that process prevented the memory from becoming permanent. There appeared to be no need for two stores with a sharp boundary or temporal transition between them. Subsequently there has been mounting evidence that information begins to enter permanent storage as soon as it comes in.

Thus, the long debate between the dual-store and the single-store hypotheses of memory seems to have been resolved in favor of the latter. The concept of consolidation of one and the same neural substrate has gradually done away with the dual-store idea. A massive amount of evidence has been accumulating, in humans as in animals, against the notion of short-term memory as a separate cognitive entity, let alone a memory system. At the same time, the evidence for the consolidation of memory in one store implicates the entire cerebral cortex as such a store and synaptic change in cortical networks as the essence of that consolidation. This view agrees fully with what in cognitive circles is known as the *unitary theory* of memory. There is no need for different neural structures to accommodate different kinds of memory if there is one store that can accommodate all memory, whatever its stage or state of development or use. What is needed, however, in light of the available physiological and clinical evidence, is a complex topography of cortical networks to accommodate the infinitely diverse contents of memory. This is the subject of the next two sections.

In sum, the concept of short-term cortical memory as a discrete system, stage, or kind of memory has become untenable. In the next chapter, the concept of time-limited memory will reemerge, however, though as an active and operant *state* of cortical memory—in other words, not as short-term memory per se but as *memory for the short term*. I am referring to working memory, a function of fundamental importance for the temporal organization of cognition, speech, and behavior that, for reasons that I hope to make clear, is more at home under the heading of attention than of memory.

Perceptual Memory

Memory, by any definition according to content, can take many forms, and any memory has a mixture of contents. Heterogeneity is a universal trait of all memories. That is the reason for the difficulty we encounter when we attempt to classify them in the search for their neural stores. In light of the discussion in previous chapters, it should be obvious that the heterogeneity of memory is a direct result of its associative nature. We are unable to classify, let alone localize in the brain, memories that are made up of diverse and distributed contents. Autobiographical memory, which is commonly characterized as *episodic* or *declarative,* illustrates both the heterogeneity and the problems of attempting to classify memories by their content. I will make my point with a literary example:

I started across to the town from a little below the ferry-landing, and the drift of the current fetched me in at the bottom of the town. I tied up and started along the bank. There was a light burning in a little shanty that hadn't been lived in for a long time, and I wondered who had took up quarters there. I slipped up and peeped in at the window. There was a woman about forty year old in there knitting by a candle that was on a pine table. I didn't know her face; she was a stranger, for you couldn't start a face in that town that I didn't know. Now this was lucky, because I was weakening; I was getting afraid people might know my voice and find me out. But if this woman had been in such a little town two days she could tell me all I wanted to know; so I knocked at the door, and made up my mind I wouldn't forget I was a girl.

—Mark Twain, *Huckleberry Finn*

Consider Twain's passage in light of some of the conventional classes of memory that some researchers attempt to localize in various brain structures or cortical areas. Certainly the entire episode would fall into the category of declarative episodic memory. Note, however, that the description is riddled with pieces of other different kinds of memory. There is memory of two sensory modalities (visual and acoustic), spatial memory, and face memory, as well as implicit references to other items of perceptual memory (e.g., the woman's features, Huck's clothing) and motor memory (e.g., steering the raft, mooring, walking to town). Then there is, of course, semantic memory, some of it almost at a conceptual level and presupposing considerable abstraction (e.g., estimate of age, gender identity). Without semantic memory, in fact, the description would be not only incomplete but incomprehensible. There is also emotional memory—of fear. And there is even memory of not recognizing and of not forgetting! It is highly implausible that, on account of its source or properties, all that memory or any of its parts would be lodged in a discrete region or component of Huck's brain, Twain's brain, or the brain of the person who reads the passage.

What seems more plausible is that the memory of the episode is represented by a heterarchical network of widely dispersed and more or less associated cortical elements of representation or cognits, each of which could serve that particular memory as well as many others.

Clearly, a connectionist model of the cortex, as I am attempting to propose in this book, makes more sense here than a modular model of "kinds" or "systems" of memory. Therefore, the relevant question before us can be formulated as follows: Is there a *taxonomy of memory* that can at the same time accommodate the brain facts, the phenomenology of memory, and our network model? The answer, I believe, lies squarely in the *biology of the cortex*. The only taxonomy of memory that seems adequate to the neuroscientist is one based on the functional architecture of the cerebral cortex, outlined in Chapter 3. That is the reason for my often repeated statement that there are no systems of memory, but there is the memory of systems (Fuster, 1995) — of neural systems, that is.

As the Russian anatomist Betz first noted long ago (1874), the entire nerve axis, from the spinal cord to the telencephalon, is anatomically and physiologically divided into two longitudinal moieties: a posterior moiety devoted to receptive functions and an anterior one devoted to motor functions. If we extend that dichotomy to the cerebral cortex we will find that, in the primate, the dividing line between the two moieties is the rolandic or central fissure, and to some extent also the sylvian fissure. The cortex behind them is broadly sensory, and the cortex in front of them is broadly motor. Thus we call *sensory* a diverse array of posterior cortical areas dedicated to the receiving and storing of information from the senses and to the cognitive functions related to them. Conversely, we call *motor* an equally diverse array of frontal areas dedicated to the actions of the organism and their related cognitive functions. Memory is stored in both sectors of cortex: perceptual memory in posterior cortex and executive memory in frontal cortex. Both sectors of cortex are hierarchically organized, as are the cognits they represent (Chapter 3).

Perceptual memory is memory acquired through the senses at any time in the life of the individual. In broad terms, this definition includes all knowledge acquired through sensory experience. Thus, the definition includes so-called semantic memory. In those broad terms, therefore, memories coincide with perceptual cognits or aggregates of them. In the present context, however, it seems more appropriate to define perceptual memory as made up of *dated* experiences. In so doing, however, we run the danger of implying a structural separation between knowledge and memory, which is indefensible on both cognitive and neural grounds. This spurious separation disappears if we anchor the memory of dated experience on prior knowledge and experience. Here I feel I have to reemphasize a critical point, namely, that all dated experience is an extension of previous experience, an expansion of old memory and of old knowledge. New perceptual memory is made up of new perception, but given that *all* perception consists of the reevocation of old knowledge to interpret and classify the new (Chapter 4), it follows that any new experience is incorporated by association into a fund of old experience. The new experience becomes an inextricable part of a vast associative cognit, a vast neural network that may contain, nevertheless, distinctive associations with space, time, and sensorium.

It also follows from our argument so far that perceptual memory, almost by definition, is essentially *heterarchical*. Any perceptual memory is an associative conglomerate of sensory and semantic features at many levels of the cognitive hierarchy of perceptual knowledge. The network representing the memory must tie together features of the same modality in unimodal association cortex and of different modalities in cross-modal association cortex. It must also tie those sensory associations with nets representing symbols, words, and concepts. As we have seen in Chapter 4, some of those representations, formed by repeated exposure to constant configurations of sensory features (e.g., faces), reside in networks of relatively low cortex of association. Others, formed by convergence and divergence of coincident and wideranging inputs, reside in wider networks of higher transmodal cortex. I need not reiterate the neuropsychological and imaging evidence on which these inferences are based (Chapters 3 and 4). Here I simply wish to highlight some corollaries of the model and of the supporting evidence with respect to the cortical distribution of the heterarchical and overlapping networks that constitute perceptual memories.

For heuristic reasons, it is useful to picture on the surface of the cortex the distribution of memories in terms of the *hierarchy* of the cognits that constitute them. Note that, according to the schema in Color Plate 1, all the perceptual memory of the individual rests on— and grows from—a layer of phyletic or innate sensory memory, by which I mean the structure of primary sensory cortices. Right above this basic sensory layer, and following the gradients of cortical development and connectivity, lie the networks of unimodal and polymodal associative memory. As noted above, certain categorical entities of memory, such as names and faces, appear represented by neuronal aggregates in those layers of sensory association. Further up in the cortex, we encounter the layers of episodic and semantic memory; here, for our purpose, they are separated from each other, although, in light of the previous discussion, it should be apparent that this separation is somewhat artificial. At the top of our schema we place conceptual memory, the highest and most integrative layer of memory. That is in reality a layer of knowledge, formed by accretion and abstraction of the common constituents (i.e., perceptual categories, general sensory impressions, spatial and temporal characteristics), of many memories. That layer comprises the concepts of general experience of the organism with its surrounding.

To summarize, on theoretical and empirical grounds, memories appear to be represented in overlapping and far-flung networks of the neocortex of the occipital, temporal, and parietal lobes. These networks contain nodes or cognits of heavy convergence and association representing categories of individual knowledge that are common components of many memories. Such nodes may be widely separated anatomically. The cortical networks of memory are essentially heterarchical, with associative components at several levels of the structural hierarchy of perceptual knowledge, and thus at several levels of the hierarchy of cognitive areas of postrolandic cortex. Consequently, the network of a memory can span wide cortical territories, from sensory cortex to the highest conceptual cortex.

Memory, like the other cognitive functions, is subject to a degree of *hemispheric lateralization*. Ever since the seminal studies of Sperry (1974) on patients with severed corpus callosum, it has been known that one cerebral hemisphere can acquire memories and motor skills independent of the other. This kind of research led to the expansion of the well-demonstrated specialization of the left or dominant hemisphere for language (Chapter 7). Many studies have shown that cognitive content and abilities are unequally represented in the two hemicortices (Rubens, 1977). Thus, some studies led to the inference of left-side specialization for logical reasoning and calculation, whereas the right cortex would specialize in nonverbal ideation, as well as in such other functions as visual imagery and memory. On the basis of neuropsychological and neuroimaging evidence, gender differences in cognitive hemispheric specialization have also been postulated. Although in almost every study the conclusions on specialization are tempered by a degree of individual variance, there seems to be little doubt that some of the interhemispheric differences are real, even for nonlanguage functions. However, there is a danger of un-justifiably inferring, from only relative differences, the categorical dedication of either hemicortex to a given cognitive function. In any case, it is clear that memories can be held in the cortex of either hemisphere, and that some memory networks extend from one hemisphere to the other through associative fibers in the corpus callosum.

Two structural factors bear on the *solidity of a memory* and on its resistance to loss by cortical injury. One is the strength of its connections, and the other is the hierarchical ranking of its contents. Synaptic strength is undoubtedly dependent on the efficiency of consolidation, which in turn depends on such cognitive operations as attention, repetition, and rehearsal. Logically, the greater the consolidation of memory, the greater its resistance to injury. Of course, not all the associations of a memory are of equal strength. Associations with specific sensory qualia, with precise spatial and temporal reference, with facial features, and with peculiar symbols (e.g., words) are weaker and more fragile that those that are based on more general features or combinations of features. The reason for their difference in strength is that the former are made up of special and unique cog-nits, whereas the latter are made up of general cognits, common to many memories and reinforced by repeated co-occurrence.

Accordingly, there is generally an inverse relationship between the hierarchical rank of memory content and the vulnerability to cortical injury. The lower the memory, the more vulnerable it is to injury; conversely, the higher the memory, the more resistant it is. By gaining breadth of distribution (note the fanning-up of memory hierarchies in Color Plate 1), memories gain solidity for two reasons. One is that their content is more redundant, supported by more lower-level networks; the loss of some connections still leaves others to carry a memory. The other reason is that at higher levels memories are accessible to more associative pathways, some of them in addition to those that contributed to their making. For similar reasons, the most concrete components of heterarchical memories are the most vulnerable. Thus, aging may lead to the forgetting of dates, names, and places, but not of the events or essential facts (Smith and Fullerton, 1981; Light et al., 1986). Individual faces may be forgotten, but not the ability to categorize faces by more or less general features. A comparable gradient of resistance to damage seems present in the frontal hierarchy with regard to executive memories.

Executive Memory

In cognitive neuroscience, the discussion of the cortex of the frontal lobe is usually framed in *operant* terms. What does the frontal cortex do? What can it not do when it is damaged? Electrical and imaging data, as well as results of cortical lesion studies, have been commonly adduced in support of one or another view of frontal function or dysfunction. With regard to motor and premotor cortices, functional discussions usually revolve around questions of neuron population dynamics in the performance of somatic or ocular movements. With regard to higher—that is, prefrontal—cortex, the critical questions commonly asked concerning the role of this cortex or its parts in cognitive functions are related to behavior or language. The integrative functions of the prefrontal cortex, notably working memory, set, attention, and act inhibition, are empirically assigned to different prefrontal areas—or vice versa, areas to the functions—in attempts to explain the role of this cortex in the working brain.

Much less consideration is given to the cortex of the frontal lobe as a neural substrate for *representation,* that is, as a store of memory—other than a transient store of short-term or working memory. The reason for the relative neglect of frontal representation obviously lies in methodology. In animals, motor memory can be tested only in operant terms. In humans, it can also be assessed phenomenologically, but humans are usually better at describing their perceptual experiences than their habits, modes of behavior, or future plans. This probably has to do with the unconscious and implicit nature of much of what we consider motor or executive memory.

Nonetheless, it is by the phenomenological study of patients with frontal lobe injury that we have come to appreciate the role of frontal cortex as the store of motor or executive memory. The inability to recount serial actions in an orderly manner is a commonly observed symptom after large lesions of the lateral frontal cortex occur. Another symptom is the inability to formulate, let alone execute, complex new plans of behavior. In fact, the *planning deficit* is an almost universal symptom of frontal damage (Fuster, 1997). Thus, the representational deficit resulting from frontal damage seems to run in both temporal directions, to the past and the future. It is a deficit of the memory of past sequences of behavior and, in addition, a deficit of the capacity to represent future actions, in other words, a deficit of *memory of the future* (Ingvar, 1985) or *prospective memory* (Dobbs and

Rule, 1987). In any case, it is a disorder of the representation of executive sequences and of what have been designated *schemas of action* (Arbib et al., 1998).

From the fine analysis of the effects of smaller frontal lesions as well as from physiological studies, a picture of a motor hierarchy of areas in the frontal lobe has emerged that matches a similar hierarchy for perceptual representation in postrolandic cortex (Color Plate 1). Clearly, however, as we ascend that hypothetical frontal hierarchy, we find the adjective *motor* increasingly inadequate. In light of the heterogeneity of schemas of action represented in higher frontal cortices, the term *executive* seems more appropriate for the entire frontal hierarchy.

That frontal *hierarchy of executive representation* is the same one I described in Chapter 3 when dealing with the cortical architecture of executive cognits. Briefly, we postulated that the most elementary aspects of executive action are represented in the motor cortex of the prerolandic gyrus (M1). That is the depository of motor phyletic memory, the innate structure for the representation of skeletal movement. Directly above motor cortex is the cortex of the premotor regions. Action is represented here more globally, in terms of trajectory and goal. Sequence and order are to some extent also represented in networks of premotor cortex (Mushiake et al., 1990; Hikosaka et al., 1999), notably in the SMAs. From the work of Rizzolatti et al. (1990), the concept of *mirror units* emerged. These are neurons in premotor areas of the monkey that respond to both the execution and the sight of an action or series of actions, even if executed by a human. Mirror units belong to networks of frontal executive memory that can be activatad (retrieved) by sensory stimuli associated with the actions they represent.

Mainly on neuropsychological grounds, the new and complex sequences of action in the behavioral and linguistic domains appear represented by networks of *lateral prefrontal cortex*. In both behavior and language, the representations in this cortex seem to consist of new schemas, plans, and programs of action. As discussed in Chapters 2 and 3, the high-level frontal networks that constitute the cognits of action—above primary motor cortex—are formed by self-organization, probably according to the same principles of synaptic modulation that govern the formation of perceptual networks in posterior cortex. Among the inputs modulating synapses between neurons of executive networks are those that carry to frontal cortex information about the course and consequences of actions. They include efferent copies

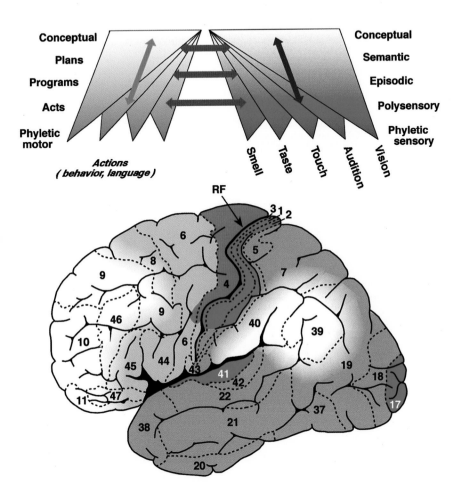

Color Plate 1. Schematic diagram of the cortical distribution of cognitive representations. The upper figure shows the hierarchical order of memories by content. The lower figure shows, on Brodmann's cytoarchitectonic map and with the same color code as in the upper figure, the approximate distribution of mnemonic contents on the lateral cortical surface. *RF,* rolandic fissure.

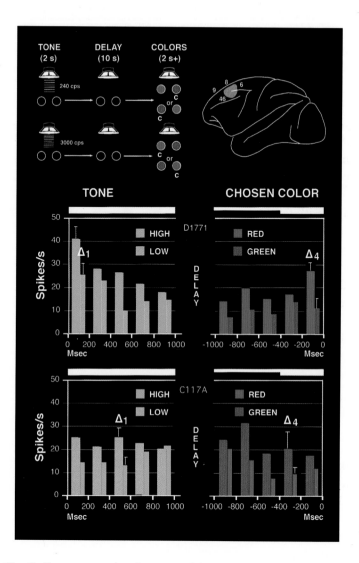

Color Plate 2. Cross-temporal and cross-modal integration in frontal cortex. *Upper left:* The behavioral task used to test it. *(1)* A tone is presented for 2 sec through an overhead loudspeaker; *(2)* a delay of 10 sec follows; *(3)* two colors are presented simultaneously; *(4)* the animal is rewarded for choosing the color (c) that matches the tone. Tone and color position change at random from trial to trial. *Upper right:* Diagram of the monkey's brain. Numbers indicate Brodmann cytoarchitectonic areas; in blue, the frontal region from which tone- and color-differential cells were recorded. *Below:* Firing-frequency histograms of two cells, one selective for high tone and red *(top)* and the other for low tone and green *(bottom).* Note the correlation of selective cell reactions to tones and colors in accord with the task rule. From Fuster et al. (2000), with permission.

of movement, kinesthetic inputs, and other carriers of *corollary discharge*. Much of that collective input is composed of feedback signals that regulate the action in the perception-action cycle. In the learning of a motor task, that input contributes to the adaptation of the motor apparatus to changing conditions and forces in the environment (Shadmehr and Mussa-Ivaldi, 1994). Those input signals are incorporated into the cognit of the task and thus, in its course, allow the organism to anticipate recurrent external conditions and forces.

The functional architecture of executive networks, as well as the cortical dynamics of the perception-action cycle, can be explored in the monkey with microelectrodes. By this method, several predictions concerning these issues can be tested. One of them is that neurons of frontal cortex will integrate sensory information for the execution of behavioral acts that are contingent on that information. We tested this prediction (Fuster et al., 2000) by recording cell discharge from the frontal cortex of monkeys that had been previously trained to perform the task depicted in Color Plate 2. On every trial, the animal was required to listen to a brief tone, to remember its pitch through a delay of 10 seconds, and to choose, from a display of two colors, the color associated with that tone. (By prior training, the animal was instructed to choose green if the tone was low-pitched and red if it was high-pitched.) The task was therefore one of associating sounds with colors across time, a test of cross-temporal and cross-modal integration. Neurons in lateral prefrontal cortex fired more spikes in reaction to one tone than to the other and more to one color than to the other. Most cells "matched" tones with colors as the monkey did; that is, cells that preferred the high tone over the low tone also preferred red over green and, conversely, cells that preferred the low tone also preferred green (Color Plate 2, lower part). Those correlations disappeared in trials ending with behavioral error (wrong color choice). It seems, therefore, that the two types of neurons, low-tone/green and high-tone/red, belonged to two different networks, each associating a tone with its corresponding color. In sum, neurons of the prefrontal cortex contribute to the behavioral integration of auditory with visual stimuli across time. They appear to belong to long-term memory networks associating stimuli of two sensory modalities as a result of learning.

Microelectrode data such as these provide a rather narrow view of the perception-action cycle. They give us useful clues, however, to the mechanisms of the cycle in higher cognitive functions. Indeed, the integrative properties of prefrontal neurons across time and across sensory modalities probably transcend the narrow context of our monkey in its matching of colors and sounds. Executive prefrontal networks and their neurons undoubtedly serve the temporal closure of the cycle, at the top, in the structuring of human behavior, reasoning, and language.

Repetition, rehearsal, and practice have effects on executive memory similar to those on perceptual memory. Through those operations, the executive memory networks of frontal cortex become consolidated. The representation of the more concrete, stereotypical, and automatic components of sequential action is relegated to lower structures of the motor system (motor and premotor cortices, basal ganglia, cerebellum, pyramidal system). This is what I meant in Chapter 3 when I referred to a *migration* of old and automatic cognits to lower structures of the executive hierarchy. Conversely, the representation of the more general, schematic, and abstract components of action becomes consolidated in prefrontal cortex. For example, the invariant movements of a monkey performing a delay task, that is, the automatic reactions to the stimuli that are similar from trial to trial, become consolidated in lower motor structures. Concomitantly, the rules and contingencies of the task, the memory of the task, and the schema of a trial are consolidated in networks of prefrontal cortex.

With practice and reenactment, the common elements of many action sequences presumably generate overarching prefrontal networks that abstract those common features in the form of global *schemas* of action. These global schemas would constitute action symbols, the equivalent of perceptual symbols in the mnemonic hierarchy of posterior cortex. In the aggregate, the networks that represent them in frontal cortex would constitute a kind of *semantic executive memory*, possibly with nodes of heavy association like those of posterior cortex for perception. Further abstraction, by dispersion and convergence of executive information, would lead to even more global frontal networks representing general *concepts* of action. In the human brain, these conceptual networks would include value systems of behavior and such concepts as those of responsibility, altruism, and the rule of law.

In sum, a large part of executive memory is represented in neuronal networks of frontal cortex. These networks are hierarchically organized by their content, conforming to connective, phylogenetic, and ontogenetic orders. The more concrete and specific cognits of motor action are represented in networks of motor and premotor cortices. The more general and abstract cognits of behavioral and linguistic action are represented in networks of prefrontal cortex. Any executive memory with some level of complexity is essentially heterarchical, in that it contains networks of different hierarchical ranks that to some degree overlap one another.

On account of their structural organization, the contents of executive memory, like those of perceptual memory, are differentially vulnerable to cortical injury. Thus, local frontal lesions at lower hierarchical levels are more deleterious to low-ranking memory than they are at higher levels to high-ranking memory. For example, lesions of motor and premotor cortices (e.g., Broca's area) are more detrimental to the representation and articulation of speech than are lesions of prefrontal cortex. Only large or diffuse lesions of the latter cortex induce disorders in the representation of complex linguistic constructs and concepts.

So far, we have mainly referred to the procedural aspects of executive memory, that is, to the memory of learned structures of action. It is the kind of memory that is commonly termed *procedural memory*. Only tangentially have we referred to the autobiographical memory of sequential actions, namely, to the memory of past sequences of behavior with specific time and space references. It seems unlikely, in the light of neuropsychological evidence, that the associative networks that represent this kind of executive memory are represented entirely in the frontal lobe. After they have been performed, behavioral sequences may also become part of perceptual memory and of the mnemonic networks of posterior cortex. The autobiographical memory of past actions may thus be largely encoded associatively in posterior cortex, where the percepts related to those actions are placed in spatial maps and linked to the clock and the calendar.

As noted earlier in this section, it is neuropsychologically evident that lateral prefrontal cortex is essential for the representation of plans. It is also evident, on physiological grounds, that its neurons are involved in the preparatory set for impending actions (Fuster, 1997). Thus, it is reasonable to conclude that, probably with the assistance of inputs from other cortical regions and the limbic system, lateral prefrontal cortex can form within itself networks that represent *future action*. The capacity to represent a rich variety of new actions is undoubtedly related to the extraordinary phylogenetic development and dimensions of that cortex in the human brain. It is for good reasons that the prefrontal cortex has been called the *executive of the brain* and the *organ of creativity*. For the same reasons, the prefrontal cortex has been found to play a crucial role in *intelligence* (Chapter 8).

Retrieval of Memory

To retrieve a memory is to reactivate the network that represents it. All phenomena related to memory retrieval are ultimately attributable to this basic assumption. Remembering, recalling, and recognizing can take many forms and differ greatly in content and context. All retrieval modes, however, essentially consist of the reactivation of a neural network that in its connective pattern defines and sustains a memory. In memory retrieval, the degree of conscious awareness may differ greatly, but conscious awareness per se defines neither the network nor the process of its reactivation. In cognitive terms as in neural terms, the process of activation of a memory network derives fundamentally from the associative character of all memory, perceptual or motor, from the simplest to the most complex. That process is in any case an *associative process:* it is the activation of the network through the activation of its associated components.

From that general assumption, it follows that the retrieval of a memory can be induced by a large variety of external and internal stimuli and by the conditions of the organism—at least as many as contributed to the associative process of forming that memory. Here we will review those stimuli and those conditions, as well as the mechanisms by which they lead to memory retrieval. To be of general relevance, our review should transcend the conscious phenomenology of human memory. This is difficult, because phenomenology weighs heavy in studies of memory retrieval, which are usually conducted in settings where recall and recognition are conscious (*declarable*) by design. Conscious awareness is a concomitant phenomenon of many acts of retrieval and of memory searches, as well as of attention and working memory (Chapter 6), but is not a necessary attribute of the stimuli that can retrieve memory or of the retrieval process itself. Perception, we have seen (Chapter 4), is essentially a process of recognition of established memory with the result of categorizing the world around us, which takes place to a large extent unconsciously. All memory is largely implicit and can be retrieved unconsciously for myriad adaptive reasons.

For a memory to be retrievable, its cognitive network must have a degree of solidity, that is, of synaptic strength. The greater that solidity, the greater its accessibility by retrieval. Some *amnesias* are wholly attributable to the loss or weakness of cortical memory networks from disuse, aging, or pathology. Other amnesias, on the other hand, are clearly attributable to a disorder of retrieval mechanisms; in these cases, the memory is there but is not retrievable. After a blow to the head, for example, memory for the events preceding and succeeding the incident may be lost. With the passage of time, the ability to recall those events recovers, and the recovery follows a converging order around the time of the incident. The amnesia "shrinks" in time: events become progressively more retrievable, from the past and from the present, toward the moment at which the concussion occurred. Although some events immediately surrounding the concussion remain irretrievable (from lack of consolidation), the bulk of the amnesia disappears. The important conclusion here is that the memory networks formed before and after the trauma were present all along but were inaccessible.

Some memories may be inaccessible to consciousness for psychogenic reasons. Dynamic defenses against anxiety (e.g., repression, denial) make those memories that are unusually laden with emotional connotations irretrievable by normal recall, at least temporarily. Again, that is mnemonic material that is present but unavailable. As we will see below, the converse may also be true. For pathological reasons, some emotional memories are *overretrieved* in the conscious state. Others are retrieved in dreams or in hypnotic states. Even motor memories may be retrieved and executed in sleep or under hypnosis.

Given that most memories are essentially heterarchical, made up of cognitive contents of different hierarchical levels, and given that the memory contents at one level are better consolidated than those at another, not all contents of a memory are equally retrievable. Further inequality of access to recall stems from differences in degree of consolidation by practice, rehearsal, or attention. We can recall general facts better than specific incidents, we can recall better the incidents that have caught our attention than those that have not, and we can play better those pieces of music we have rehearsed than those we have not. Finally, it is well known that memories can be more easily retrieved by recognition than by recall. In *recognition,* the stimuli or *prompts* are present and usually more numerous; in *recall,* they are indirect and sparser, at least partly internal. In either case, the retrieving stimuli have associative links to the memory and, through them, activate it. The difference between the two retrieval modes is conveniently illustrated by analogy with the hand that reaches into the basket of cherries. In recognition, it grabs a bunch of them; in recall, it pulls only one or two, and the others follow as their stems are interlocked.

The *hippocampus* has been implicated in the conscious retrieval of certain kinds of memory, notably the kind of perceptual memory called *declarative* (facts and episodes). On close examination (Sagar et al., 1985), H.M. was found to exhibit amnesia extending into long periods of his life before the temporal-lobe surgery (Figure 5.4). Thus, in addition to being unable to form new memories (anterograde amnesia), he was unable to remember established memories from the past (retrograde amnesia). Other patients with hippocampal damage exhibit what amounts to global amnesia extending to infancy (Schnider et al., 1995). It is a reasonable assumption that these patients, as well as H.M., suffer from a memory retrieval deficit caused by the absence of intact hippocampi. Further evidence of a role of the hippocampus in memory retrieval comes from a PET imaging study (Schacter et al., 1996). Presumably, the hippocampus exerts its memory-retrieval role via its reciprocal connections with the neocortex.

To the reader who has followed the discussion of relationships between old memory and new memory, the dual role of the hippocampus in the formation and retrieval of memory must appear logical, although the mechanisms for either remain obscure. We said that new memory is formed on old memory. Thus the acquisition of new memory presupposes the retrieval of the old. If the hippocampus is essential for the formation of a new memory, it must almost necessarily play a part in the retrieval of the long-term memory in which the new memory is going to lodge. Not surprisingly, some patients with hippocampal damage have difficulty assessing the novelty or familiarity of new happenings.

Three categories of neural input can lead to the activation (retrieval) of a cortical memory network:

a. sensory stimuli;
b. inputs from other memory networks; and
c. inputs from the internal milieu, including influences from visceral systems and the neural substrates of instinct and affect (limbic system).

Despite the attempts to dissect them experimentally in humans and animals, there are good reasons to assume that inputs in all three categories intervene in the retrieval of *any* memory, whether perceptual, executive, or both. We need not discuss again the connective lines of access of those inputs to the cortex (Chapter 3). Nor do we need to belabor the point that memory retrieval occurs as much top-down as it occurs bottom-up. Here, however, with our neural model in mind, it seems appropriate to briefly discuss those categories of inputs and some of the neuropsychological aspects of the memories they help retrieve.

A sensory stimulus can retrieve a memory inasmuch as that stimulus has been previously associated with others in the formation of that memory. The best evidence for the neural transactions of *sensory retrieval* comes from microelectrode studies in the monkey. In the inferotemporal cortex of this animal, which contains associative networks of the visual modality, neurons respond in similar manner, that

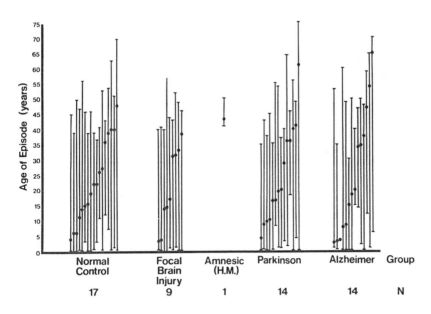

Figure 5.4. Age of the episodes (median and range) recalled or recognized by subjects of various groups on Crovitz's Test. In this test, the subject is prompted by associations to retrieve episodes from a previous period of life. The patient H.M. limited his production of memories to a period of about 41 years ago, when he was 17 years old, some 11 years before he underwent temporal lobe surgery. He had difficulty retrieving events from other periods. From Sagar et al. (1985), with permission.

is, with similar firing changes, to two visual stimuli that have been associated by training (paired associates) and have become components of the same cognitive network (Sakai and Miyashita, 1991). In somatosensory cortex, cells have been found that react similarly to the touch of an object and to a visual stimulus that has been behaviorally associated with it (Zhou and Fuster, 2000). Evidence of this kind demonstrates not only the access of different associated sensory stimuli to the same memory network, but also the heteromodal and heterarchical character of some networks. Some of them appear to reach down into primary sensory cortex. Thus, in the act of retrieval they are probably reactivated, at least in part, in top-down fashion.

In memory retrieval, as we noted in the context of perception (Chapter 4), sensory stimuli can act as surrogates for each other, whether on account of similarity and perceptual constancy or as members of the same category. This interchangeablility of memory retrieving stimuli results from the associative structure of memory networks and from the fact that, as in perception, a stimulus can access a memory at several hierarchical levels. That multilevel access to memory networks is the reason that, when the access to one level of memory is reinforced, the access to another becomes facilitated. Therein also lies the reason why the cueing or organizing of memory items by category (animals, tools, metals, etc.) facilitates their recall (Tulving and Pearlstone, 1966; Bower et al., 1969) (Fig. 5.5). That is also a reason for the success of some common mnemonic strategies.

In neural terms, the multilevel access of stimuli to memory networks implies that the retrieving associations take place at several levels of the perceptual or executive hierarchies. Within each level this can be accomplished through collateral connections. As discussed in previous chapters (2 and 3), this type of connectivity is pervasive in both cortical hierarchies, perceptual and executive. Through collateral connections, sensory inputs arriving at one level can activate associated memory contents at the same level. In addition, upward and downward connections can spread the activation from a given sensory source to the contents of the memory it evokes at other levels, in other words, to higher and lower components of the memory network.

A second category (b) of memory-retrieving inputs is internal, consisting of outputs from *other memory networks*. An active network can act as the retriever of another network through connective links that associate the two. The first may have been activated by an external stimulus or as part of a chain of associative retrievals. Or else the

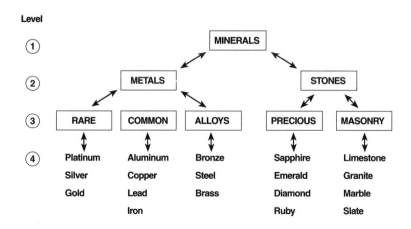

Figure 5.5. The conceptual hierarchy for minerals. Mentally organizing the items into classes facilitates their recall. From Bower et al. (1969), with permission.

retrieving network may have been activated in another cognitive process, such as reasoning or imagination. As a result, excitation can spread from one network to another through common associative links. At the same time, some of the networks previously active may be inhibited or become inactive. Thus, any memory retrieval operation initiated externally or in the cortex itself can act as the source of further retrievals. In this manner, any stimulus, external or internal, can unleash a wave of spreading associative activations in vast regions of the cortex. This would be the neural basis for the spreading activation of memory postulated by some cognitive psychologists (Anderson, 1995). It would also be the basis of the free-association method of the psychoanalyst—assisted by inputs of emotional memory (c, below).

A third source of memory retrieval is the *internal milieu* (c). The diencephalon and the lower brain stem integrate a host of visceral influences. These are transmitted through the limbic system to cortical areas, where they modulate the activity of memory networks. Those inputs from the internal milieu are associated in cortical networks with external stimuli, thus forming the neural substrate for such behavioral phenomena as state-dependent learning and fear conditioning. In both of these conditions, external stimuli are probably processed in the amygdala at the same time as, or before, they reach the cortex, where they activate motor networks mediating aversive behavior (Gustavson et al., 1974; Le Doux, 1993). The aggregate of visceral and emotional inputs associated with external stimuli, and the networks that associate them, constitute what we call *emotional memory*. Some networks of emotional memory extend into the prefrontal cortex, especially its orbital aspect, where they contribute to the structuring and activation of executive networks to meet the challenges of the environment to homeostasis and to social order.

In certain conditions, however, emotional memory, presumably through overactive inputs to the cortex from limbic structures, can lead to distorted or maladaptive memory retrieval. The distortion of memory, otherwise called *false memory* (Schacter and Curran, 2000), has lately attracted a great deal of attention, among other reasons because of its legal implications (witness accounts). The phenomenon is manifested as severe and unwitting alterations or recreations of past events in the recollection of long-term memories. Often the distortion is easily attributable to psychodynamic defenses. In this respect, it is akin to the confusion between fantasy and past reality that is common in some neurotic disorders (e.g., hysteria). In neural terms, it is unclear whether false memory is due to a change of the mnemonic networks that represent memories or to a faulty retrieval mechanism.

Other pathological conditions of emotional memory lead to the internally generated and uncontrollable retrieval of either perceptual memory or motor memory. Thus, for example, the obsessive-compulsive disorder leads to both. The patient is besieged by perceptual representations that intrude repetitively into his or her consciousness and cause unbearable anxiety. Concomitantly, the patient is driven to execute compulsive acts and routines to obtain relief from that anxiety. In the Gilles de la Tourette's syndrome, an inherited autosomal genetic disorder, the patient is uncontrollably compelled to proffer inappropriate verbal utterances; here only a fragment of motor memory seems to be repetitively retrieved and stereotypically enacted. There is some evidence (from imaging studies, e.g., that of Baxter et al., 1987) indicating that these conditions are accompanied by abnormal excitability of orbital prefrontal cortex. This cortex is closely connected to the amygdala and basal ganglia and plays a critical role in the regulation of emotional behavior.

Whereas we may be fully conscious of a retrieved memory— sometimes painfully so—the vast majority of the memories that we retrieve remain unconscious. As I remarked in the previous chapter, we are unconscious of most of what we perceive in our daily lives; similarly, we perform myriad acts automatically and without being aware of them. In fact, the awareness of all that is declarable or semantic in our innumerable daily retrievals from memory would be an enormous burden on our minds and an encumbrance to our behavior. Thus, most memory retrieval is *implicit*. At one time or another it may have been explicit, but as it is retrieved and put to use, it is not. Thus, the phenomenological distinction between implicit and explicit memory, as if we were dealing with two different categories of memory or memory systems, is somewhat artificial. In neural terms, the distinction can only properly refer to relative differences in consolidation, strength of connection, and state of activation.

One state of memory activation that has received considerable attention is the one that underlies the phenomenon of *priming*. Priming is the facilitation of retrieval from memory by previous exposure to a stimulus that is at some level related to the memorandum. The relationship may be sensory, perceptual, semantic, logical, or executive. For example, the subject is presented with a small fragment of an object that does not per se evoke a specific memory, and then is requested to memorize or recognize a series of objects that includes that object in its entirety or another fragment of it. The object will be recalled or identified with higher probability, speed, and accuracy than the others in the series. Essentially, the first stimulus, even though unrecognized, has implicitly primed the retrieval of the second. By the ingenious experimental use of semantic inferences and relationships, priming can be shown to bias the choice between alternative mnemonic representations (Anderson, 1995). In any case, priming need not be considered a kind of memory or a memory system, let alone one with a neural location. It can be appropriately understood, instead, as the result of the preactivation of a memory network—at a *subliminal* level of conscious awareness—through an associative link within itself or with other networks. The heterarchy of established memory makes any memory network accessible to plentiful priming influences.

Executive memory is retrieved in much the same way as perceptual memory. Here the associative retrieving inputs to the executive networks of the frontal lobe are of categories b and c (above), that is, from networks of posterior cortex and the limbic system. Again, retrieval can be heterarchical, inasmuch as executive networks can be accessed at various levels: motor, premotor, and prefrontal. The networks retrieved by association may represent specific motor acts, programs of behavior, schemas of action (motoric or linguistic), and con-

cepts of action. Imaging studies indicate that prefrontal cortex, especially on the right, is activated in the retrieval of various forms of perceptual memory (e.g., episodic). The activation is most conspicuous
in lateral prefrontal cortex when the subject is obliged to organize
the mnemonic material retrieved (Fletcher et al., 1998a,b). It is unclear, however, whether the role of this cortex is to retrieve memory
or to assist the executive function of integrating and organizing the
cognitive information retrieved.

The organization of behavior requires the continuous, orderly activation of networks of executive memory represented in the cortex of
the frontal lobe and lower structures of motor systems. That recruitment of executive networks can only take place through the functional interplay of frontal with posterior cortices in the perception-
action cycle (Chapters 3 and 4). The operation of this cybernetic
cycle between the organism and its environment implies that the
frontal cortex receives a constant flow of perceptual information
from posterior cortex to guide the action. That information includes
feedback from the effects of previous action on the environment. The
perceptual flow into executive systems also includes sensory stimuli
associated with behavioral action by prior learning. After learning,
such stimuli reach the frontal lobe through memory networks of posterior cortex. The resulting networks linking posterior with frontal
cortex represent the sensory–motor sequence toward a goal. In the
pursuit of that goal, those networks enter the perception-action cycle,
whereby their activity becomes orderly and distributed in time and in
cortical space.

To summarize, these are the principal concepts developed in this
chapter:

1. Memories are formed in cortical networks by associative principles and mechanisms.
2. Perceptual memory networks are hierarchically organized in
   posterior cortex of association.
3. Executive memory networks are hierarchically organized in
   frontal cortex.
4. The retrieval of a memory consists in the associative reactivation
   of its network, that is, the increased excitability and firing of its
   neurons.
5. Organized behavior results from the joint activation of perceptual and executive memory networks.

Throughout this chapter, in consonance with these ideas, I have repeatedly referred to the heterarchy of memory networks, in other words, to the heterogeneity of the hierarchical rank of their component cognits. I will conclude the chapter with a few remarks on the retrieval of the most heterarchical of all memories, namely, the episodic autobiographical memories. In addition to its heterarchical nature, the memory of an episode in one's life has the essential associative features of *temporality*. The temporality of episodic memory has two aspects. One is the time frame in which the remembered episode occurred, that is, its associations with chronological age, clock, and calendar. The other is the temporal order of the events that constituted the episode. We do not know the neural basis of either time or temporal order, that is, of the cognits that encode them. However, a faith-

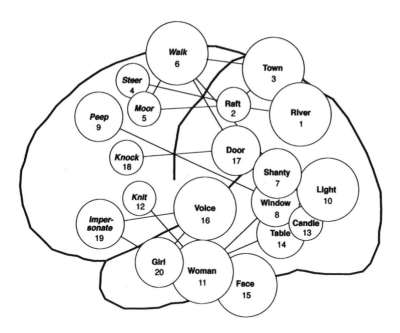

Figure 5.6. Hypothetical connectionist map of the memory network of the episode remembered by Huckleberry Finn, as recounted by Mark Twain (p. 122). The circles represent 20 nodes of the cognits that constitute the network. Other than by separating verbs (frontal) from nouns (posterior), cortical localization is not attempted. The nodes' relative size is roughly proportional to their assumed importance in Huck's life and/or the episode recounted. Numbers represent the approximate order of their activation in the recall.

ful recall of the episode preserves temporal associations. It is reasonable to suppose, therefore, that in the act of recalling the episode, its
component cognits are activated in the order in which they occurred
in the formation of the network that encoded the episode as it was experienced. Thus, we can tentatively estimate the cognitive components of the vast memory network that represents an episodic memory and the order of the activation of its components in the recall of
the episode (Fig. 5.6).

In conclusion, because of the absence of sharp boundaries between cognits and between memory networks, we might construe the
entire cerebral cortex as an all-encompassing web to accommodate
any cognitive memory of any kind. The empirical evidence discussed
in this chapter indicates that, within such a global cortical web, there
can be exquisite specificity of representation. This specificity derives
from two basic assumptions: (*1*) any neuron population within the
web can be connected, directly or indirectly, with practically any other
and (*2*) the strength of connectivity between them can vary greatly in
terms of number of fiber connections and in terms of synaptic bond.
Thus, from the enormous richness of anatomical relations between
cortical neurons and the wide range of the strength of those relations
derive the immense capacity and specificity of human memory. With
the retrieval of memory, whether in free recall, in recognition, or in
the pursuit of a behavioral goal, cortical activation would spread from
one part of that global web to another as a wave of association in a
giant connectionist network.

6

Attention

*I*t is the taking possession by the mind, in clear and vivid form, of one out of what seem several simultaneously possible objects or trains of thought. Focalization, concentration, of consciousness are of its essence. It implies withdrawal from some things in order to deal effectively with others. With these now famous words, William James (1890), the dean of American psychology, defined attention at the end of the nineteenth century. For a long time thereafter, however, the prevalent schools of psychology, behaviorism in particular, considered attention an irrelevant or intractable subject. It was not until the 1950s, with the advent of information theory, that attention reemerged as a worthy subject of experimental psychology and, eventually, of cognitive science. Still, James' definition of attention, with its critical attributes of focus, selectivity, and exclusiveness, remains valid to this day. The only unnecessary attribute in it is consciousness, for the processing of information under attentional control need not be conscious. The hallmark of attention is the allocation of neural resources to that processing. At lower levels of the nerve axis, the resources consist of specialized neuronal assemblies and the pathways between them. In the cerebral cortex, however, the resources expand enormously, as they become a massive array of overlapping and intersecting networks, where specificity is defined by multiple alternate relationships between neurons. Since those relationships are potentially infinite, selective attention becomes crucial in cortical processing. Here, resource allocation is the orderly activation of certain networks in the midst of a myriad. The role of attention is to select one of those networks at a time and to keep it active for as long as it serves a cognitive function or the attainment of a behavioral goal. This chapter deals with the neural mechanisms by which this is accomplished.

Biological Roots of Attention

In lower animals, the adaptation of the organism to its environment is based on a continuous flow of information from sense organs to motor effectors and back through the environment to sense organs. Action is essentially reaction, processed by specialized receptors at one end and specialized effectors at the other. The sea anemone lives by reaction, without internal feedback control from effector organs upon receptors or upon any processing stage in between. All feedback is external. Such a simple cycle (Fig. 6.1A) is the evolutionary precursor of the processing depicted by clockwise-oriented arrows in the perception-action cycle of Figure 4.7 (Chapter 4). In higher animals, internal control emerges in the form of neural feedback from action organs upon sensory organs (Fig. 6.1B). Thus, in these animals, motor organs provide regulatory signals to sensory organs that will set the latter for improved receptivity and analysis of the world's impressions; thereby better, more adaptive, reactions will ensue. Those regulatory signals are a kind of *corollary discharge* upon sensors or upon sensory processing stages, ostensibly with the function of refining adaptation. This form of internal feedback in higher species is represented by counterclockwise connections in our picture of the perception-action cycle (Fig. 4.7).

Internal feedback has enormous biological implications. Consider the interactions between eye movement and retinal input. An unexpected stimulus of possible behavioral significance appears in the periphery of the visual field. The retinal image of the stimulus will cause an orienting movement of the eyes toward it. This will have the effect of foveating the stimulus, that is, bringing it to the center of the retina, where receptors are more tightly packed and the stimulus can be best analyzed. The more refined image will activate, by association, posterior cortical cognits in inferior temporal cortex, where the stim-

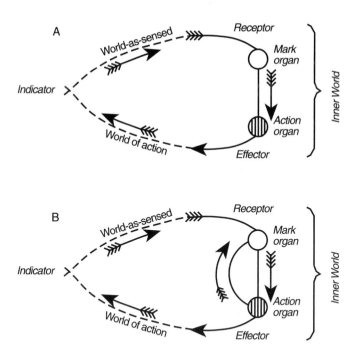

Figure 6.1. The flow of processing between the organism and its environment, according to Uexküll (1926). *A:* Primitive organism: reaction to external stimuli without internal feedback between the action organ and the receptor organ. *B:* Higher organism: the receptor organ is modulated by internal neural feedback from the action organ.

ulus will be further scrutinized for behavioral significance in the context of past experience. At the same time, the spatial characteristics of the stimulus will be analyzed in posterior parietal cortex. Outputs from both cortices will reach executive networks of the frontal lobe, including the prefrontal eye fields, which in turn will generate top-down controlling signals upon lower levels of the visual processing hierarchy. These include regions of the temporal and parietal lobes, the basal ganglia, the thalamus, the amygdala, the superior colliculus, the cerebellum, and the mesencephalon. This extensive frontal feedback will have the effect of enhancing the analysis of the stimulus at all levels and from all relevant perspectives, including its history.

The essence of attention is the *selective allocation* of as many neural resources as are available and necessary to the analysis of a discrete stimulus of biological relevance. The attentional control allocating

those resources need not come from the very top. Under ordinary circumstances, to treat ordinary stimuli, rapid and automatic control
may come from lower structures, without involvement of the executive networks of the frontal lobe. In any case, attention per se does not
generate new sensory inputs. It does, however, set and modulate receptors as well as the neural analyzers behind them, whereby present
inputs can be better analyzed and subsequent ones brought in for
analysis.

Feedback control is accompanied by feedforward control, the
latter as much an essential component of attentional mechanisms as
the former. Whereas feedback modulates sensory processing stages,
feedforward modulates proactively motor processing stages, priming
the motor systems for more efficient action. Consider again the frontal
cortex in the adaptive cycle after reception of a visual stimulus that
engages the attention of the animal. While feedback signals from the
frontal cortex reenter sensory cortices for enhancement of sensory
analysis, the frontal cortex also feeds signals forward to lower motor
stages to prepare motor systems for anticipated motor action. Some
such signals fall upon nuclei of oculomotor integration for better
control of eye movements. Others fall upon skeletal motor systems, to
prepare them for locomotor action if the visual stimulus calls for it.
In either case, feedforward to motor systems serves what later in this
chapter will be characterized as motor attention or preparatory set.

The sensory and motor mechanisms that attentional control facilitates have both excitatory and inhibitory components. Both operate at all levels of the central nervous system. One universal role of
inhibition is to enhance the role of excitation. In some structures, the
effects of excitation cannot take place without the inhibition of other
structures. Figure 6.2 illustrates examples of the function of inhibition in sensory and motor systems. In panel A, the figure shows the
reaction of a neuron in the lateral geniculate body—the thalamic
relay nucleus for visual information—to discrete light stimuli falling
in its receptive field. Light in the center of the receptive field induces
in the cell a brisk discharge of action potentials. Conversely, an an-
nulus of light in the periphery of the field induces an inhibition of
firing—and a brisk off-reaction. In the diffuse illumination of the entire field, the two effects on the cell, excitatory and inhibitory, antag-
onize and cancel each other. The important points here are that the
cell's reaction to illumination of the center of the field benefits from
absence of light in the periphery and, further, light in the periphery

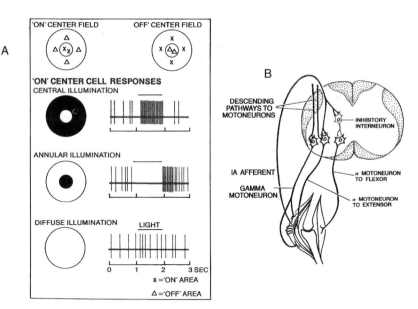

Figure 6.2. Reciprocal interplay of excitation and inhibition in sensory and motor systems. *A:* Reactions of a cell in the lateral geniculate body to light in different parts of its receptive field: the cell is excited by central illumination and inhibited by peripheral (annular) illumination; thus, the illumination of either the center or the periphery inhibits input from the other, enhancing contrast. *B:* Reciprocal spinal innervation of flexor and extensor muscles facilitating extension of the knee. From Kuffler and Nicolls (1976), slightly modified, with permission.

inhibits the cell. The end result of the opposite effects of central and peripheral illumination of receptive fields is to enhance the spatial and temporal contrast of geniculate cell responses to discrete stimuli in the center of their receptive field.

Sensory contrast is thus achieved by mechanisms that are reminiscent of those that Sherrington described in motor systems. One such mechanism is reciprocal innervation, shown on panel B of Figure 6.2. It illustrates the reciprocal innervation of the extensor and flexor muscles of the knee. Two motoneurons of the spinal cord innervate respectively two muscles, one flexor and the other extensor. When the extensor muscle is contracted, its muscle spindles send afferent sensory signals that maintain contraction—despite the shortening of the muscle—by exciting the extensor motorneuron (stretch reflex). At the same time, those same afferent signals inhibit the flexor motorneuron through an inhibitory interneuron. In this manner, by their reciprocal innervation, the two antagonistic muscles cooperate for effective extension of the knee.

It is from that *cooperative duality of excitation and inhibition* in sensory and motor systems that the two basic operations of attention seem to emerge. The two are (*1*) enhancing the processing within a discrete sector of sensorium, motility, or cognition and (*2*) reducing or suppressing the competing others. In the cerebral cortex, because of the massive interconnectivity and overlap of cognitive networks, those two operations become critical; they have to be highly selective, as the alternative neuronal paths and the networks they define become practically infinite. In any case, at a given time, attentional control in the cortex implies the selection and enhanced activation of one network, while other networks, which may or may not share with it common neuronal elements, are suppressed. At cortical levels, the two basic operations of attention, enhancement and suppression, support mechanisms of reciprocal innervation that are similar to those present in lower levels of the nervous system. In the cortex, however, attentional control is generated and sustained in the cortex itself by the intervention of hierarchically higher networks.

The foregoing discussion has led us, from a biological perspective, to the two fundamental processes of attention or resource allocation. The first is the selectively inclusive process commonly understood as the focus of attention. It is usually defined, in phenomenological terms, as the awareness of a limited sector of sensorium or of sensory perception at a given moment. This narrow concept of the focus of attention constitutes basically what cognitive psychology considers *selective attention* (with obvious redundancy, for all attention is selective). The concept practically ignores the existence of motor attention, that is, the selective allocation of motor structures and mechanisms to the execution of orderly goal-directed behavior, much of which takes place outside of conscious awareness. The second attentional process is exclusionary, consisting of the suppression of sensory or motor contents—cognits in the cortex—that interfere or are incompatible with the contents that are in focus at the time. This process is the essence of the control of distractions. Such control complements the inclusive process of focusing attention.

In any case, attention is inherent in the neural processing of sensory and motor information for adaptive purposes (Neisser, 1976). Nowhere in the central nervous system is there evidence of a separate structure or group of structures dedicated to attention as a separate function. Nor is one needed from a biological point of view. Attention, with its qualities of selectivity of resources and biased competition (Desimone and Duncan, 1995), is identical to specificity in sensory and motor systems. In the cortical stages of these systems, attention is the process of timely and selective activation of cognits to attend to the ever-changing cognitive demands of adaptation to the environment.

Perceptual Attention

To interact adaptively and selectively with the environment, the cerebral cortex requires the functional integrity of subcortical sensory and motor systems. In addition, it requires the continuous inflow of nonspecific activating influences from several structures of the brain stem. This kind of activation is the neural basis of arousal and of the state of vigilance; a base minimum of it is indispensable for attention to any sector of the environment. Nonspecific cortex-activating inputs originate in a series of brain stem nuclei that are the source of major excitatory neurotransmitter systems, cholinergic and monoaminergic. They innervate the neocortex diffusely, although each terminates predominantly in certain cortical layers.

Arousal and vigilance depend in large measure on the activation of the neocortex by those diffuse projecting systems of the brain stem, especially the *reticular formation* of the mesencephalon, which generates mainly cholinergic influences. In arousal from sleep to wakefulness, that activation increases more or less abruptly; in the maintenance of vigilance and general alertness, the activation is tonic and sustained. That tonic activation of the neocortex by subcortical projection systems is a necessary condition for the selective cortical processing of sensory and motor information. There is evidence that the degree of activation of the cortex by structures controlling arousal and wakefulness bears on the efficiency of attention mechanisms in perception as well as action. For example, in the monkey, the mild electrical stimulation of the mesencephalic reticular formation facilitates the discrimination of tachistoscopically presented visual stimuli and the motor responses to them (Fuster, 1958).

Attention-enhancing influences also come to the neocortex from the *limbic system*. Some of these influences are mediated by the anterior nuclei of the thalamus and the entorhinal and cingulate cortices.

In this manner, inputs from structures encoding mood and affect, such as the hypothalamus and the amygdala, probably modulate the effectiveness of neocortical dynamics in the selective processing of sensory stimuli and motor acts. In that processing, limbic structures would interact with both sensory and motor areas of the cortex, and thus with perceptual and executive cognits. We know that, after a degree of processing through sensory association cortex, sensory stimuli gain access to limbic structures, especially the amygdala and the hippocampus (Chapters 2 and 3). There the stimuli presumably undergo analysis of their motivational and emotional connotations, and the output of that analysis feeds back into the perceptual cortex, reinforcing or gating the response to further sensory stimulation.

In sum, by mechanisms that are still poorly understood, limbic and diffusely projecting subcortical structures serve attention by modulating sensory systems. The control of attention itself, however, that is, the selective enhancement or inhibition of component structures of sensory systems in the attentive processes, takes place within those systems themselves. In selective processing, the highest cortical levels (that is, cortices of association) control one another. To reiterate a point made earlier, the cortical networks dedicated to perceptual attention are the same networks that are dedicated to the processing of sensory information. Thus, for example, the so-called top-down control of attention can be understood as the selective modulation that higher cortical networks exert upon lower ones in the processing of structured behavior or cognition. There is no need to attribute to those higher networks a special or exclusive role in attention. Both high and low cognits are selectively and jointly involved in attentional processing.

At any level of the cortical processing hierarchy for perception, the attentional selectivity of information processing is subject to control both from below and from above, one usually predominating at a given time over the other. From below, the cortical networks of sensory and associative cortices are subject to the structure of sensory stimulation in its spatial-temporal context. The saliency and novelty of stimuli determine the extent to which they are to be selected against competition. Salient or novel stimuli are more likely to be detected and selected by automatic bottom-up processing than are stimuli embedded in a clutter or in a monotonous sequence. In vision, this is epitomized by phenomena such as *pop-out* (Treisman and Gelade, 1980), a typical manifestation of control from the bottom. This kind of bottom-up control of attention is what has been characterized as *preattentive* processing (Julesz, 1984), which is executed speedily and in parallel. Most of it takes place in primary sensory and parasensory cortices (in vision, V1–V4 and interotemporal and posterior parietal cortices). It is reasonable to assume that the perception of salient stimuli is in large part the result of the local mechanisms of specific excitation of certain neural networks and the inhibition of others, the functional tandem of excitation and inhibition that prevails throughout sensory systems.

Some of that preattentive and parallel processing, however, while still mostly controlled bottom-up, is also subject to varying degrees of *top-down control*. In Chapter 4, I emphasized the automatic aspects of perception. I noted that perception consists largely of a continuous, parallel, and automatic matching of sensory inputs to internal cognits. This matching is the basis of Grossberg's (1999) *adaptive resonance theory* (ART). According to it, inputs from external receptors gain fast access to *lists of categories,* where they are filtered and where they find their match or *resonance* in preestablished networks. The result of that matching is the generation of feedback in the form of top-down expectation, or set, for further match and continued—now serial—analysis. Thus, rapid parallel processing (bottom-up) leads to match and recognition, which lead to top-down feedback, which leads to focusing and further analysis. In this interplay of bottom-up and top-down controls that characterizes the attentive processes in cortical networks, the reader undoubtedly recognizes again the circular operation of the perception-action cycle. For in cortex, attention is essentially no different than it is elsewhere: it is the optimization of adaptive processes to accommodate new experience on a base of old experience.

The role of experience and top-down control on attentional neuronal processes has been exposed in the *inferotemporal cortex,* which is associative cortex dedicated to the analysis of visual information. There it has been observed that the attention that a monkey directs to the location or quality of a visual stimulus results in the enhancement of the reactions of neurons to that stimulus. Attention to a spot of light within the receptive field of an inferotemporal cell will enhance the response of the cell to that spot while suppressing the response to other, unattended, spots in the field (Moran and Desimone, 1985). Thus, both aspects of attention, inclusion and exclusion, seem to take place within the receptive field of the same neuron. The effect of at-

tention focused on sensory quality can be observed in inferotemporal
cells when the animal has to attend selectively to different features of
a complex visual stimulus (Fuster, 1990). Monkeys trained to attend
to either the color or the pattern of such stimuli reveal the presence
of units that respond more to one or the other feature if the animal
must attend to it to perform a task correctly (Fig. 6.3). If the animal
must first notice a pattern to decide whether color is relevant, then
the cells that select color show strong and differential long-latency
(150–500 ms) responses to colors. The long latency of the attention-
dependent responses of inferotemporal cells—also in Chelazzi et al.
(1993) (Fig. 6.4)—indicates that the inferotemporal cortex is subject
not only to bottom-up sensory inputs, but also to top-down control
dependent on the focus of attention. In other words, inferotemporal
cells are subject not so much to preattentive influences from the environment as to the attention control from higher cortical levels. In
sensory cortical areas, therefore, it seems that bottom-up influences
operate largely in parallel and with short latency, whereas top-down
control operates in series, with longer latencies after stimulus appearance.

In the human, as in the monkey, attention focused on the location or quality of a stimulus enhances the electrical response to the
stimulus in posterior cortex; this has been well established by scalp-
recording of evoked potentials (Näätänen, 1992; Luck and Hillyard,
2000). Also as in the monkey, the top-down effects of attention take
place on the long-latency components of the evoked response potentials. A clear implication of these phenomena is that attention facilitates the activation of perceptual cognits in posterior cortex. The
source of that facilitating modulation can be reasonably assumed to
reside in higher cortex, that is, in the cognitive networks of long-term
memory established by experience, which contain associations with
the stimulus.

It appears, therefore, that top-down attentional control is essentially made up of feedback from higher cognits upon lower ones. In
the attentional processing of perception, cortical networks do a kind
of continuous "turning upon themselves" and upon lower networks
to better analyze the surrounding world. No specialized controlling
structures are needed for that processing, because the processing networks control themselves. Thus, in the processing of perceptually
guided executive sequences, the prefrontal cortex, which harbors the
highest networks for the representation and execution of novel and
complex actions, is apparently the source of the modulating influ-

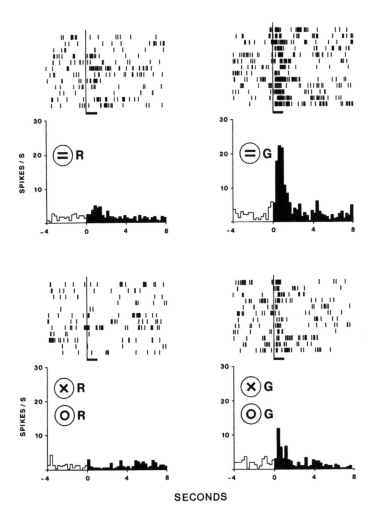

Figure 6.3. Reactions of an inferotemporal cell to a visual stimulus (a pattern inside a round colored disk) in a delayed matching task. The task requires that the animal pay attention to, and retain, the color if the pattern is =, and the pattern itself if this is X or O. The cell reacts more to green (G) than to red (R), especially when green is relevant (=) and must be attended to and remembered. From Fuster (1990), with permission.

ences upon lower-level networks of frontal and posterior associative cortices engaged in those sequences. Let us briefly review some of the supporting evidence.

In principle, because the attentional facilitation of electrical responses to a stimulus in a behavioral task is best observed when the subject must focus on the stimulus for correct performance of the

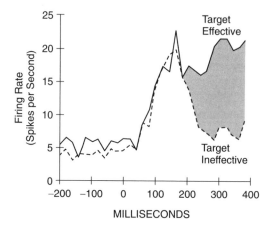

Figure 6.4. Responses of inferotemporal cells of the monkey to visual stimuli in the focus of attention. Some cells (*continuous line*) show elevated long-latency firing after the stimulus; others (*broken line*) do not or are suppressed. From Chelazzi et al., (1993), modified, with permission.

task, we can infer that the facilitation results from executive frontal feedback. Clinical and experimental data point to the prefrontal cortex as the origin of such feedback. Patients with large lesions of lateral prefrontal cortex have considerable difficulty in attending to environmental changes or in shifting attentive set from one aspect of the sensory environment to another. Some patients manifest complete neglect of events in large sectors of the environment. Concomitantly with these difficulties, the patient with a frontal lesion shows a diminution of the normal attentional capacity to modulate sensory evoked responses in perceptual cortex (Knight, 1984; Daffner et al., 2000).

Imaging further supports the functional interaction between prefrontal and posterior cortices in perceptual attention. Humans performing visual attention tasks, for example, exhibit concomitant activation of prefrontal and inferotemporal cortices (Kastner et al., 1999). In the monkey performing a visual attention task, it has been possible to demonstrate—with the aid of selective cuts of the corpus callosum—the prefrontal modulation of inferotemporal cells in the recognition of visual stimuli (Hasegawa et al., 1998; Tomita et al., 1999).

In conclusion, perceptual attention is the selective processing of sensory stimuli as a function of their physical context and prior history. That selectivity takes place at all stages of sensory processing and is enhanced by neural influences that run in two directions along the sensory processing hierarchy: bottom-up and top-down. The bottom-up control of attention derives largely from the physical properties of the stimuli and the physiological properties of sensory systems. The top-down control is the modulation exerted by higher cortices upon the responses of perceptual cognitive networks to sensory stimuli. In the execution of perceptually guided tasks, that control comes from prefrontal cortex.

Working Memory

Working memory is attention focused on the internal representation of a recent event for a pending action. The term *working memory* originated in cognitive psychology, where it referred to the temporary memory of sensory stimuli utilized by humans in the process of solving problems and executing cognitive operations (Atkinson and Shiffrin, 1968; Baddeley, 1986). It applied to information held in the mind as needed for prospective action. Baddeley (1986) incorporated the concept of working memory into an elaborate theoretical construct of executive functions that included certain specific linguistic operations that he and his colleagues considered essential to that form of memory—for example, the *articulatory loop*.

In behavioral neurophysiology, the concept of working memory has been given a more general meaning, deprived of linguistic constraints and extended to the nonhuman primate. It still retains its character of short-term memory, but this is well differentiated from the concept of new memory in the consolidation process, that is, from the conventional view of short-term memory as the gate to long-term memory. Working memory is, rather, *active memory* for the short term (Chapter 5). The distinctive properties of working memory are not those of a new memory in formation, but rather those of a cognit, new or old, which is held active in the focus of attention as required in the processing of information for prospective action. The content of working memory essentially consists of long-term memory that has been activated for the processing of actions. That content may include new items, which by virtue of association, perceptual constancy, and categorization (Chapters 4 and 5), can be readily incorporated into an activated, and attended-to, old network for the processing of new action. Again, also in the form of working memory, attention is inseparable from selective neural processing.

Working memory is the first cognitive function to have been substantiated at the neuronal level. In prefrontal cortex of monkeys performing a delayed-response task, cells were found that maintained an elevated level of discharge during the delay or *memory period* of the task, while the animal had to retain a sensory stimulus for prospective use (Fuster and Alexander, 1971). Such cells were subsequently called *memory cells.* Their discharge during the delay period was higher than in periods between trials, when the animal did not have to retain any particular item of information in short-term memory (Fig. 6.5). Those intertrial baseline periods were essential to the method for demonstrating the phenomenon, because they allowed the comparison of firing frequencies between memory and nonmemory states. The delay-period activation of memory cells had several important characteristics (Fuster, 1973): (*1*) it was strictly dependent on the need to perform an act contingent on the signal in memory; (*2*) it was not induced by the mere expectancy of reward; (*3*) it was correlated with the monkey's ability to remember the signal; and (*4*) it could be obliterated by distraction. These characteristics made memory cells the likely constituents of frontal networks engaged in the process of attending to a memorandum for consequent and subsequent action.

Indeed, the prefrontal cells active in working memory appear to reflect the sustained attention to a sensory stimulus after it has disappeared from the animal's environment. Their persistent discharge is selective, related to the efficacy of stimulus retention and vulnerable to distraction. It is reasonable to infer that the network to which they belong represents the cognit of the stimulus, that is, a network that represents the associated properties of that stimulus in the context in which the animal makes use of it. On a given trial, maximum activation may take place in the part of the network that encodes the stimulus properties that change from trial to trial and that are the focus of attention in the memory period of that particular trial. Thus, prefrontal memory cells have been found for stimulus position (Fuster et al., 1982; Funahashi et al., 1989), color (Fuster et al., 1982; Quintana et al., 1988), acoustic tone (Bodner et al., 1996), and tactual features (Romo et al., 1999). It is also reasonable, however, that many delay-activated cells, while not in the focus of attention, are in parts of the activated network that encode associated stimulus properties that are constant for all trials and that categorize the stimulus at a somewhat higher, more general, level.

With her colleagues, Goldman-Rakic (the first neurobiologist to characterize memory cells as the neural substrate of Baddeley's working memory) contributed decisively to our understanding of the to-

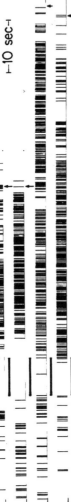

Figure 6.5. Discharge of a prefrontal cell in the course of five delay-response trials. During the delay (30 sec in the upper three trials, 60 sec in the lower two), the monkey must remember the cue for the correct response (at the *arrow*). From Fuster and Alexander (1971), with permission.

pography of working memory in the prefrontal cortex of the monkey (Goldman-Rakic, 1987, 1995). Her group made two especially significant findings in animals performing visual delayed-response tasks. The first was the presence, in lateral prefrontal cortex, of memory cells exquisitely attuned to the position of light spots in the two-dimensional visual field. The second was the functional dissociation of two subareas of that cortex seemingly specialized in working memory of two different categories of visual memoranda. Neurons for working memory of spatially defined stimuli predominate in the dorsal aspect of lateral prefrontal cortex, whereas neurons engaged in the memory of objects predominate in the ventral aspect of this cortex. Those two prefrontal fields are known to hold reciprocal connections with posterior cortical fields specialized in the processing of spatial and object-visual information (Chapter 3). In the anatomical evidence of the corticocortical connectivity of the lateral prefrontal cortex, to which she and her collaborators contributed (Schwartz and Goldman-Rakic, 1984; Cavada and Goldman-Rakic, 1989a,b), Goldman-Rakic (1988) recognized indications of the distributed, network-like nature of working memory.

Physiological data substantiate that notion. The wide distribution of the cognits activated in the state of attention that we identify with working memory is clearly evinced physiologically by the presence of memory cells in regions outside of the prefrontal cortex, notably in posterior association areas. Visual memory cells have been found in the inferior temporal cortex (Fuster and Jervey, 1981; Miller et al., 1993), spatial memory cells in posterior parietal cortex (Andersen et al., 1990), and tactile memory cells in somatosensory cortex (Zhou and Fuster, 1996). Thus, in the execution of a memory task, it appears that a large network of cortical neurons is activated. The executive aspects of the task activate assemblies in frontal cortex, whereas its perceptual aspects activate neuron assemblies in assorted areas of posterior cortex, depending on the modality of the sensory components of the task's sequence. In the course of that sequence, the maximum of the network's activation probably shifts from one region of the cortex to another in accord with the task's immediate demands—that is, with the focus of attention.

Imaging studies in the human also provide evidence of prefrontal activation in working memory and of the wide cortical distribution of working memory networks. The lateral prefrontal cortex has been shown to be activated during working memory of visual

stimuli (Jonides et al., 1993; Swartz et al., 1995) and verbal stimuli
(Grasby et al., 1993; Petrides et al., 1993b). Some of these activations
extend to areas of sensory association cortex in the parietal and temporal lobes. Tasks that call for high levels of attention, whether they
require working memory or not, are shown to activate areas of anterior cingulate and lateral prefrontal cortex in addition to parietal or
temporal areas (Posner and Petersen, 1990; Corbetta et al., 1993;
Kastner et al., 1999).

When a task demands the retention of a piece of sensory information in working memory, the activation maximum—focus of attention—must remain in the network's components that represent
that information for as long as needed. Because the information is
held for the bridging of a cross-temporal contingency of action, neurons of a lateral prefrontal net remain active. At the same time, because the information is of a sensory nature and is part of perceptual
memory, neurons of a posterior cortical net also remain active. Based
on these assumptions, two inferences may be drawn: (1) working
memory consists essentially of the joint activation of the neural components of a large cognitive network of perceptual and executive
memory, and (2) the selective attention on the memorandum in
working memory consists essentially of the sustained and selective activation of that network. There is experimental support for those two
inferences and for a mechanism of sustained network activation in
working memory—that is, sustained network activation during the
focusing of attention on the cognit held in working memory. The support comes from two sources: evidence of functional interactions between cortical areas in working memory and computational evidence
of reverberation of excitation in active neuronal networks during
working memory.

Monkeys were trained to perform a delayed matching task for
color (Fuster et al., 1985): (1) presentation of a sample color; (2) delay or memory period; (3) simultaneous presentation of two or more
colors; and (4) choice (rewarded) of the sample color. Thus, the experimental animal had to retain the sample color in working memory
for the duration of the delay or memory period—10 to 20 seconds
long. The animals had implanted devices that allowed the cooling of,
or cell recording from, lateral prefrontal and inferotemporal cortices.
As they performed the task, one of the two cortices was cooled to 20°C,
while units were recorded with a microelectrode from the other. The
bilateral cooling of either cortex induced a deficit in the performance

of the task, to wit, a sharp deficit in the number of correct responses; this occurred without any overt sensory or motor deficit and without any performance deficit in the task without delay. Such observations indicated that the functional depression of neuronal activity in either prefrontal or inferotemporal cortex induced a reversible deficit in the animal's ability to retain information (color) in working memory. In other words, the cooling appeared to depress critical components of the cortical network or cognit of the memorandum, which in this case was a color in the executive context of a memory task. The inferotemporal deficit could be understood as the result of depression of the perceptual component, which included the representation of the color and the other sensory attributes of the memorandum. The prefrontal deficit, on the other hand, could be attributed to the depression of the executive components of the network.

While one cortex—prefrontal or inferotemporal—was being cooled, and the animal's performance dropped, cells in the other cortex were affected in several ways. Many showed increases or decreases in their reaction to the sample color, either while this was present in front of the animal or during the delay, when it had disappeared from view and had to be retained for the choice. The most characteristic finding was that of some cells that, under remote cortical cooling, showed a diminution in their capacity to distinguish the colors in memory—judging from their firing frequency during the delays. It appeared that their working-memory role had deteriorated. In cells that could be recorded long enough to test them after rewarming the remote cortex, that degradation of discriminant cell function was shown to be reversible, as was that of the monkey's behavioral performance. In sum, surface cortical cooling seemed to hamper the activation of the underlying portion of the network supporting visual working memory and, at the same time, the ability of neurons in other portions of the network to discriminate visual memoranda. A reasonable conclusion is that prefrontal and inferotemporal neurons are part of the same network, which represents the cognit of the task with its perceptual and executive components. In visual working memory, they are jointly activated in *reverberating excitation* through reentrant circuits. The cooling of either cortex interrupts those circuits and prevents the network from adequately maintaining the memorandum in the focus of attention and working memory.

Computational methodologies also provide evidence that the reentry of excitation within cortical networks is the primary mechanism of working memory. In collaboration with David Zipser (Zipser et al., 1993), we developed a computer network whose connective architecture was characterized by layers of processing units, between input and output, and full recurrence between layers. We then trained the network to perform the sample-and-hold operation of a monkey performing a working-memory task. On completion of training, while the network performed its operation, units were observed within it (*hidden units* in intermediate layers) with patterns of activity extraordinarily similar to those of memory cells in the real brain (Fig. 6.6). A legitimate inference from those observations is that working memory is basically sustained by reentrant or reverberating activity within recurrent networks, as suggested by the cooling-microelectrode experiments outlined above.

Electrical *oscillation* is one of the features of recurrent activity in neural networks. Cortical HF oscillations (20–60 Hz) have been described in visual perception (Chapter 4) and states of heightened attention (Llinás and Ribary, 1993). They have been interpreted as evidence for the binding of features, in neural networks, that are essential to perception (Singer and Gray, 1995). Thus, HF in working memory would be an indication of the binding of the associated features of the cognit in the focus of internal representation. A recent study of somatosensory cells in a tactile memory task (Bodner et al., unpublished) indicates, however, that HF oscillations are the exception rather than the rule. The analysis of patterns of spike discharge shows that, during the memorization of a tactile stimulus, cells tend to drift between periodic patterns of firing, or *attractors*. Because of the variability in the frequency of those attractors and their shifts, HF oscillations—as revealed by autocorrelograms—tend to decrease rather than increase. The washout of oscillations in working memory is the result of a proliferation of fixed attractor frequencies. We are led to the conclusion that, in that state, the shifts between attractors reflect the shifts of the focus of attention between different aspects of the cognit of the memorandum. In other words, it would appear that in working memory that focus shifts from one part of the network to another, each representing a different feature of the cognit and characterized by a different attractor frequency. That frequency might reflect the reentry of excitation between the neuronal elements that encode that particular feature in the cortical network.

Reentry of excitation within an active memory network may be local or may span widely separated sectors of the network, and thus

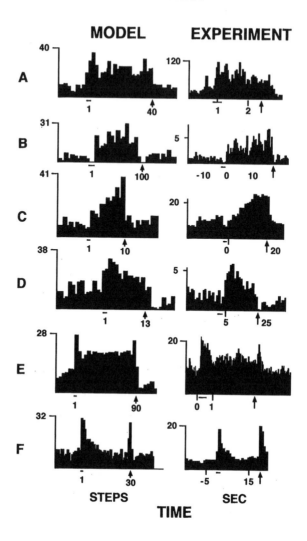

Figure 6.6. Comparison between the activity of selected units in a recurrent computational model of working memory and the activity of real cells experimentally encountered in studies of working memory in the monkey. From Zipser et al. (1993), with permission.

widely separated areas of the neocortex. The cooling and imaging studies mentioned above suggest that the loops of reentrant excitation tie together different areas of posterior and frontal cortices, depending on the nature of the information that constitutes the active network or cognit. Inasmuch as the information is needed for execution of prospective action, executive components of the network are activated in frontal cortex. Inasmuch as the information is perceptual, network components are activated at the same time in posterior cortex. Figure 6.7 illustrates areas presumed activated, and tied by reentry, in the memory period (delay) of four working memory tasks. Reentry through prefrontal cortex is present in all, insofar as they require the executive mediation of cross-temporal contingencies. Reentry through perceptual cortex is also present insofar as that mediation requires the sustained attention on a recent percept. But note that reentry obviates the need for any cortical or subcortical structure extrinsic to the network for attentional control. The network is selectively recruited and activated by itself, bottom-up and top-down, through the associative paths that constitute it and that were formed when it became long-term memory. Attention is part of the processing that takes place with the ad hoc activation of that network and is not the result of control from an attention-dedicated structure outside of the network.

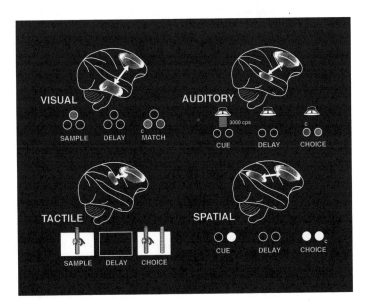

Figure 6.7. Cortical interactions in the brain of the monkey during working memory. Reentrant connections link the prefrontal cortex with a different area of posterior cortex, depending on the sensory modality of the active cognit: inferotemporal if visual, superior temporal if auditory, anterior parietal if tactile, and posterior parietal if spatial (c, correct response).

Working memory, as any form of attention, involves not only the selective activation of certain cortical networks, but also the concomitant *inhibition* of other networks. We can only speculate on how that exclusionary aspect of attention is implemented. Based on our introductory reasoning with regard to the basic neurobiology of attention, lateral inhibition probably plays an important role in that exclusionary operation. Its effect would be to attenuate or suppress activity in cognitive networks that can interfere in some way with the cognit in focus. In working memory we have observed inhibition or deactivation in and around activated areas, both in monkeys with microelectrodes (Fuster and Jervey, 1982) and humans by tomographic imaging (Swartz et al.. 1995). It is not unreasonable that such effects are induced by lateral inhibition originating in the active networks on focus at the time.

In conclusion, working memory is attention focused on the internal representation of a cognit recently activated for executive function. The activated cognit consists mainly of long- term memory in a widely distributed network of associative cortex. During working memory, the sustained and selective activation of the network, that is, the sustained and selective attention on the cognit, is the result of continued reentry of excitation within that network. This attentional process, which is based on reentrant excitation, is presumably complemented by the exclusionary inhibition of networks that are extraneous to the cognit temporarily in focus and extraneous to the task at hand.

Executive Attention

The processing of actions requires the selective allocation of neural resources, much like the processing of sensory perception. Thus, in the cognitive sphere, there is executive attention just as there is perceptual attention. Yet, in cognitive neuroscience, executive attention and its neural correlates have been largely neglected or inadequately treated. To be sure, neuropsychology has dealt with the issue for a long time using a variety of terms and concepts, mainly in the context of frontal-lobe function. Nonetheless, the neuroscientific study of attention that is directed to and focused on movement, and more generally action, has suffered from the pervasive tendency of cognitive scientists to reserve the term and concept of *attention* for sensory systems and processes. Most people, in general, associate attention with the choice between sensory alternatives, not with the choice between motor alternatives. This bias obviously parallels a comparable bias in the study of executive memory, as we saw in the previous chapter. The neglect of executive attention is most curious, as sensory attention depends to a large extent on the allocation of very important motor resources, namely, the neural apparatus for the motility that controls the direction of gaze and the orientation of the head.

As with perceptual attention, there is no conceptual or empirical reason to construe a special neural system, structure, or group of structures dedicated to executive attention. Executive attention, like perceptual attention, has its roots in the elementary biology of the adaptation of the organism to its environment. It is inherent in the processing of adaptive action at any level of the central nervous system. It is the neural extension, on a large scale, of the effector mechanisms of homeostasis that operate at the most elementary physiological levels of the organism. In the cerebral cortex, which incorporates the highest and most specific executive processing, the selective allocation of executive cognits and effector networks is essential for purposive action. In sum, attention in the executive domain, like attention elsewhere, is generated and guided within processing systems; it is an integral part of their operation. No neural structure, separate from those systems, has been found or appears necessary for the control of executive attention.

From this reasoning, it follows that the prefrontal cortex, which is the highest and most integrative stage in the hierarchy of cortical regions dedicated to action, should constitute the highest level of executive attentional control. There is considerable evidence for this assumption. Such evidence has led many investigators to attribute to the prefrontal cortex the function of *executive control*, which is another term for executive attention. The empirical origin of this concept lies in human neuropsychology. It has long been known that humans with large prefrontal lesions, especially if they affect the lateral convexity of the frontal lobe, suffer from the inability to formulate, initiate, and execute plans of action, especially if they are novel and complex (Luria, 1966; Fuster, 1997). They suffer from what has been characterized as the *dysexecutive syndrome* (Baddeley, 1986). Such a syndrome is directly attributed to the failure of executive control, in other words, the failure of attention to the schema, initiation, and course of sequential action toward a goal. From the same neuropsychological evidence derives the notion of prefrontal cortex as the seat of a *supervisory attentional system* (Norman and Shallice, 1986).

In the context of executive memory (Chapter 5), we discussed the presence of executive networks in the cortex of the frontal lobe that represent the elements, schemas, and plans of action. Those networks, or executive cognits, were hierarchically organized. At the base of the executive cortical hierarchy we found the primary motor cortex (phyletic memory), which represents elementary movements. Above it, in premotor cortex, we found more complex cognits of action defined by goal and trajectory. At the summit of the hierarchy, in prefrontal cortex, we assumed the presence of networks for the representation of sequential actions defined in more abstract terms than at lower levels; in other words, the programs, schemas, plans, and concepts of goal-directed action. We specified that the sequential actions apparently represented in the prefrontal cortex had the attributes of novelty and complexity. We noted that such high-level cognits were derived from and associated with networks of posterior cortex. We also noted that many high-level frontal cognits could be assumed to be heterarchical, their networks spanning several levels of the executive hierarchy.

Executive attention consists in the process of selection of alternatives among those executive networks and their inputs and outputs. In consonance with the views expressed at the beginning of this chapter, it is a self-generated process operating without need for a *central executive* or an agent independent of the action-processing systems themselves. Thus, executive attention is as widely distributed in frontal cortex as are the networks involved in the process of selection of inputs and outputs underlying executive action. If the inputs are simple, and the goal-directed actions associated with them are also simple, the executive cognits selected may be represented in lower or intermediate levels of the frontal executive hierarchy—in premotor cortex, for example. The best available evidence for retrieval and enactment of intermediate-level executive cognits comes from microelectrode recording in the awake and behaving monkey. Rizzolatti and his colleagues (Di Pellegrino et al., 1992) discovered in premotor cortex a category of neurons that they called *mirror units*. Mirror units are activated not only during the execution of an action (e.g., grasping an object or pushing it away), but also during the visual observation of the same action being executed by another subject (e.g., the experimenter). Clearly, in the latter case, the premotor network is activated by inputs from perceptual—that is, visual—networks of posterior, probably inferotemporal, cortex. In my view, mirror neurons epitomize the attentional, selective activation of the cells of an executive network.

If the sensory inputs or actions are complex, ambiguous, or embedded in a cluttered field, then executive attention and the selective processes that underlie it involve networks of higher, prefrontal, cortex. The prefrontal region or regions activated will depend on the aspect or aspects of attention most heavily challenged. In this regard, neuroimaging studies point to three major regions: anterior cingulate cortex, the cortex of the lateral prefrontal convexity, and orbital prefrontal cortex. The cingulate cortex appears activated mostly by tasks that require high motivation or the resolution of conflict, the Stroop task for example (Pardo et al., 1990). This is a task in which the subject is required to name, within time limits, the color of a word printed with a color different from the one signified by the word (e.g., the word *Red* printed in green). Areas of the lateral prefrontal convexity are active mainly in set or gaze shifting and in the necessity to integrate information across time (next section). Because the lesion of cingulate and lateral areas commonly leads to attention deficits (e.g., neglect, set-shifting difficulties), and because they are activated in spatial-attention tasks, those areas have been ascribed to a widely distributed cortical *network for spatial attention* (Mesulam, 1981; Posner and Petersen, 1990). Orbital areas are activated in tasks that require the suppression of interference. This is in line with the assumption, based on lesion studies, that the orbital prefrontal cortex plays a crucial role in inhibitory control or the exclusionary aspect of attention. Remarkably, all three regions are activated in a variety of behavioral paradigms that, to one degree or another, depend on those three aspects of executive attention (Duncan and Owen, 2000).

Set and Expectancy

The overriding function of the lateral prefrontal cortex is the *temporal organization* of behavior (Fuster, 1997) — not of any behavior, however. Routine, instinctual, or well-rehearsed behaviors, however lengthy and complex, can be integrated at lower neural stages. In these behaviors, one act leads to the next in chain-like fashion to form goal-directed sequences of sensory–motor integration mediated at lower levels of the perception-action cycle (e.g., premotor cortex, basal ganglia, hypothalamus, or other subcortical structures). It is only when the behavior requires the mediation of contingencies across time, and the resolution of uncertainties or ambiguities, that the temporal organizing role of the lateral prefrontal cortex becomes essential. This applies to practically all novel and temporally extensive behaviors.

The crucial function of the prefrontal cortex, at the foundation of its temporal organizing role, is *temporal integration*. Temporal integration consists of the structuring of behavior on the basis of information that is temporally discontinuous. The essence of the process, therefore, is the mediation of contingencies between elements of information that are separate in time ("if now this, then later that; if earlier that, then now this"). It is this process of continuous mediation of cross-temporal contingencies that imparts order and timeliness to successive actions in a behavioral sequence toward a goal (Fig. 6.8). The mediation of cross-temporal contingencies is the critical role that the lateral prefrontal cortex performs at the summit of the perception-action cycle. This role is supported by two complementary and temporally symmetrical functions of that cortex: one is working memory, that is, attention to the internal representation of a stimulus; the other is preparatory set, that is, priming of perceptual and motor systems for expected information. In the previous section, we discussed the first, the temporally retrospective function. The subject of this section is the second, the temporally prospective function.

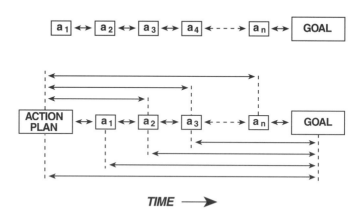

Figure 6.8. Top: A routine and well-rehearsed series of acts ($a_1 \ldots a_n$) toward a goal. Contingencies (*arrows*) are present only between successive acts. *Bottom:* A complex new sequence in which acts are contingent across time on the plan, the goal, and other acts. Prefrontal cortex is essential for the mediation of contingencies across time and, therefore, for the structuring of the sequence.

Preparatory set is executive *attention directed to the future* —much as working memory is a form of attention directed to the past. It is attention focused on expected events and on the anticipated consequences of present events and actions. It is part of the processing of anticipated actions and inseparable from it. This *set* function of the lateral prefrontal cortex is in all likelihood the physiological foundation of the ability to make plans of action, for which this cortex has been shown to be indispensable. In the human, planning is the neuropsychological function most consistently disrupted by large lesions of the lateral prefrontal cortex. The functional relationship between set and planning is obscure, however. If that relationship is a causal one, the direction of causality is difficult to discern in it. On the one hand, the preparation for actions requires a degree of prior planning. On the other, the planning of actions requires the motivation and initiative that are inherent in the ability to prepare for them.

Set, like working memory, has its electrical correlates in the frontal lobe. In both the human and the monkey, set and working memory are accompanied by sustained neuronal activity in the lateral frontal cortex. In the interval between a percept and a subsequent motor act that depends on it, humans exhibit slow potentials on the surface of the frontal scalp (Brunia et al., 1985; Singh and Knight, 1990) that appear to reflect the sustained and accelerating discharge of underlying neuronal assemblies. The best-known and most conspicuous of these potentials is the *contingent negative variation* (CNV), a slow surface-negative potential that can be recorded in the frontal region during that interval (Fig. 6.9). Because it occurs concomitantly with expectancy, that potential has also been called the *expectancy wave*. It increases in size with the passage of time toward the motor response and as a function of the speed with which that response will be performed when it is due. In posterior aspects of the frontal lobe, premotor cortex and the supplementary motor areas, another potential appears 1–2 seconds before the motor act: the *Bereitshaftspotential* or *readiness potential*. Both the CNV and the readiness potential appear to be part of a continuum of electrical activity that originates in the prefrontal cortex during the percept-to-action interval. This activity progresses in the posterior direction, down the executive hierarchy, toward motor areas in charge of executing the movement. Thus, a spatial-temporal progression of underlying neuronal discharge seems to take place in frontal regions during the expectation of, and preparation for, a motor action. It is reasonable to assume that such a pro-

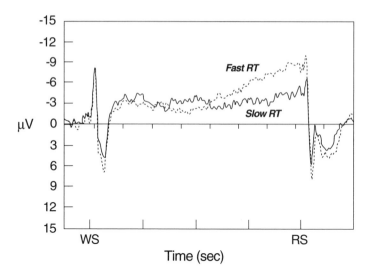

Figure 6.9. Surface-negative potential from human frontal cortex in the interval between a signal (WS) and a motor response (RS). The potential is greater when the reaction time (RT) of the subject is fast than when it is slow. This difference is probably related to the degree of motor attention and readiness to respond. From Brunia et al. (1985), modified, with permission.

gression or wave of neuronal discharge represents the correlate of both, set and expectancy—the latter being, at least in part, the sub-jective experience of the former.

Cells most likely related to set and expectancy have been re-corded in the prefrontal cortex of monkeys performing delay tasks, where a sensory signal presages by a few seconds a perceptual deci-sion or motor act dependent on that signal. Such cells show increas-ing discharge as the action nears, anticipating that action like the slow field potentials that, in the human, presumably reflect their ac-tivity (Niki and Watanabe, 1979; Fuster et al., 1982). Preparatory neu-ral activity has also been inferred from the activation of prefrontal areas observed by neuroimaging in humans during the performance of *planning tasks* (Partiot et al., 1995; Baker et al., 1996). In sum, the preparation for action, whether that action is the interpreting of a perceptual signal for a subsequent motor act or the motor act itself, elicits the activation of frontal networks. There is no reason to suspect that the activated networks are different from the cognits of the ac-tion themselves. Their activation before the action can best be un-

derstood as the priming of their neuronal elements for the performance of the action. In other words, it would appear that those neuronal elements, which are members of vast representational networks
of executive memory, are activated and become functional as those
networks cease to be just representational and also become operant.

Preparatory set, therefore, complements working memory in
temporal integration. Whereas working memory is attention focused
on a recent signal, preparatory set is attention focused on expected
events and actions contingent on that signal. In the lateral prefrontal
cortex of the monkey (Quintana and Fuster, 1999), set cells have
been found in close proximity to working-memory cells (Fig. 6.10).

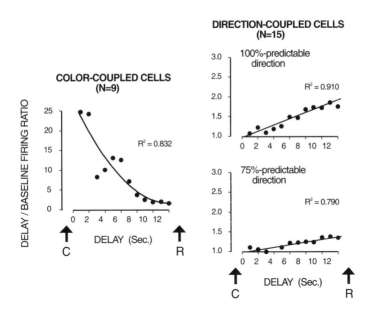

Figure 6.10. Activity of lateral-prefrontal cells of the monkey in the interval (delay) between two visual stimuli. The combination of the two stimuli determines
the direction of a manual response after the second. Depending on the color of
the first stimulus, the monkey can predict the second and the consequent direction of the response (the level of predictability is 100% if the color of the first
stimulus is blue or yellow, and 75% if it is red or green). Some cells (working-
memory cells, color-coupled) respond selectively to color, and their discharge de-
scends in the course of the delay. Others (set-cells, direction-coupled) accelerate
their discharge in the course of the delay. The acceleration of direction-coupled
cells is greater if the animal can predict the direction with 100% certainty than if
it cannot. From Quintana and Fuster (1999), with permission.

Set-cell discharge accelerates as a function of the probability with which the animal can predict precisely the motor act to be performed—paralleling the slow potential difference as a function of reaction time in the human (Fig. 6.9). In conclusion, it appears that, in this part of the cerebral cortex, temporal integration is based on direct transfer of information from cells representing a signal in the recent past to cells that prepare the consequent response to that signal in the near future. Imaging studies reveal the activation of lateral prefrontal cortex in tasks that challenge the ability to plan ahead and to prepare for appropriate responses, such as playing chess (Nichelli et al., 1994).

Execution and Monitoring

In the performance of motor actions, executive attention is conceptually and empirically inseparable from the processing of the actions. Both motor attention and motor execution consist in the selective allocation of the components of motor systems indispensable at a particular time for the action in progress. Nowhere is the identity of executive attention and executive processing more evident than in ocular motility and in the orientation movements of the head and the body. The reason is that such forms of motility are themselves dedicated to the focusing of attention. It is therefore understandable that certain regions of executive cortex of the frontal lobe, notably the eye fields of area 8 and the SMA, are critically involved and invariably activated in behavioral tasks that require a high degree of spatial attention. Those regions control attention, and thus perception of the visual environment, by controlling the direction of gaze. It is, however, useful to view that kind of motor control as consequent, even subordinate, to the inputs from perceptual cortex. Thus, the executive control of action, in this case ocular motility, does not originate in frontal cortex but in the environment and the perceptual cognits that process information from it. In this light, visuospatial attention appears to be a clear example of the cortical operations of the perception-action cycle, the continuous circular interaction of the organism with its environment.

As we have seen, the frontal representations of action (executive cognits) are hierarchically organized. From motor cortex up to prefrontal cortex, executive cognits become progressively broader and more abstract. Programs of sequential action have more distant goals and become more schematically represented, although the networks that represent them keep associative connections with their lower, more concrete motor components and, of course, with their perceptual components in posterior cortex. Although this hierarchical arrangement is generally correct, however, the executive representations in the frontal lobe are to a certain degree heterarchical. There is evidence that, even at lower levels of the frontal hierarchy, there is a degree of global representation; ensembles of neurons in primary motor cortex represent and enact movements defined by direction (Georgopoulos et al., 1982). Further, the participation of frontal areas in the execution of movements does not follow a rigid top-down hierarchical order. Prior to a movement, prefrontal, premotor, and motor neurons do not become activated in a strict temporal sequence (Kalaska et al., 1998). Thus, it appears that the execution of any program or schema of action involves the concurrent participation of components of representation at all levels of the executive hierarchy. Executive attention goes with the action, shifting between levels and domains of executive representation in the cortex of the frontal lobe as well as in lower structures of motor systems. This determines the highly distributed nature of executive attention in both the spatial and the temporal domains.

In the execution of sequential goal-directed actions, the prevailing trends of neural processing are from prefrontal cortex to motor cortex and from global to concrete representations and actions. Along with these trends, the allocation of executive structures (executive attention) becomes progressively more selective. Here it must be emphasized that selective focusing is accompanied, and thus enhanced, by the *inhibitory processes* of filtering and suppression. Executive attention, like perceptual attention and the processes they support, are achieved to a high degree by reciprocal inhibition, that is, by exclusionary mechanisms. Even at the highest levels of cortical execution, in the prefrontal cortex, we encounter the basic biological interplay of excitation and inhibition.

Serial processing is a requirement for the timely and selective allocation of neural resources in the orderly execution of sequential actions. However, in all neural systems, the emphasis on serial processing easily leads to the underestimation of parallel processing. In motor systems, as in perceptual systems (Chapter 4), *parallel* processing must occur on a large scale to complement serial processing. Despite the imponderables, ambiguities, and uncertainties of any new motor task, that task contains a considerable body of actions that are automatic, well rehearsed, and strongly based on experience. The processing of those actions may be to some extent serial, but also to a large extent parallel. Those actions need minimal attention and can be performed outside of awareness. In fact, as almost any typist or pianist can attest to, excessive attention can be an impediment to good performance. There is good reason to believe that those automatic actions can be executed at relatively low levels of the perception-action cycle, through lower frontal-striate loops, mostly in parallel (Alexander et al., 1992). At the same time, actions necessitating high executive attention require serial processing and the temporal integrative capabilities of the prefrontal cortex.

In order to perform its role in executive attention, whether serially or in parallel, the prefrontal cortex requires feedback from receptors and from posterior areas of associative cortex in order to close, at the top, the perception-action cycle. Decision making at any point in a sequence of actions is predicated on that feedback as well as on the anticipated consequences of the actions. That feedback is the basis of what has been termed *monitoring*. It may be generated internally, in the form of proprioceptive inputs and *efferent copies* of current motor action; or it may be generated externally and come to higher cortex through the senses. In any case, internal and external feedback allow the prefrontal cortex to perform its function of monitoring ongoing action. Monitoring is, in sum, one of the temporal integrative functions of the lateral prefrontal cortex, which has been ascribed to a portion of it on the basis of lesion experiments (Petrides, 1991) and neuroimaging (Petrides et al., 1993a; Fletcher et al., 1998b). Long ago, Hans-Lukas Teuber (1972) construed the aggregate of monitoring and internal feedback as the source of a key prefrontal function that he called *corollary discharge*. By that he meant a form of output to sensory systems from voluntary movement that prepared—premodulated—those systems for the consequences of further anticipated movement. Consequently, monitoring and corollary discharge can be viewed as tools of executive attention, and thus as means by which the frontal "executive" controls the actions, as they occur, and prepares the organism for prospective events. Thus, when these events occur, they will be incorporated into the gestalt of the action to ensure that it remains on target.

At all levels of the perception-action cycle, the feedback from sensory systems on motor systems is reciprocated by inhibitory feedback in the opposite direction. This motor–sensory feedback is an essential support of the *inhibitory control* over sensory systems that constitutes the exclusionary component of attention. Thus, at the top of the cycle, the prefrontal cortex not only integrates and monitors sequential actions—including internal actions, such as reasoning—but also protects those actions from extraneous influences. Included among such extraneous influences would be a host of distracting sensory stimuli and schemas or *models* of action that are incompatible with the current action and its goal. There is good evidence (reviewed in Fuster, 1997) to suspect that the orbital prefrontal cortex is an important source of inhibitory control of both internal and external interference. On those grounds, it is reasonable to speculate that laggard maturation of the frontal mechanisms of inhibitory control lies at the root of certain attention disorders of childhood.

7

Language

anguage is the ultimate source and product of civilization. Curiously, even though neurolinguistics is still in its infancy, language is the first cognitive function to have been "localized" in the cortex. For more than a century, two discrete portions of the cortex of the left hemisphere, Broca's area and Wernicke's area, have been considered the seat of linguistic functions; supposedly, the first is in charge of the production and the second the comprehension of speech. Despite a mound of conflicting evidence, that pair of cortical areas, working in tandem, remains as close to a *speech module* as anyone has ever been able to identify in the brain. Some language scholars, however, keenly aware of the limits of those assumptions and the evidence on which they are based, have proposed a broader cerebral module for language. Such a module, yet to be defined anatomically, would be genetically inherited and operate separately from general cognition. Recent evidence, however, seriously challenges any kind of modular localization of language. It is beyond question that language is a means of communication unique to our species (which does not mean that language is *only* a means of communication). That fact by itself at least implies an enormous evolutionary increase in the complexity of the neural substrate of animal communication. It is questionable, however, that language rests on a cortical foundation that differs from that of all other cognitive functions. Language has been rightfully called the *mirror of the mind;* indeed, there is no mental operation that language cannot reflect. Conversely, there is no language without the support from the functions I have discussed in previous chapters. In this chapter, I reason again for the pivotal role of cortical networks in all cognition, now especially with regard to language. Linguistic representations essentially consist of cognits, and linguistic operations such as syntax, comprehension, reading, and writing consist of neural transactions within and between cognits.

Neurobiology of Language

It is uncertain when, in prehistory, language made its appearance. Anthropological estimates vary widely, between 250,000 and 40,000 years ago—the former figure approximately coinciding with the transition from *Homo erectus* to *H. sapiens.* Despite the early archeological evidence of graphic symbolic depictions, speech seems to have preceded writing. Undoubtedly, both inventions took place gradually, in some communities earlier than others. The term *invention* is appropriate for both speech and writing, but it needs qualification. Clearly, language was a new development, a new function that primitive man discovered in a relatively short time—short, that is, in evolutionary scale. Yet that relatively abrupt development of a new form of communication can be best understood as the culmination of an evolutionary process of progressively better adaptation of the organism to its environment. It was a massive expansion of a preexisting system of cognitive communication with conspecifics. That linguistic expansion has been called *arbitrary,* in that it was based on symbols of largely arbitrary selection (Deacon, 1998). The new system vastly extended the repertoire of acts and gestures that nature had selected in some species to communicate symbolically instincts and emotions (Tinbergen, 1951). Language, in this sense, complemented the rich repertoire of facial and bodily expression that many mammalian species possess and Charles Darwin (1998) so well described. In any case, language is the most advanced and effective instrument ever devised for adaptation to the social environment. However, it is probably erroneous, in evolutionary terms, to dissociate linguistic functions from other forms of adaptation to the environment. All are part of a developmental continuum. This view certainly makes sense in neurobiological terms.

In evolution, and also to some degree in ontogenesis, all means of communication develop pari passu with the development of sensory and motor systems. In the salamander (Herrick, 1948), movement is mostly reflex and massive, involving almost the entire body, and is integrated in the central neuropil of the brain stem. Also centralized—in the diencephalon—are the basic neural mechanisms of homeosthasis. The communication with conspecifics is minimal. In higher animal species, the neural substrate for communication expands in two directions: (1) upward, by growth of limbic structures and of paralimbic cortex, such as the cortex of the medial/cingulate and orbital frontal regions; and (2) laterally, by expansion of the neocortex of the two hemispheres. The first evolutionary trend provides the organism with the means to communicate instinctively and emotionally with others. The second mediates the development of language.

However, insofar as the neocortex develops out of the paleocortex and archicortex (Chapter 2), language remains functionally dependent on *limbic structures*. This dependency has three major implications. The first implication is the prominent role of motivation in language. Both the initiation and the course of language are heavily influenced by internal drives as well as by emotional state. The second implication is the overriding role of strong emotions on linguistic expression, especially as a result of the pathological weakening of neocortex or the hegemony of limbic-subcortical circuitry. Hence the *subcorticalization* of language after massive cortical lesions, with its reduction to primitive affective expression. Hence the explosive vocalizations of patients afflicted by the Gilles de la Tourette syndrome or the obsessive-compulsive syndrome—both presumably involving orbitofrontal pathology. (Hence, also, the linguistically bare expletives of normal demeanor.) The third implication is that, in nonhuman primates, where the neocortex is underdeveloped, vocal communication is to a large extent controlled by limbic structures or paralimbic cortex. According to the research conducted by Ploog (1981, 1992) and his collaborators, the limbic control of communication appears prevalent in monkeys, especially the squirrel monkey, an animal with a rich repertory of species-specific vocalizations. In nonhuman primates, as in the human, the orbitomedial prefrontal cortex, the amygdala, and some anterior nuclei of the thalamus form a system of interrelated structures dedicated to emotional and social behavior. In harmony with this concept, these structures constitute the substrate for emotional and social expression, including the rudiments of oral communication.

With the development of the neocortex in larger apes (chimpanzee and orangutan), symbolic communication in the cognitive sphere becomes possible (Premack, 1976). Such animals are capable of learning the bare essentials of sign language to symbolize nouns and actions. Attempts to teach them syntax, however, have proven unsuccessful. The syntax of semantic elements does not make its appearance until evolution produces the human brain with its large cortex, one-half of which is dedicated to language and its related cognitive functions. However, as we will see, the evolutionary advent of linguistic syntax is closely correlated with the development of the capacity for complex motor sequencing (Kimura, 1979, 1993), in other words, for what Lashley (1951) called the *syntax of action*. Linguistic syntax and motoric syntax seem to have a common phyletic origin. The first makes its appearance, and the second reaches its apogee, in the left frontal lobe of the human.

In phylogeny as in ontogeny, the development of the receptive and productive aspects of language is correlated with the development of the cortices of association. In the human, the associative neocortex of the temporal, parietal, and occipital regions accommodates mainly the semantic aspects of language, whereas that of the frontal lobe accommodates its productive aspects. Especially significant in this respect are the large increases in neuron numbers and connections taking place in those cortical regions in the course of evolution. In the development of the individual, those regions are the latest to mature in terms of axonal myelination and dendritic branching (Flechsig, 1920; Conel, 1963; Gibson, 1991). The ontogenetic maturation of axons and dendrites in associative neocortex comes on top of the vast evolutionary increase of subcortical white matter (Chapter 2), which is to a large extent composed of corticocortical connections. All in all, the enormous phylogenetic and ontogenetic expansion of *connectivity* in cortex of association undoubtedly leads to the flourishing of language, as well as cognition, in the adult human brain. The combinatorial power that connectivity adds to neuronal assemblies is the basis for the specificity of associative cortical networks. It explains the practically infinite variety of cognits possible and the idiosyncrasy of individual memories. It also explains the creative po-

tential of language. Most certainly, the additional connectivity opens
a wealth of new long-distance cortical paths. Those new paths, in addition to the proliferation of myelin sheaths, are bound to facilitate
the speedy processing of information, much of it in parallel, that language necessitates.

The question now before us is, how much of that connective apparatus is ready-made for language at birth? The question is important because it bears directly on the issue of the genetic aspects of language, which is a strongly debated issue. Clearly, the phylogenetic
development of the supralaryngeal tract and the telencephalization
of the neural structures supporting vocalization have provided the
human with a unique genetic foundation on which to develop language under appropriate environmental conditions. Spearheaded by
Noam Chomsky (1975, 1986), however, a highly influential school of
modern linguistics takes a more radical position. According to its proponents, language itself is genetically inherited and the foundation
of all cognition. The empirical base for this position is the evidence of
the speed and ease with which children acquire the structural rules of
language, that is, the rules for the formation of new and meaningful
phrases and sentences. By the age of 10, a normal child has mastered
those rules spontaneously, unwittingly, and without aid. To be sure,
those rules vary somewhat from language to language. For example,
word order is much more important in English than in Finnish. Besides, the child unquestionably acquires the phonetics, vocabulary,
and prosody of the native language by imitation and learning from
others, notably the mother. But phonetics, vocabulary, and prosody
may be considered peripheral and conventional aspects of language.
Its essence is structure; its meaning depends mainly, if not exclusively,
on the spatial-temporal structure in sequences of words with their inflections. Accordingly, the essence of Chomsky 's empirical theory is
that the child develops from within, as if expressing an innate instinct, the grammatical structure of language, the so-called *universal
grammar.* Again, the fundamental support of the theory is the child's
proven ability to create completely new language with proper grammatical structure. Of course, the inherent creativity of language is to
stay and expand into adult life.

Is there, then, such a thing as phyletic memory for language
somewhere in the cortex, much as there is phyletic memory for sensations and movements in sensory and motor cortices? The answer is,
probably, a qualified yes. Here it is helpful to view Chomky's "revolu-

tion" as the challenge that it was, and still is, to behaviorism and learning theory in all their forms. Indeed, correct language cannot be
learned by the conditioning of stimulus–response links, by reinforcement of verbal expressions, by mere imitation, or by rote memorizing. As Lashley (1951) remarked long ago in a classic publication, the
mere chaining of words by superficial associations does not make language. Language is learned and made by creating, with spoken words,
grammatical structures of meaning according to a well-defined set of
rules—largely unknown to the child. Language is strictly a structure-
dependent function, and the structure of language must conform to
grammatical rules. In accord with these rules, a sentence can undergo
innumerable changes in its *superficial structure* while preserving its
meaning. Hence the epithet *transformational,* which has also been applied to universal grammar.

Unquestionably, however, children learn a large vocabulary before they undergo formal education. Along with it, they learn a large
fund of relationships of meaning between words and objects, as well
as between words and between objects. They also learn to categorize
words and the objects they represent. In addition, they establish associations between words, objects and affects, or needs. Likewise, they
learn to use words and to manipulate objects to satisfy those needs.
Almost all of that *learning* essentially consists of the formation of cognitive networks in cortex of association, as described in previous chapters. Whether the learning process takes place by selectionist or constructivist synaptic mechanisms at the neuronal level is unclear. Both
probably intervene. In any case, the acquisition of language makes extensive use of synaptic plasticity, probably in accord with hebbian
rules (Pulvermüller, 1992). It stands to reason, nonetheless, that the
mechanisms of associative learning take place on a template of preexisting or innate connectivity linking neuronal assemblies in the
highest—semantic and conceptual—levels of association cortex. It
also stands to reason that such a template contains the potential for
plastic relationships of meaning at the highest level. The connective
architecture of such a template, together with its synaptic substrate,
may be there from birth, genetically inherited and ready for pheno-
typical realization under the necessary environmental conditions.
Much as the perceptual and executive cognits of posterior and prefrontal cortices are ready to implement the syntax of motor action,
they are also ready, with the aid of symbolic cortical representations,

to implement the syntax of language. Thus, inasmuch as rules are contingencies of association between cognits, there may be an innate cortical apparatus for the rules of grammar. There is some evidence—reviewed by Pinker (1991)—that both, symbolic computation by genetic rules and associative memory, operate in the processing of different grammatical forms (e.g., regular versus irregular verbs). Once again in neuroscience, two apparently opposite views of the same order of phenomena may turn out to be complementary to each other.

In children, the development of language correlates with the development of motor skills. The ability to organize behavior sequentially is both a harbinger and a correlate of the ability to organize the spoken language (Kimura 1993). Both types of ability are clearly dependent on left-hemisphere dominance. Greenfield (1991) argues that Broca's speech area is the homologue of a phylogenetically older region of the left frontal lobe specialized in the manipulation of tools and instruments. This comparative homology is functionally reflected in ontogeny. The child develops the ability to articulate meaningful sequences of words concomitantly with the ability to manipulate objects in an orderly and purposeful manner. Nevertheless, even though nonhuman primates (e.g., the rhesus monkey) exhibit hand preferences, they do not exhibit functional hemispheric lateralization as clearly as does the human.

In the adult, nothing illustrates better the *plasticity* of the neural apparatus for language than the functional recovery of language after large lesions of the left cortex. Typically, depending on the extent and location of one such lesion, a global, semantic (fluent), or expressive (nonfluent) aphasia ensues. With time and rehabilitation, the patient may recover much of the lost linguistic ability. Except in cases of proven functional recovery of the damaged tissue, it has been repeatedly demonstrated that other cortical or subcortical regions take over that ability. In this manner, it has been shown that the right hemisphere can become a surrogate language hemisphere, albeit with considerable limitations (Cummings et al., 1979; Ogden, 1988). Conclusive evidence of that interhemispheric transfer of language is the observation that, after the recovery from a left-hemisphere lesion, the unilateral narcotization of the right hemisphere with intracarotid sodium amytal (Wada test), or a subsequent right-hemisphere lesion, reinstates the aphasia (review by Kinsbourne, 1998). However, right-hemisphere language is in no case quite the same as left-hemisphere language (next section). For one thing, the "restored" right-hemisphere language is never as competent phonologically, semantically, or syntactically as the preexisting language of the normal individual.

Hemispheric Lateralization

It is an established fact that most people use mainly or exclusively the *left hemisphere* of their brain for processing language. The bulk of the evidence comes from studies of the disorders of language (aphasias) resulting from brain injuries. In evolutionary and neurobiological terms, the reasons for the emergence of a dominant left hemisphere and for the lateralization of language to it are unknown. They probably have to do, though it is unclear how, with morphological differences between the two hemispheres: certain anatomical features are larger or more developed on the left than on the right. It has long been surmised that such asymmetries are related to linguistic functions. In human evolution, however, cerebral asymmetries seem to have appeared very early. By study of endocasts, they have been traced back to *Pithecanthropus erectus* (Australopithecine), a genus still supposedly deprived of language. Further, morphological asymmetry and lateralization of function are not limited to the cerebral hemispheres. It has been proposed (Tucker, 1993) that the lateralized dominance of the controls of communication is widely distributed along the nerve axis, possibly related to lateral differences in the distribution of neurotransmitter systems, notably DA and NE (Luu and Tucker, 1998).

Left-leaning *asymmetries* also have an early origin in ontogeny; they have been found to be present before birth (Witelson, 1995). In any case, there is no convincing morphological evidence that one hemisphere matures more slowly than the other (Hiscock, 1998). The left hemisphere specializes at an early age in a variety of perceptual and motor functions, some of which are related to language. In infants below the age of 3 months, studies of dichotic listening (Entus, 1977; Best, 1988) show a right-ear advantage for phonetic discriminations—and, conversely, a left-ear advantage for musical discriminations. One of the earliest manifestations of motoric left-hemispheric dominance is the tendency of neonates to turn to the right spontaneously or in response to sensory stimuli (Liederman, 1987), a tendency that has been found to correlate highly with a right-hand preference later in life (Coryell, 1985). The results of surgical hemispherectomy at various ages provide additional evidence of the early specialization of the left hemisphere in several functions, including language use (Spreen et al., 1995).

In the adult human, interhemispheric asymmetries have been recognized in clinically defined language areas since the classic publication of Geschwind and Levitsky (1968). By anatomical measurements in 100 brains, they found that, in the majority of cases, a cortical field in the posterior wall of the Sylvian fissure, called the *planum temporale,* was larger on the left than on the right. This finding, which was subsequently confirmed by a number of studies (review by Galaburda, 1995), is of singular significance for language. The planum temporale is located within a cortical region that has been characterized as the *posterior language area.* This area comprises parts of Brodmann's area 22 (area of Wernicke, 1874) and areas 39 through 42 (Fig. 7.1). Recent studies by magnetic resonance imaging (MRI) confirm the asymmetry not only in Wernicke's area (Kertesz et al., 1992), but also in Brodmann's areas 44 and 45, which include Broca's area (Broca, 1861), the anterior language cortex (Foundas et al., 1995). The left-side volumetric advantage is correlated with right-handedness and left language dominance. Hemispheric asymmetries in language areas have also been described at the microscopic level. Pyramidal cells in language areas have been found to be larger on the left than on the right (Hayes and Lewis, 1995; Hutsler and Gazzaniga, 1997). The dendritic trees of pyramids in language areas have been found to extend further than those of pyramids in homologous areas of the right hemisphere (Jacobs and Scheibel, 1993). Studies of the corpus callosum (Aboitiz and Ide, 1998) reveal an inverse relation between the size of the callosal cross section and behavioral laterality, especially in males; this inverse relation indicates decreased interhemispheric communication as a function of hemispheric specialization.

The left or dominant hemisphere seems to have overriding, though not necessarily exclusive, control of all aspects of linguistic function: semantic, syntactic, and phonological. This control extends to the lowest cortical levels of the language processing system. Thus, the lateralization of auditory discrimination in infants, mentioned above, appears to extend to the adult. PET shows an equal bilateral activation of auditory cortices in the discrimination of slow acoustic frequencies (Belin et al., 1998). It also shows, however, a left-biased asymmetry of activation in response to higher frequencies; this asymmetry can be explained as the reduced (inhibited?) response of the

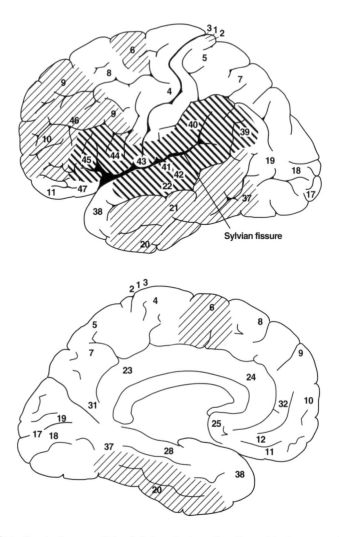

Figure 7.1. Cortical areas of the left hemisphere implicated in language by the study of the effects of cerebral lesions. Heavy crosshatching marks the posterior and anterior (frontal) language areas, lesions of which often result in severe language disorders. Lesions in lightly crosshatched areas result less frequently in less severe language disorders. Areas are numbered according to Brodmann's cytoarchitectonic map.

right auditory cortex to those frequencies. In a linguistic task with phonological and semantic demands, an fMRI study (Binder et al., 1997) shows metabolic activation strongly lateralized to the left cerebral hemisphere (frontal, temporal, and parietal lobes). The study also reveals, however, that the activation extends cortically beyond the language areas (Wernicke's and Broca's); further, the activation extends to a number of subcortical structures on the left and to the right cerebellum. The activation of cerebral structures on the right, although minor, is not negligible. In sum, this study illustrates the left cortical dominance in language. In addition, however, it illustrates the widely distributed nature of linguistic functions. The wide distribution of both the content and operations of language challenges the classical model of two discrete areas in the left hemicortex—one sensory and the other motor—in the tandem control of language. That model is further challenged by the results of direct experimental stimulation of the neurosurgically exposed cortex in the awake subject. Electrical stimuli to the cortex have been shown to block linguistic operations selectively and reversibly (Ojemann, 1983). Thereby it has been possible to assess the contribution of neuron assemblies to those operations. Electrical blockage shows (1) large individual variation in the topography of language-active cortical assemblies; (2) wide cortical distribution of those assemblies—some of them outside of the classical language areas; and (3) participation of other cognitive functions—attention, perception, and memory—in the recognition and naming of lexical entities.

Clearly, then, imaging and stimulating studies, and to some degree lesion studies as well, point to the wide and idiosyncratic distribution of language networks in operation. Most of them are lateralized to the left and have nodes in the classical language areas. The emerging picture of the cortex in language, however, is one of widespread active networks defined by their cognitive content and by the demands of cognitive operations that are essential to the comprehension and expression of language. These operations include attention, working memory, auditory and visual perception, and access to long-term memory (perceptual and executive). It is no longer plausible to construe a set of language-dedicated areas or networks— that is, a module (Fodor, 1983)—outside of the sphere of general cognition. It is plausible, however, to view language as a set of information processing operations in an immense substrate of overlapping and intersecting cortical cognits of both hemispheres. We do not know the neural mechanisms that mediate these operations. We do know, however, that language makes use of the available cognits to construct ever-new forms of linguistic expression.

In brief, it seems reasonable that the constructive process of language relies largely on two major areas of the cortex of the left hemi-

sphere: one posterior (Wernicke's) for the processing of relationships of meaning, and the other anterior (Broca's) for syntactic expression. Both kinds of processing are hardly conceivable, however,
outside of the informational context of the cortex at large and without the contribution of cognitive functions other than language itself.
Further, both kinds of processing probably take place through multiple networks, in series as well as in parallel. At all times, both the
cognitive substrate and the operations of language remain amenable
to plastic change.

The apparent capacity of the right hemisphere to restore language after left-hemisphere damage has led many to question the
normal role of the *right hemisphere* in language. A way to examine this
question is to study subjects who for remedial reasons have under-
gone the surgical severance of interhemispheric commissures, including the corpus callosum, the anterior commissure, and the hippocampal commissure (Zaidel, 1990). For all practical purposes, in these
patients the two hemispheres are disconnected from each other, and
the function of either hemisphere can be examined separately by
presenting sensory stimuli and queries only in its hemifield. The right
hemisphere disconnected in this manner possesses considerable capacity for perceptual functions, notably in the visuospatial domain.
In the language domain, it possesses a degree of comprehension of
speech as well as lexical and pictorial semantics. However, it can barely
read—one letter at a time—and cannot generate or organize either
speech or writing. It is practically deprived of syntax. On the basis of
such findings, and the effects of left decortication, it has been suggested that the linguistic competence of the right hemisphere is re-
stricted to the use of visuospatial representations, intonation, prosody, and emotional tone. The competence of the right hemisphere in
these aspects of language would complement that of the left hemisphere in others, especially syntax. At a more general level, it could
be argued that normally some of the complementary linguistic functions of the right hemisphere remain latent, or even inhibited, under
the dominance of the left hemisphere. In any case, with the emphasis on left dominance, the contribution of the right hemisphere to semantics may be injudiciously neglected.

A special issue is that of *bilingual* subjects and polyglots. Do these
individuals store more than one language in one hemisphere? Do the
two hemispheres store different languages? To what extent do different languages use the same neuronal resources? There are no defi-

nite answers to these questions, but the study of those individuals' aphasias provides valuable insights. After substantial damage of the left hemisphere, people who speak two languages generally lose both (Berthier et al., 1990; Junqué et al., 1995). More than two languages seem to suffer the same fate (Paradis, 1998). However, the pattern of recovery from the resulting aphasia, as reported in the literature (reviewed by Paradis, 1998), varies greatly between subjects. Some patients recover more than one language in parallel, others recover one before another, and still others follow a pattern of temporally alternating recovery from one language to another. The reasons for the absence of uniform recovery are obscure. Preferential recovery of one language over another appears related to its being the native language, the most practiced language, or the language invested by the patient with the highest degree of affectivity, and thus presumably with motivation to relearn it. From differential patterns of recovery in bilinguals, some investigators have drawn the inference that each language has a different cortical representation, possibly one language in one hemisphere and the other in the other. However, that both languages are represented in the same (left) hemisphere is borne out by the evidence from cortical stimulation (Ojemann, 1983; Rapport et al., 1983), PET imaging (Klein et al., 1995), and Wada testing (Rapport et al., 1983). By the Wada test, both sign language and English have been found represented in the dominant hemisphere (Homan et al., 1982; Mateer et al., 1984), though sign language seems to have greater bilateral representation than English. An imaging study (Neville et al., 1998) substantiates the contribution of the right hemisphere to sign language (this study is discussed further below).

In conclusion, it appears that, in bilinguals and polyglots, all the languages mastered by the individual reside essentially in the dominant hemisphere. Interhemispheric differences in representation, as suggested by asynchronies in recovery from aphasia or by functional tests, may be attributable, in part, to differences in the contribution of each hemisphere to each language. Paradis (1998) has proposed that the left or dominant hemisphere contributes to any language the basic and implicit linguistic competence—possibly including, as we discussed in the previous section, such innate components as an essential grammar. The right or nondominant hemisphere, on the other hand, would contribute much of what he calls *metalinguistic* knowledge, that is, the explicit component of language largely acquired by learning and education. Thus, whereas linguistic operations depend on the cortex and subcortical structures of the dominant (usually left) hemisphere, the cognitive content on which those operations take place is probably distributed widely and to some degree redundantly in both hemispheres.

Hemispheric lateralization also seems to apply to music, which is a kind of language. It has prosody, temporal order, and "syntax." Like language, music is communicable graphically by written symbols. It is also an artistic form that reflects and evokes affect and emotion in the composer as well as the listener. By lesion studies or the Wada test, certain musical abilities, such as the recognition of melodies, have been ascribed to the superior and middle temporal gyri in the nondominant, commonly right, hemisphere (Kimura, 1964; Bogen and Gordon, 1971; Critchley and Henson, 1977; Brust, 1980). The more analytical abilities of musicians, however, seem to be lateralized to the left, or dominant, hemisphere. Thus, the pitch of experienced musicians has been related by MEG to increased auditory discrimination of left auditory cortex (Pantev et al., 1998). This increase is correlated with the years of prior musical experience. Neuroimaging shows that musical sight-reading is accompanied by the activation of cortex in the vicinity of Wernicke's area, whereas keyboard performance activates cortex near Broca's area (Sergent et al., 1992). In sum, musical memory seems to depend at least in part on the functional integrity of temporal cortex of the right hemisphere, whereas the analysis and performance of music seem to depend on the cortex of the left hemisphere. In any case, music, like language, is a widely distributed function of cortical and probably noncortical structures. Its neocortical substrate consists of cognits distributed in the nondominant hemisphere but also possibly extending to the dominant one. The neural operations of listening to and playing music depend on the processing role of cortical areas of the dominant hemisphere adjoining the classical language areas.

Neuropsychology of Language

Heretofore, the principal source of knowledge on the neural foundations of language has been the clinical study of cortical *aphasias*, the disorders of language that result from lesions of the cortex (Wernicke, 1874; Brown, 1972; Benson and Geschwind, 1985). Lesions of the posterior association cortex, especially Wernicke's area (posterior half of the superior temporal gyrus, area 22), tend to cause deficits in the semantics of language. The patient has difficulty understanding the meaning of words and sentences but little difficulty articulating them; in fact, the patient may spontaneously engage in profuse and illogical speech production. For these reasons, Wernicke's aphasia has been characterized as *semantic, sensory* or *fluent*. Conversely, Broca's aphasic, from damage to the inferior frontal gyrus (usually also affecting the surrounding cortex of the frontal operculum), has difficulty articulating words and sentences (*motor* or *nonfluent* aphasia). The most characteristic feature of this aphasia is the absence of *function words* (e.g., articles, pronouns, conjunctions, and prepositions). Thus, to the listener, the speech of Broca's aphasic sounds *telegraphic* and agrammatical. Global aphasia results from lesions affecting both areas, Wernicke's and Broca's, whereas the conduction and transcortical aphasias result from lesions of the underlying or intermediate white matter. These aphasias have mixed features of the former two.

In any case, pure aphasias of any kind are rare. The reason, to put it simply, is that language is an eminently integrative function and none of its components, phonological, semantic, or syntactic, can operate normally in isolation from the others. This is also the case for the cortical areas that support them. Thus, a patient with Wernicke's aphasia is deprived of the ability not only to comprehend language but also to construct it with meaningful syntax, despite the patient's loquaciousness. Conversely, a patient with Broca's aphasia lacks the ability not only to articulate elaborate language but also to give it the full meaning that syntax provides. In a sense, therefore, all aphasias can be considered conductive, and included within the category of disorders that Geschwind in his classic and insightful publication (1965b) called *disconnection syndromes*.

Nonetheless, it is unquestionable that the two cortices, Wernicke's and Broca's, participate differently in the operations of language. Whereas the former mediates access to the meaning of words and sentences, the latter mediates the construction, that is, the syntax, of speech. Hence the classical language model proposed early on by Lichtheim (1885), which is still largely correct today, albeit only in the broadest terms (Fig. 7.2). The model consists of an *acoustic center* connected to a *motor center*, and above them a *conceptual center* to which both are connected. A more apt scheme would have the conceptual center, the assumed substrate of meaning, divided into the two large moieties of association cortex, one postrolandic and the other prerolandic, that are the substrates for perceptual and executive cognits,

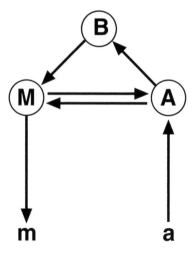

Figure 7.2. Lichtheim's model of interactions between cortical centers in language. A, acoustic center; B, conceptual center; M, motor center; a, acoustic input; m, motor output. From Lichtheim (1885), slightly modified.

respectively. A further refinement of the scheme, more in accord with clinical observations, would conform the acoustic center to a broader definition of Wernicke's area (Damasio, 1989b) to include cortex of the angular gyrus (areas 39 and 40). Thus this broader Wernicke's area would include associative cortex for stimuli other than those of the auditory modality.

Note, therefore, that the two cortices, Wernicke's—broadly defined—and Broca's, lie at relatively different levels in their respective hierarchies of cognition. Wernicke's cortex lies high in the perceptual hierarchy, situated above unimodal association cortex and including portions of *transmodal cortex* (Mesulam, 1998). Broca's cortex, on the other hand, lies relatively low in the executive hierarchy, in premotor cortex and possibly also in motor cortex at the foot of the precentral gyrus, which controls the oral musculature. In other words, Broca's area is closer to speech output than Wernicke's area is to speech input. This hierarchical asymmetry of the two areas in terms of cognitive representation has two important implications. One implication is that the lesions of Wernicke's area can, and do, cause deficits not only of language (e.g., semantic aphasia, anomia), but also of higher cognitive—that is, conceptual—functions (e.g., agnosias). The other implication is that, with the emphasis on the executive role of Broca's area and the effects of its injuries on speech formalities, the more subtle roles of higher frontal areas in the representation and execution of language are generally underestimated.

Despite considerable problems of individual variability, the lesions outside of those classic language areas provide useful, though sketchy, information on the distribution of semantics. As lesions encroach on cortex beyond area 22 of the dominant hemisphere, into the areas of the broadly defined Wernicke's area, they are likely to induce *agnosia* (lack of recognition, the term coined by Freud, 1953) for both words and sentences (Penfield and Roberts, 1966; Geschwind, 1970). The patient cannot retrieve the meaning of structured language. If the lesion affects the homotopical cortex of the right hemisphere, it may cause agnosia for nonverbal auditory material (e.g., music). As we enter the higher association cortex of the posterior regions of the hemisphere, we find that lesions ostensibly affect the linguistic manifestations of cognits of higher order in the perceptual hierarchy. These include (1) cross-modal cognits, as patients are unable to name visually presented objects or their features (Luria, 1966; Walsh, 1978; Davidoff and Ostergaard, 1984); (2) lexical cognits, as patients cannot understand written words and language (Geschwind, 1965a); and (3) categorical cognits, as patients fail to identify object categories, or objects by category—for example, animate, inanimate, fruits, animals, vegetables (Warrington and McCarthy, 1983; Hart and Gordon, 1992).

In sum, it would appear, from lesion studies, that the semantic substrate for language is the same substrate that serves perception and perceptual memory (Chapters 3, 4, and 5). As we will see below, functional studies support this view. That substrate consists of the cortical hierarchy of cognitive networks representing all the cognits accessible to language. At the lowest stage of that hierarchy, in auditory association cortex (area 42), are the phonological cognits or networks formed by associations between vocal sounds; at higher cortical stages are the cognits formed by associations between phonemes and stimuli of other modalities, especially visual, to constitute words; and in the highest areas of transmodal association cortex are the categorical and conceptual cognits. The words for them are probably represented in parallel lexical networks (next section) with a degree of heterarchical association.

Conversely, the productive substrate for language seems to coincide with the substrate that serves action and executive memory.

Frontal lesions expose the *frontal linguistic hierarchy.* Above motor cortex and Broca's area, other speech areas have been identified in the frontal lobe by lesion studies. One is the premotor cortex of area 6, especially the SMA of the dominant hemisphere. Lesions of this area result in aphasias of motor character, similar to Broca's aphasia but less conspicuous, that is, with lesser disruption of syntax and grammar (Luria, 1970; Goldberg et al., 1981). Medial prefrontal lesions, especially those affecting the anterior cingulate area, induce a speech impediment that—when the lesion is large—may reach mutism, that is, the absence of spontaneous or elicited speech. The cingulate area, however, on account of clinical manifestations and its connections with limbic structures, appears involved primarily in the attentive and motivational aspects of speech, rather than in its semantic or syntactic aspects. Lesions of lateral prefrontal cortex induce disorders of language of varying degree, depending on the extent and location of the lesion. An extensive lateral prefrontal lesion in either hemisphere leads commonly to what has been termed *central motor aphasia* (Goldstein, 1948) or *frontal dynamic aphasia* (Luria, 1970). This kind of aphasia is characterized by low spontaneity and fluidity of speech and by general impoverishment of the structure of language (Lhermitte et al., 1972; Barbizet et al., 1975). On close analysis, what seems most affected is the capacity to conceptualize complex propositions and to make use of the recursive and sentence-embedding capacity of language (Chomsky, 1975). In other words, the patient with a prefrontal lesion is unable to conceptualize, plan, and execute complex structures of language, much as he or she is unable to do those things with actions of other kinds.

Thus, to sum up in light of the results of lesion studies, the cognits supporting the productive aspects of speech appear hierarchically organized in lateral frontal cortex in a manner similar to that of the semantic cognits in posterior association cortex. At the top of the frontal hierarchy, in lateral prefrontal cortex, lie the representations of learned or intended propositions of some complexity in more or less schematic form. Under them, in premotor cortex, lie simpler propositions with some syntax. At the bottom, in Broca's area and neighboring motor cortex, lie the simplest propositions, with only the most elementary syntactic structure.

In harmony with these interpretations is the evidence, also stemming from clinical analysis of cortical lesions, for a characteristic double dissociation of linguistic categories in frontal and posterior cortices. It is now well established that *verbs* and action words are generally represented in frontal cortex, whereas *nouns* and names for objects are represented in posterior associative cortex. Goodglass et al. (1966) were the first to document this dichotomous topography of semantic categories. They observed that Broca's aphasics had difficulty naming verbs and words for actions, whereas Wernicke's aphasics had difficulty naming objects. These observations were replicated by a number of other investigators (Miceli et al., 1984; Caramazza and Hillis, 1991; Damasio and Tranel, 1993; Gainotti et al., 1995). Because of the variability of lesion sites in different studies, the precise cortical topography of the two categories—verbs and objects—remains unclear, however. In any case, there appears to be a focal region for the representation of verbs in lateral frontal cortex and another for nouns in superior temporal cortex. The latter area seems to extend into the cortex of the angular gyrus, thus involving a sensory convergence area that has been associated with naming (Geschwind, 1967). As I briefly mentioned before, lesions of this area commonly result in anomia. In any event, the inference of different cortical distributions for nouns and verbs—in posterior and frontal cortices, respectively—is evidently compatible with my view of the distribution of perceptual and executive cognits. What is not evident and remains to be clarified, however, is the precise distribution of the words that symbolize categories and concepts, that is, the lexical support of cognits. As I discuss in the next section, it seems parsimonious and correct to assume that the semantic cognits and their symbolic word representations share to some degree the same networks, in posterior cortex for objects and in frontal cortex for actions.

Functional Architecture of Semantics

Semantics is the meaning of language. Both language and its semantic content conform to a hierarchical order. At the lowest level of that order, spoken or written language is made up of sounds or letters forming the symbolic units of meaning called *words*. Some words (onomatopoeic) derive their meaning from phonic similarities to the sounds of the real objects they symbolize. Others, the vast majority in any language, have acquired their meaning arbitrarily in the evolution of that language. Some words symbolize concrete entities, whereas others symbolize classes of entities and still others classes of classes of entities, and so on up the semantic hierarchy ascending to the level of words that symbolize abstract concepts. The structure of language derives from the union of words forming phrases and sentences, a union called *syntax*. Thus, phrases and sentences derive their meaning not only from the symbolic meaning of the words that constitute them but, most essentially, from the spatial–temporal relationships between those words (inflections taken into account), that is, from syntax. The phrase structure of a sentence is also organized hierarchically, with small pieces combined into larger pieces of increasing size and specificity of meaning. Thus, the semantics and syntax of language are intimately entwined, and any search for the neural base of either has to take this fact into consideration. This section deals with the neurophysiological correlates of semantics in cerebral cortex.

Functional studies support the cortical dissociation of semantic representations of word categories that lesion studies indicate and were discussed in the preceding section. Category- and area-related differences have been detected in the amplitude of cortical field potentials (ERPs) elicited by the presentation of words in lexical decision tasks (Preissl et al., 1995; Pulvermüller et al., 1999). Reportedly, these differences occur mainly in long-latency potentials, that is, in potentials recorded 200 ms or more after the visual presentation of a word. Verbs elicit larger potentials than nouns in anterior (frontal) regions, whereas nouns elicit larger potentials than verbs in posterior (occipital) regions.

Another anterior-posterior difference in ERPs predicted from aphasias has been observed with regard to so-called open-class (OC) and closed-class (CC) words. OC words are content words, consisting of nouns, verbs, and adjectives; CC or function words include articles, pronouns, prepositions, and conjunctions. Whereas OC words carry semantic meaning, CC words by themselves do not, although they are essential for syntax. Neville et al. (1992) recorded field potentials evoked by both OC and CC words embedded in visually presented sentences. They found that CC words elicited a negative potential 280 ms after presentation that was largest in frontal regions. Conversely, OC words elicited a later negativity (350 ms) that was largest in posterior regions—occipital, temporal, and parietal. (Differences between verbs and nouns could not be probed in this experiment, as both were treated as OC words.) These observations are congruent with the inferred role of frontal cortex and CC words in syntax, as well as the role of posterior cortex and OC words in the representation of semantic contents. The role of posterior cortex in semantics is fur-

ther supported by other ERP studies in subjects presented with words
and sentences (Kutas and Hillyard, 1983; Posner and Pavese, 1998).
In one of these studies, words are placed out of syntactic or semantic
context in the middle or at the end of a sentence (Kutas and Hillyard,
1983). When the linguistically anomalous word is a content word (semantic anomaly) but not a function word (syntactic anomaly), it elicits a large long-latency (400 ms) negative potential in posterior cortical locations (Fig. 7.3).

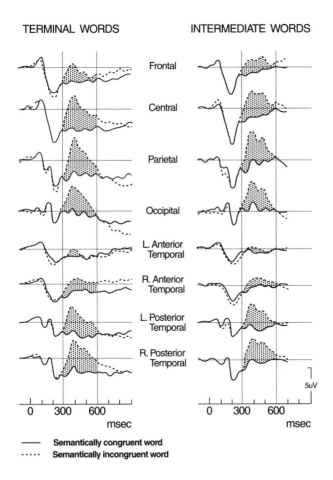

Figure 7.3. Average potentials elicited by semantically congruent content words
(solid lines) and by semantically anomalous content words *(dashed lines)* placed at
the end (terminal) or middle (intermediate) of a sentence. From Kutas and Hillyard (1983), with permission.

The search for the semantic structure of language in cerebral cortex has greatly expanded with the advent of *neuroimaging* methods. In this search, reading is commonly used to access meaning. Typically, metabolic activations are correlated with the reading of words or sentences in order to unravel the cortical topography of their meaning. The approach is useful despite considerable methodological difficulties. The principal difficulty is the limited resolution, in space and time, of the most widely used imaging methods, PET and fMRI. In both methods, there is a mismatch between the resolving power of the machine and the spatial and temporal scales of cognition. Another difficulty is the large individual variability in intensity and distribution of the observed activations. Both difficulties tend to distort the pictures of semantic structure. Such pictures typically consist of (*1*) spatial and temporal averages of peak activation and (*2*) areas of overlapping activation—within or across subjects. In either case, the extent of the activated cognits tends to be underestimated. Nonetheless, imaging during word or sentence reading reveals the most elementary features of cortical lexical maps.

A survey of the peak activations reported in a number of articles on brain imaging (Cabeza and Nyberg, 2000) shows that, generally, the areas activated by written words coincide with the areas activated by spoken words (Fig. 7.4). These areas include, most prominently, the classic language areas of the left hemisphere. Unlike spoken words, written words tend to activate visual (occipital) areas in addition to language areas. As already noted, however, peak activations represent only average maxima ("tips of the iceberg"). The activated networks are probably idiosyncratic and extend into higher cortices of association, largely undetected under the statistical threshold or criterion of activation set by the investigator. In any case, the reviewed studies strongly suggest that the same cognits can be accessed through the eye as through the ear. They also indicate that the meaning of words activates language-production areas. Another interesting and related finding is the activation of the cerebellum (e.g., Fiez and Petersen, 1998), a structure that, like motor and premotor cortices, takes part in the orderly execution of purposeful actions. The activation of executive structures by word meaning reveals the participation of these structures in the perception-action cycle, which serves language as well as other forms of behavioral expression (next section).

An fMRI study by Neville and her collaborators (1998) further illustrates the participation of areas beyond language areas in the de-

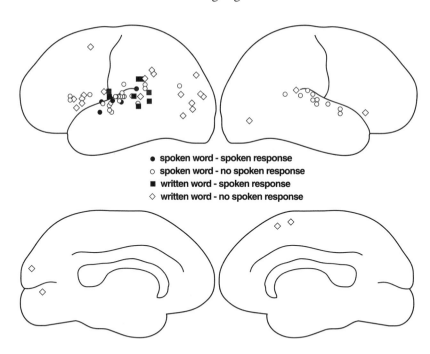

Figure 7.4. Peak activations elicited by recognition of spoken and written words (with or without a spoken response). From Cabeza and Nyberg (2000), with permission.

coding of semantic meaning. Three groups of subjects are investigated: (*1*) normally hearing monolingual speakers of English, (*2*) deaf users of American Sign Language (ASL) — the native language — who have learned English late and imperfectly, and (*3*) bilinguals for whom both English and ASL are native languages (native signers). All subjects are requested to read silently both English and ASL sentences (nonsigners merely observe ASL). Controls include the presentation of consonant strings and post hoc tests of comprehension. Both English and ASL elicit strong activation of classical language areas (Wernicke's and Broca's) in native speakers of those languages (Fig. 7.5). In addition, both English and ASL activate the cortex of the angular gyrus, of the anterior and middle superior temporal sulcus, and of several dorsolateral prefrontal areas. In deaf, late learners of English, English activates only areas on the right hemisphere. ASL activates those areas of the nondominant hemisphere in all signers. Evidently, as we saw in the previous section, early in life the two languages de-

Written English

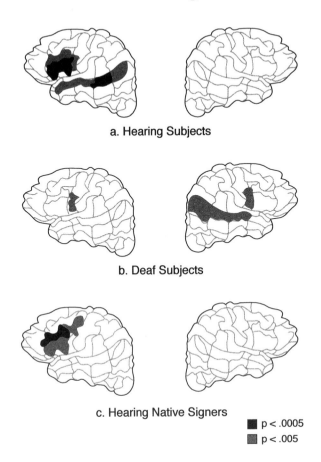

a. Hearing Subjects

b. Deaf Subjects

c. Hearing Native Signers

■ p < .0005
▒ p < .005

Figure 7.5A. Cortical areas activated by English sentences (vs. nonwords) for each subject group (see text). From Neville et al. (1998), slightly modified, with permission.

velop the cognitive substrate for language in the left hemisphere. Apparently as a result of experience, that substrate grows to include associative convergence areas in that same hemisphere (dominant). By repeated association, the semantic cognits in these areas become multimodal and heterarchical (Chapter 5). In signers, the learning of ASL recruits from the beginning areas of both the left and right hemispheres that are involved in processing the visual and motor information essential to this language. With learning, the use of this in-

American Sign Language

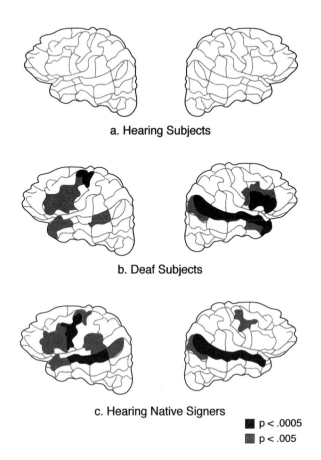

a. Hearing Subjects

b. Deaf Subjects

c. Hearing Native Signers

■ p < .0005
▨ p < .005

Figure 7.5B. Cortical areas activated by ASL sentences (vs. nonsigns) for each subject group (see text). From Neville et al. (1998), slightly modified, with permission.

formation presumably shapes the cognits that come to represent it in perceptual and executive memory.

In conclusion, as far as can be determined by clinical and functional data, the semantic substrate of language contains an essential core of cortical areas around the Sylvian fissure of the left hemisphere, including Broca's and Wernicke's (the latter, by narrow definition, is the posterior half of area 22). The synaptic and connective architecture of these areas is probably determined genetically to accommodate the elements of semantics and syntax of language. Perhaps in the neonate these areas support the primitive form of vocalization called *babbling*. Pulvermüller (1992) speculates that, on the neural base of that primitive form of vocalization, networks are successively formed to represent syllables, words, and syntax. That progressive process of network formation would occur in accord with hebbian principles, as discussed in Chapters 2 and 3.

With experience, the networks emanating from the core language areas would establish associations with higher cognitive networks in association cortex of the posterior and frontal regions. Thus, expanding into the higher cortex of both hemispheres, the networks would be established to constitute the lexical and semantic base of language. Failure of those networks to develop, even in the face of a relatively well-developed cognitive structure, would result in certain selective disorders of language. One such disorder is *dyslexia*, which has long been considered a developmental deficit. A recent PET study (Paulesu et al., 2001) substantiates the diminished proportions of the cortical networks that are activated by reading in dyslexics from three different countries (Fig. 7.6). Despite differences in lexical background, all three groups show the "shrinkage"—compared with normal subjects—of frontal, parietal, and temporal areas of the left hemisphere implicated in the processing of language.

Earlier, with regard to perception (Chapter 4) and memory (Chapter 5), I noted that in higher—that is, conceptual—levels of cortical association, cognits adopt schematic or symbolic form. They become categorical prototypes of the classes of cognitive experiences they represent. Their networks link neuronal assemblies and networks that represent lower classes of cognits. At those levels, as at others below in the perceptual and motor hierarchies, cognitive networks develop by associations of co-occurrence and similarity. Interlevel connections (convergent and divergent) mediate the formation of progressively higher, more *abstract cognits*. In this manner, the cognitive networks of conceptual cortex develop, bottom-up, over lower-level networks that represent their common features as well as repeated experiences with common features. Thus, the networks of conceptual cortex come to represent, in symbolic or schematic form, the most abstract categories of cognition: symbolic percepts in transmodal posterior cortex and schemas of action in prefrontal cortex. In all cortical areas of association, however, there is considerable topographical overlap between the networks that represent abstract cate-

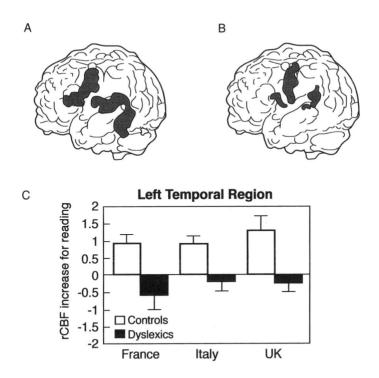

Figure 7.6. Areas activated during reading in normal and dyslexic readers from three countries. *A:* Normal controls. *B:* Dyslexics. *C:* Graphic display of activation differences between controls and dyslexics. (rCBF, regional cerebral blood flow). From Paulesu et al. (2001), modified, with permission.

gories and those that represent their more concrete constituents (Price et al., 1999). As in our model of perceptual organization (Chapter 4), and in many models of the conceptual information that governs language (e.g., Allport, 1985), the distribution of concepts and their constituents depends on the sensory or motor modality of their origin (Fig. 7.7).

The upward formation of higher cognitive categories in cortex of association is probably accompanied by the formation, also by associative principles, of a parallel *lexical-semantic system* of neural networks. This second, parallel system of networks would represent the words for the corresponding cognitive categories of equivalent hierarchical rank. The two systems, cognitive and lexical, would develop alongside each other and intertwined with each other. Thus, there would be a lexical hierarchy of verbal symbols alongside and inter-

Non-linguistic attribute-domains

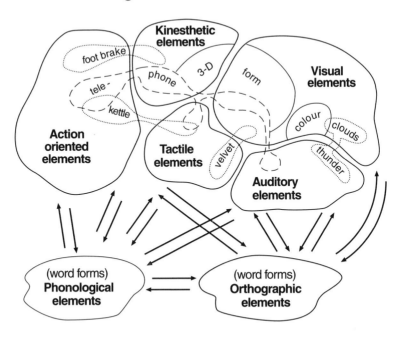

Figure 7.7. Diagram illustrating how concepts of objects *(dotted and dashed outlines)* may be represented by association across representational domains for sensory and motor attributes. Similarly, word forms may be represented by association across phonological and orthographic domains. From Allport (1985), slightly modified, with permission.

twined with the perceptual memory hierarchy, and a comparable action-related lexical hierarchy in parallel with the executive hierarchy. Both pairs of lexical and cognitive hierarchies, perceptual and executive, would develop side by side and upward, from the specific to the general, from the concrete to the abstract. With their upward expansion, both would become progressively more widely distributed, each with varying degrees of associative strength between component assemblies. Both would contain, at various levels and between levels, nodes of heavy convergence and representation (Fig. 7.8). Because of their parallel, overlapping structures, the two systems, cognitive and lexical, would coexist in the same areas of cortex and would activate each other. Thus, the lexical system would activate the cognitive system and vice versa. In many cognitive operations, one

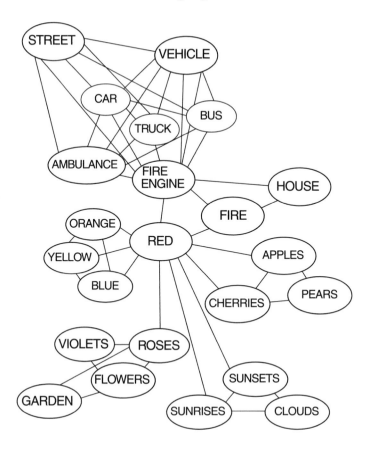

Figure 7.8. Schematic model of representations of word meaning. Each node represents a concept and is linked to other nodes by semantic associations. From Collins and Loftus (1975), with permission.

system could stand for the other: the cognitive for the lexical and the lexical for the cognitive. These theoretical propositions receive considerable support from the observation that the cortical areas activated by pictures of objects are the same ones activated by the words that symbolize them (Vandenberghe et al., 1996).

In conclusion, then, we can reasonably hypothesize a lexical system that represents perceptual cognits in posterior cortex and executive cognits in frontal cortex. At lower levels of the perceptual hierarchy, symbols represent elementary phonemes (letters and syllables) and the names for sensory qualia. A collateral system might develop by associative principles to represent digits and numerical values

(Polk and Farah, 1998). At higher levels, words represent progressively more complex and conceptual cognits. By similar reasoning, the cortex of the frontal lobe contains a hierarchy of symbolic representations *of and for action*. At the bottom of that hierarchy, in Broca's and neighboring cortices, the function words are represented (articles, prepositions, etc.), which are crucial for syntax and which are missing in the expressions of Broca's aphasics. At higher levels of the frontal executive hierarchy, in ample networks of premotor and prefrontal cortices, verbs and action words are represented that symbolize higher cognits of action. Only further functional research can validate these assumptions.

Cortical Dynamics of Syntax

The word *syntax* derives from the Greek verb *syntassein,* which means to join or put together. Thus, the source of the word is an active, transitive verb. The word and its origin imply an agent. To the grammarian, of course, the agent is the speaker or writer, who arranges words in sentences according to a set of rules. To us here, the agent is the brain of the speaker or writer. How does the brain, in accord with those rules, impart order to the structure of phrases and sentences to give them precise meaning? The thesis of this section is that the ordering function of syntax is largely the work of the cortex of the frontal lobe—thus, an agent within an agent within an agent.

The order of syntax is a *temporal order.* The speaker or writer provides meaning to sentences by ordering words in the temporal domain. That temporal ordering is the essence of syntax. Semantics and lexicon provide the elements to be ordered for meaning. Prosody is an important coadjutant. Our basic problem here, therefore, is to understand how cognits and verbal symbols, which have the distributed cortical topography we outlined earlier, are timely selected and ordered to impart meaning (deep structure) to language. The critical question, then, is how spatial order in the brain is converted into temporal order in language. That conversion is what Lashley (1951) called "the translation from the spatial distribution of memory traces to temporal sequence."

Let me briefly review the *brain space of syntax* as it can be gleaned by the analysis of aphasias. Of course, analyzing aphasias and their brain pathology cannot yield understanding of brain function in syntax, but it can identify the main players. Such kinds of analysis, as we have seen, unmistakably identify Broca's area and the surrounding opercular cortex as one of those players. The most characteristic trouble of Broca's aphasic is the inability to make syntax, a deficit that Zurif et al. (1972) characterized as the "central syntactic deficit." This deficit lies not in the absence of temporal order per se but, more basically, in the absence of lexical elements that are indispensable parts of that order. Without them the proper relationships between words cannot be established in an orderly way. Most obviously missing are the function words (*the, a, but, over, before, as, in, though,* etc.) and the inflexions, prefixes, and suffixes of content words. The result is agrammatical and scarcely productive speech. Aphasics with premotor or cingulate lesions—barring a large injury that leads to mutism—are verbally more productive, but their syntax is limited to the formation of short, simple, and automatic speech. In addition, that speech lacks spontaneity and prosody.

Less conspicuous is the speech disorder of the prefrontal patient (*dynamic aphasia* of Luria), which may result from extensive injury to either hemisphere. Here the capacity to *propositionise* (Jackson, 1958) is compromised. The patient's speech is superficial and structurally weak, with few dependent clauses or subtle qualifications. The syntax may be essentially correct, but it is rarely utilized to bridge substantial gaps of time or of associated meaning. The underlying syntactic disorder of the prefrontal syndrome transcends language, however. After careful analysis of frontal-lobe patients' behavior as well as language, Luria (1966) concluded that the disorder lay in the capacity to organize behavior. He did, however, attribute to language, in some kind of internalized form, a crucial role in organization. That role of the prefrontal cortex in the temporal organization of behavior has now been extensively documented not only in the human but also in the nonhuman primate (review in Fuster, 1997). We can, therefore, conclude that the syntactic disorder of the prefrontal patient is an expression of a general disorder of the *syntax of action* (Lashley, 1951).

In brief, the disorders of linguistic expression after frontal lobe damage provide a veiled view of the hierarchical organization of syntactic functions in the lateral cortex of the frontal lobe. In very general terms, it appears that Broca's area plays a key role in elementary grammatical syntax. Conceivably, this role is to some degree innate and thus part of what has been characterized as a universal grammar. It serves to provide cohesion to speech by functional words and proper inflections to related words, at least at the level of the single phrase or simple sentence. Some parts of the premotor cortex, also in the left or dominant hemisphere, seem to provide coordination (praxis) of more complex, though largely routine, automatic speech. The lateral prefrontal cortex, bilaterally, not only constitutes a reservoir of executive cognits (Chapter 5), but also serves as the means to access those cognits in the construction of novel and elaborate language. Its role transcends speech and writing and extends to the temporal organization of behavior in general.

Neurophysiological studies of brain function in speech production are hampered by technical problems, among them the difficulty of screening out movement artifacts. Such studies, however, have been helpful to clarify the cortical dynamics of cognitive functions that mediate language. This dynamics has been discussed in previous chapters with regard to perception, memory, and attention, functions involved in the comprehension and expression of language. The rest of this chapter will be dedicated to a brief discussion of the neural mechanisms supporting two cognitive operations that depend on those functions and that are essential to syntax: (*1*) access to lexicon and (*2*) working memory. Both operate in speaking, reading, and writing. Both involve the cortex of the frontal lobe in a major way.

The purposeful expression of language, like the execution of goal-directed action, is preceded by the mental formulation of a broad plan or schema of the intended production, however simple or ill-defined. Such a plan or schema is probably represented in a cortical network of frontal cortex and is made up of lexical components of executive cognits, notably verbs. That network can be activated by associated inputs from other cortical or subcortical structures or from the environment (e.g., an interlocutor). When it surpasses a certain threshold of activation, that executive-linguistic network will activate lower executive networks, thus initiating the expression of language and the syntactic process. This process requires continued access of frontal networks to the semantic-lexical networks of executive and perceptual cortices. Unless the expression is brief, routine, or well rehearsed, its syntax will continue to require that access until completion of the expression. In my theoretical framework, that access to memory and lexicon implies the associative activation, in an orderly manner, of a set of cognits and their lexical counterparts. Figure 7.9 depicts schematically the orderly interplay of posterior and frontal lexical networks in the syntax of a simple expression.

The efficacy of the frontally driven access of syntax to lexicon de-

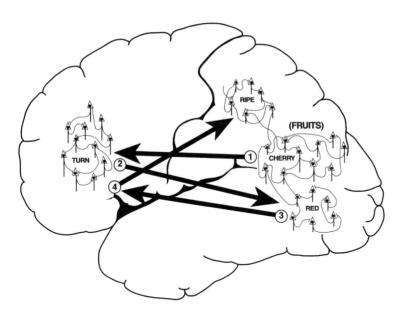

"CHERRIES TURN RED AS THEY GET RIPE"

Figure 7.9. Highly schematic diagram of hypothetical interactions between networks of posterior and frontal cortices in the construction of a simple sentence.

pends on the strength of the connections within and between the lexical networks of association cortex. Each of these networks, when active, will tend to gravitate into *fixed-frequency states*. In those states, its neurons will fire at more or less regular frequencies determined by the recurrent connectivity that constitutes the network. The strength and stability of its fixed-frequency states will determine whether or not at a given time a lexical network enters the syntactic process. Through extrinsic connections, the activation of a semantic network may be primed or facilitated. Thus, the prior or concomitant activation of associated networks may lead to the priming of others in the lexical domain, as in the cognitive retrieval of memory (Chapter 5). Disorders of memory (e.g., dementias) may entail the loss of access to lexical networks and result in paraphasias, that is, in the activation of associated words but not the most appropriate word at the moment. However, whereas a cognit or the word that represents it may appear inaccessible, it may be retrieved by priming through another associated cognit or word (Hagoort, 1998). This explains why amnesics appear to have lost cortical representations when, in reality, they have only lost *access* to them. Comparable processes of access to lexicon probably take place in reading. Here the access to cognits occurs through the visual perception of orthographic and lexical items. Similarities between percepts of either kind may compete for semantic meaning (Fig. 7. 10). Graphic and semantic priming through associated networks may also play a role in the comprehension of the written language. Paralexias or dyslexias may result from faulty connective access to lexicon.

In syntactic construction, frontal networks interact with posterior cortical networks in a continuous interchange. Whereas both frontal and posterior networks provide the lexicon, frontal networks, in addition, provide the grammar. The frontal contribution to syntax takes place at various levels. Broca's cortex contributes the most elementary syntax, whereas higher-level frontal cortices contribute propositional syntax. As the syntactic process is engaged in the integration of longer and more elaborate speech constructions, *working memory* becomes a syntactic function. Syntax is temporal order, and temporal order in speech requires the temporal integrative functions of the frontal cortex. These functions are essentially two, working memory

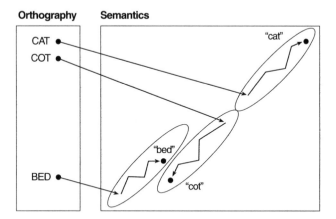

Figure 7.10. Two layers, orthographic and semantic, of a theoretical attractor network for reading. In reading, words are converted from the orthographic layer to topologically corresponding basins of attraction *(ovals)* in semantic space. By certain network operations, each word is drawn to its closest meaning within its basin. Words that are orthographically close (*cat* and *cot*) may compete for distant positions in semantic space. From Plaut and Shallice (1993), slightly modified, with permission.

and preparatory set, both discussed in Chapter 6, as both are forms of attention (one retrospective and the other prospective). Both are prefrontal functions that mediate contingencies across time. In linguistic syntax, working memory plays its role when attention to a word, a phrase, or a sentence needs to be maintained over time for its integration with subsequent expressions. It plays a similar role in the comprehension of language, as it assists in the temporal integration of auditory information across time. Working memory is also necessary in reading and writing, especially when these require the integration of information across substantial text— and time.

In conclusion, the syntax of language shares cortical areas with the integration (the syntax) of actions in nonlinguistic domains. Widely distributed in the same areas, we postulate a system of lexical-semantic networks paralleling the cognitive networks and interacting with them in the syntactic process at all levels of the perceptual and executive hierarchies. At the summit of those hierarchies, the executive networks of the lateral prefrontal cortex interact with lexical-semantic networks in the construction of complex language. Thus, the syntax of such language is the equivalent, in the language domain, of the integrative operation of the *perception-action cycle* in complex behavior and cognition (Chapter 4). That cycle, it will be remembered, is the cybernetic flow of information from the environment, through sensory and motor processing structures, back to the environment in the form of actions; actions produce changes in the environment, which lead to new sensory information, and so on. Also in the case of language, lexical information flows from posterior perceptual cortex into frontal executive cortex, especially in the left or dominant hemisphere, where the information is integrated in time and into linguistic expression in the form of speech or writing. That expression will generate new sensory impressions in the form of self-monitored auditory or visual signals; those sensory impressions may include reactions from the interlocutor. The new sensory information will generate subsequent language, and so on. Thus, the prefrontal cortex, with its temporal integrative function of working memory, plays a crucial role in bridging temporal gaps at the top of the linguistic cycle.

Thus, although we have no direct evidence of the neural mechanisms of syntactic order, the neuropsychology of language disorders that result from brain lesions strongly indicates that the ordering agent is the cortex of the *frontal lobe*. Further, by extrapolating to language what we know of the role of frontal cortex in the temporal organization of sequential actions, the following tentative picture of the cortical dynamics of syntax emerges. In neural terms, the making of syntactic order is hierarchically organized. The most basic syntactic order is established by lower frontal cortex (Broca's and vicinity) interacting with low-level associative cortex, notably auditory (Wernicke's). That interaction ensures the articulation of words and short phrases in essential grammatical order, which includes function words. More complex syntax, with recursiveness and embedded sentences, requires higher frontal cortex, notably prefrontal, in close interaction with posterior cortex of association. Those two cortices contain the lexical-semantic representations that prefrontal cortex accesses and selects for syntax. At that level, syntax is established by the successive mediation of contingencies across time: (1) contingencies between the words in the series and (2) contingencies between words, phrases, and sentences on the one hand and the linguistic schema on the other. The mediation of those contingencies is a function of the perception-action cycle. Syntactic order results from the serial operation of that cycle. By continuous internal and external feedback, the cycle ensures the order of words, phrases, and sentences in accord with the intended meaning.

8

Intelligence

*A*mong the five cognitive functions considered in this monograph, intelligence is the most complex and the most difficult
to define. The complexity derives from the close relationships
between intelligence and all other four functions—perception, memory, attention, and language. All four contribute to intelligence, though
each does it in a different way and to a varying degree, depending on
the individual and the circumstances. The difficulty of defining intelligence derives from the almost infinite variety of its manifestations.
Here it is defined as the ability to adjust by reasoning to new changes,
to solve new problems, and to create valued new forms of action and
expression. This definition is broad enough to reach into the biological roots of cognition, as I have tried to do with every other cognitive
function. At the same time, it is broad enough to reach up to the
heights of human achievement. In both depth and height, the definition suits our goal of identifying the cortical correlates of intelligence. The pertinent data from cognitive neuroscience indicate that
intellectual performance can be best understood as the result of neuronal transactions between perceptual and executive networks of the
cerebral cortex. Because these networks also serve other cognitive
functions, this chapter must deal again, albeit lightly, with some subjects already covered in previous chapters.

Development of Intelligence

Human intelligence is the culmination of the evolution of the cerebral mechanisms dedicated to the adaptation of the organism to its environment. Intelligence thus emerges from biological imperatives and reaches its apogee in the human. Much of the debate about whether or not other animals have intelligence is idle. Surely it can be argued that the appearance of human intelligence constitutes a quantum leap of cognitive evolution. It can also be argued that animals do not have certain intellectual abilities that humans have (abstraction, use of tools, language, etc.). Nonetheless, as prominent scholars and researchers have remarked (e.g., Köhler, 1925; Janet, 1935; Von Frisch, 1993; Tomasello and Call, 1997), it is beyond dispute that animals are capable of intelligent behavior and of certain essential cognitive functions that mediate it. The shepherd's dog displays unquestionable intelligence as it tends to its task of protecting the herd and helping it reach its destination. To the careful observer, that task involves much more than chasing predators and forcing sheep in a certain direction. It involves the use of a spatial map of a commonly rugged terrain, the successive attention to many individual animals, the prediction of their movements, the finding of detours around obstacles for itself and for those less agile animals, and sometimes the selective yielding of logistic responsibilities to other dogs. The fox shows no less intelligence—we may call it guile—as it tries to rob the farmer of his fowl. Further, do not certain insects such as ants or bees display marvelous examples of collaboration, which is the hallmark of social intelligence?

In any case, intelligence is too complicated to be approached by the neuroscientist as a unitary function with a uniquely human make-up. Some of its essential supports consist of such other cognitive functions as attention and memory, which clearly have a cortical substrate in both humans and animals. The monkey that bridges time with working memory for the purpose of integrating information across time is clearly exercising intelligent behavior—and solving a problem. Reasoning may be the outstanding characteristic of human intelligence, but we can hardly altogether deny it to animals. The animal that learns to discriminate and categorize sensory stimuli, extracting from them essential features despite wide variations (perceptual constancy), uses the essentials of both inductive and deductive reasoning. Animals that use their pincers or antennae to reach their sometimes elusive goals can be said to use tools (their own tools!). The same can be said of Sultan, the ape that telescopes two bamboo canes into each other to reach a banana (Köhler, 1925).

In more general terms, to attribute intelligence only to humans is to ignore its profound biological foundation. It is to ignore not only that intelligence has a biological origin, but also that the development of human intelligence has occurred in a continuum of evolving means to adapt to the world. The study of the development of intelligence is in many respects the study of the development of adaptive behavior. In the human, however, adaptation to the world involves, even requires, the pursuit of goals that transcend the individual and that are based on the processing of large amounts of information extending over large expanses of space and time. Much of that information consists of existing cortical cognits, and the processing of those cognits is the essence of goal-directed reasoning and behavior. Thus, in principle, the development of human intelligence is the development of cortical cognitive networks and of the efficiency with which they process information. This was a subject of previous chapters with regard to the cognitive functions that support intelligence; it is now the subject of this section with regard to the more global function they support.

If intelligence is the processing of cognitive information toward cognitive or behavioral goals, the degree of intelligence is the *efficiency* with which it can process that information. Efficiency, therefore, refers here to the ability to use available means, including prior knowledge, to attain a goal such as the solution of a problem. Hence the emphasis of intelligence tests on the efficiency of performance, although such tests notoriously ignore certain forms of knowledge and the ways to handle it. In evolution, animals have become progressively more efficient at processing more information in the pursuit of their goals. As intelligence tests show, the same thing is true for a human in his or her formative years.

In phylogeny as well as ontogeny, the development of intelligence is closely correlated with the development of the cerebral cortex, in particular those cortical areas that are designated *cortex of association*. This assumption is mainly based on (*1*) the large evolutionary expansion ("explosion") of the cerebral cortex in the species with the highest cognitive ability, especially the human primate, and (*2*) the ontogenetic parallelism between the maturation of cortical areas, especially the areas of association, and the development of cognitive ability. In human adults, however, rigorous studies have failed to show any clear correlation between measures of intelligence and measures of cortical structure, either at the microscopic or the macroscopic level. This lack of correlation can be attributed to either of two factors, or both. First, the measures of intelligence may be flawed. Second, the structural measures fail to reflect the true structure of intelligence, as this may reside in imponderable elements of cortical circuitry (e.g., synaptic density). Thus, by contemporary methods of measurement, the cortex of the genius does not differ significantly from that of the average human being.

Nonetheless, the study of intellectual development in the child provides valuable insights into the adaptive nature of intelligence, its hierarchical organization, and the parallel development of the cortical organization that supports it. Probably no one has had a more decisive impact in this field of study than Jean Piaget (1952), especially in Europe. His lesser impact in American developmental psychology is probably attributable in large part to the mostly observational character of his work. It makes little use of statistics, thus incurring the criticism of lack of rigor from experimentalists who rely only on quantification for the assessment of psychological functions. A further target of criticism has been his emphasis on the verbal aspects of intellectual development, with perceived neglect of its behavioral aspects. In later years, however, his approach included increasing attention to behavior (Inhelder and Piaget, 1958). That approach is fundamentally genetic in that intelligent language and behavior are analyzed as expressions of innate tendencies in a growth continuum (Halford, 1993).

According to Piaget, the intellect of the child undergoes four distinct stages of development, each within a well-defined period of chronological age. The first, between birth and 2 years, is the *sensory–motor* stage. In it, the child learns to integrate complex sensations and movements, thus extending in terms of complexity the basic adaptive reflexes present at birth. During that stage, the child begins to form schemata of sensory–motor integration, that is, of motor reactions to objects in the immediate environment. Symbolic expressions of such schemata begin to appear in the form of brief stereotypical pantomimes. The second stage, from 2 to 7, is the *representational* stage, in which the child extends the use of symbolism to the verbal domain in order to represent the external world. Manipulation of objects becomes progressively more regulated by feedback and by trial and error. The feedback includes progressively more language from other persons. The third stage, from 7 to 11, is that of *concrete operations*. In it, the child becomes less *stimulus-bound* and more capable of independently organizing the means—including language—toward goals. Improvisation and creation make their appearance or increase markedly. This is the period of erector sets, skillful games and sports, and the onset of artistic and problem-solving abilities. The fourth, from 11 to 15, is the stage of *formal operations*. Now the child begins to utilize hypothetical reasoning and to test alternatives. Both inductive and deductive logic flourish. The means to a goal become more numerous and more complex. Most important, the child becomes capable of temporally integrating information, and thus capable of constructing temporal gestalts of logical thought and action toward distant goals. Language has now become essential for the formulation of propositions in the construction of those goal-directed gestalts.

Although in general terms it is methodologically useful, Piaget's scheme needs several important qualifications prescribed by later work. His structuralist approach, based on the development of progressively higher constructs (categories) of perception and sensory–motor integration, is insufficient cognitively and neurobiologically. For one thing, it needs to incorporate *inhibition* in the first stage of development (Houdé, 2000). In other words, it requires the exclusionary aspect of attention (Chapter 6) that we deem essential for the formation of percepts, memories, and patterns of relation with the world. The development of logical constructs in the child, as in the adult, must proceed pari passu with the development of inhibitory suppression of distracting sensory inputs, of alternate constructs (or hypotheses), and of conceptually competing categorizations. For another thing, there is increasing evidence that children can reason with numbers at a much earlier age than Piaget and others had concluded (Dehaene and Changeux, 1993; Houdé, 2000).

Nonetheless, in the properly qualified developmental scenario outlined by Piaget, it is easy to intuit the sequential engagement of progressively higher levels of a *hierarchy* of neural structures that are dedicated to the integration of cognits and actions. In other words, the stages of development of the child's intellect readily suggest the recruitment of increasingly higher levels of integration. It appears that, at the appropriate age, the neural substrate for a given developmental stage takes over the integrative functions of others that supported cognition in previous stages. That taking-over may not necessarily involve the suppression of lower levels but, rather, their subordination to the neural structures of higher levels in the pursuit of higher goals. In the process, whereas some constituents of those lower levels may be inhibited, others may be used to contribute the integration of the more automatic actions to the higher gestalt of behavior, language, or logical thinking.

The serial recruitment of hierarchically organized neural structures in the cognitive development of the child can be best understood in the context of the *perception-action cycle* (Chapters 4 and 6). This is the circular processing of information between posterior and frontal cortices (Fig. 4.7) in the integration of sensory–motor behavior, as well as in higher cognitive activities such as language. A posterior tier of hierarchically organized associative sensory areas is reciprocally connected with a corresponding frontal tear of associative motor areas. In the integration of behavioral or cognitive actions, a continuous flow of neural processing takes place through and between those areas at various hierarchical levels. Goal-directed actions of progressively higher complexity are integrated at progressively higher levels of the cortical hierarchies of the cycle. The feedforward integration of those actions is assisted by continuous feedback signals from the environment through posterior (sensory) areas. These signals provide frontal areas with the necessary inputs for monitoring action sequences to the attainment of their goal. Reciprocally connected at the top of the perception-action cycle, it will be recalled, are the lateral prefrontal cortex and posterior cortical areas of polymodal sensory association. It is through that connectivity at the top that the prefrontal cortex plays its temporal integrative role in the construction of novel plans of behavior. It is also through that connectivity, as well as through outputs to lower motor structures, that prefrontal cortex controls the execution of those plans.

At every stage of intellectual development, therefore, it would appear that a higher level of the perception-action cycle is brought into play. It is reasonable to suppose that the onset of participation of each level of the cycle occurs with, and as a result of, the *structural maturation* of its areas (Chapters 2 and 3). The operations of sensory–motor integration of the first stage (birth to 2 years) are supported by subcortical structures, as well as sensory and motor cortices. At the representational stage (2 to 7), the child experiences an enormous growth of his or her cognitive fund. This growth probably involves the formation of a vast array of new cognits in posterior cortex, notably the symbolic cognits of language. The stage of concrete operations (7

to 11) undoubtedly engages the circuitry between areas of sensory association and premotor cortex, as well as between higher polysensory
and prefrontal areas. These areas, which are of late maturation, most
assuredly intervene in the cognitive operations of the fourth stage (11
to 15), when their role becomes crucial for the integration of complex structures of behavior, reasoning, and language. It is the functional cooperation of cognits at the top of the perception-action cycle
that enables the formation of intricate behavioral sequences, logical
constructs, and elaborate sentences. That functional cooperation
takes place under the control of the prefrontal cortex. Therein lies
the reason not only for the developmental correlation of intelligence
with prefrontal maturation, but also for the large phylogenetic expansion of the prefrontal cortex (Fig. 8.1).

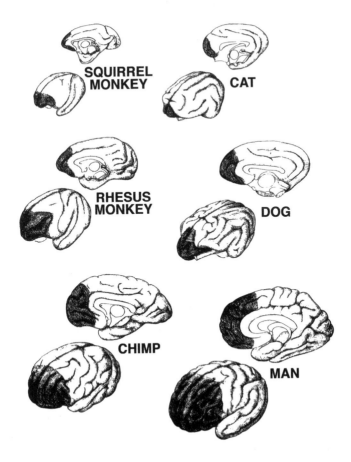

Figure 8.1. The prefrontal cortex *(shaded)* in six species.

Anatomy of Intelligence

Like every other cognitive function, intelligence has both a *structural anatomy* and a *functional anatomy*. The first consists of the individual's base of knowledge, that is, the aggregate of cortical cognits or networks acquired by experience. The second consists of those cortical cognits that at a given time process knowledge in the exercise of intellectual activity. The first substrate is subject to individual variations, the second to variations that depend on the type of intellectual activity that the individual exercises at a given time. Confusion between the two substrates and their sources of variance leads to errors or contradictions in many of the attempts to identify the neural correlates of intelligence.

We need not belabor the correlation between the growth of information storage capacity of the cerebral cortex and the measures of its phylogenetic and ontogenetic development. In human adults, however, the correlation between information storage capacity and cortical structure is questionable, except in cases of severe mental retardation or general cognitive deficit from extensive cortical malformation, disease, or trauma. This is true whether the structural measurements are made at the macroscopic or the microscopic level. It is possible that the correlation exists, but at a level of analysis inaccessible by current methods. All the evidence we have about the cortical anatomy of the fund of knowledge derives from physiological and neuropsychological studies in monkeys and humans. That evidence pertains to the *distribution by areas* of the different categories of cognits, as discussed in Chapters 3, 4, and 5. With regard to the lexical aspects of cognition, it has been discussed in the previous chapter.

What I have called the functional anatomy of intelligence is very different from the cortical fund of knowledge or structural anatomy, though the two overlap to some degree. The reason for the overlap is that the first (function) always uses part of the second (structure) — the computer analogy is compelling. The cortical topography of functioning intelligence, that is, the part of the cognitive fund engaged at any given time in intellectual dynamics, depends strictly on the kind of information under process at that time. Before discussing the neural aspects of that dynamics, let us briefly consider the forms of intellectual performance commonly investigated by cognitive scientists. Sternberg (1985) proposes a useful classification: (*1*) *analytical* intelligence, based essentially on reasoning; (*2*) *practical* intelligence, based on problem-solving abilities largely acquired by ordinary life experience; and (*3*) *creative* intelligence, based on conceiving, imagination, and intuition. There is considerable interaction, overlap, and trade-off between those three kinds of intelligence. Individual humans vary with regard to the use and command of each. Only the first two, analytical and practical intelligence, lend themselves to measurement by intelligence tests. Because these tests are often used in neuroscience, it seems useful to consider briefly their general features and constraints.

Since 1905, when Binet issued his famous test for French schoolchildren, a variety of psychometric instruments have been developed to measure intelligence. Most of them are intended to rate intelligence with reference to standardized scales of a person's *mental age*— from which, in combination with chronological age, the intelligence quotient or IQ derives. Intelligence tests have been used principally for scholastic and clinical purposes. In the United States, the tests most widely used are the Stanford-Binet and the Wechsler-Bellvue, the latter with two versions, the Wechsler Intelligence Scale for Children (WISC) and the Wechsler Adult Intelligence Scale (WAIS). Some tests challenge mainly reasoning and others problem solving. Some challenge mainly verbal intelligence and others performance (including motor skills). In addition to testing intellectual performance, all test to some degree the subject's fund of knowledge. None is culture-free. Because most measures of intellectual ability tend to correlate with one another, many attempts have been made to extract a common factor that could serve as a measure of *general intelligence.* From several metrics, including a test devised by him for that purpose, Spearman (1927) derived such a factor, which he called the *g-factor.* The g-factor can also be derived by factor analysis from many tests currently in use, notably the Raven's Progressive Matrices (RPM) test (Raven, 1941), an analytical test of so-called "fluid intelligence" which is relatively exempt of linguistic influences. (The term *fluid intelligence* is commonly used to characterize the performance of tasks that require manipulation of novel information, whereas *crystallized intelligence* refers mostly to tasks—commonly verbal—that are performed by retrieval of existing knowledge from long-term memory.) The RPM test has been used in a number of studies of the neural dynamics of analytical intelligence.

Attention is the cognitive function most critical to intellectual performance, certainly in reasoning, problem solving, and creative language. Thus the cortical physiology of intelligence largely coincides with the cortical physiology of attention (Chapter 6). This appears especially true at high levels of the cognitive organization of the neocortex. At those levels, intelligence, like attention, ensures the selective allocation of cognits to the processing of information in new situations, as in the solution of new problems. Both attention and intelligence rely heavily on the executive networks of the prefrontal cortex. On the one hand, as we saw in Chapter 6, prefrontal networks provide attentive control to posterior cortices, which is necessary for the selection of perceptual cognits in intellectual performance. On the other, prefrontal networks play a crucial role in working memory, the sustained attention to selected cognits that is a pivotal element of the brain mechanisms of temporal integration in reasoning, problem solving, and other intelligent operations.

The study of the electrocortical correlates of intellectual performance yields only a sketchy picture of the engagement of cortical networks in that performance. There appears to be a relationship between IQ and the presence of frequencies in the upper alpha range (12–20 Hz) of the cortical EEG (Martindale and Hines, 1975; Vogel and Schalt, 1979; Earle, 1988; Wszolek et al., 1992). After extensive parametric analysis of electrocortical variables at rest and during the performance of an intelligence test, one study (Anokhin et al., 1999) concludes that coherence in the theta range, between frontal and posterior cortical areas, is the most consistent correlate of cognitive abilities. In general, therefore, it seems that intellectual capacity and performance are associated with the tendency to *synchronicity* in wide cortical areas. This general inference agrees with the notion of reentrant activity in the cortical networks that support intelligence.

Neuroimaging provides abundant evidence of the activation of prefrontal networks in intellectual performance. A review of a large number of studies (Duncan and Owen, 2000) indicates that the performance of a variety of behavioral tasks (perceptual difficulty, novelty, working memory, etc.) is accompanied by the activation of the anterior cingulate cortex as well as the cortex of the lateral prefrontal convexity. The close analysis of those tasks reveals that they all share the attention and temporal-integration requirements for which those two cortices have been shown essential (Chapter 6). Both attention and temporal integration are at the foundation of intellectual performance and of the role of the prefrontal cortex in it. On the basis of neuropsychological work (Duncan et al., 1995), it has been proposed (Duncan et al., 1996) that this role can best be characterized as one of general intelligence, as defined and measured by Spearman's statistic, the g-factor. The g-factor is common to many of the tasks that are impaired by a prefrontal lesion and that activate the prefrontal cortex in the normal subject.

To further test by functional means the role of the prefrontal cortex in general intelligence, Duncan et al. (2000) devised several problem-solving tasks assumed to be high in g-factor and investigated cerebral blood flow (by PET) during their performance (Fig. 8.2). Their study revealed that, as predicted, those tasks activated areas of

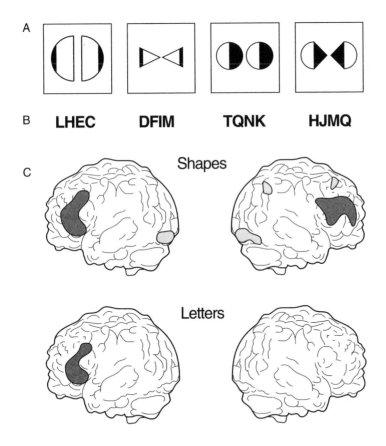

Figure 8.2. Cortical activation in problem-solving tasks challenging general intelligence (g-factor). *A:* Example of a spatial problem (find the set of shapes that does not belong with the other three; answer, item 3, asymmetrical). *B:* Example of a letter-order problem (find the letter set that does not belong with the other three; answer, item 3, different alphabetical progression). *C:* General intelligence tasks (such as *A* and *B*) induce prefrontal activation. From Duncan et al. (2000), modified, with permission.

lateral prefrontal cortex. From this observation, the authors concluded that these areas contributed the general intelligence (g-factor) critical for performance of the tasks. However, whereas this inference may be correct for the executive side of intelligence, the results do not exclude a contribution to intellectual performance from dispersed perceptual cognits of posterior cortex. The probable contribution of active posterior networks to intellectual performance may have a more widely distributed base than that of executive frontal networks and, thus, may have passed undetected by the threshold set for detecting changes in cerebral blood flow. In other words, the prefrontal activations may reflect the contribution to intellectual performance by executive networks near the common output path of cortical cognition. The contributions of perceptual cognits, on the other hand, may originate in more widely distributed networks whose activation eludes detection by imaging methods.

Reasoning

Reasoning is the formation of new knowledge from prior knowledge, that is, the making of new cognits with existing cognits. The new cognits, which are called *inferences,* may derive exclusively from preexisting knowledge or from both preexisting knowledge and new or recent sensory information. This definition of reasoning includes logical thinking, both deductive and inductive, and a wide range of cognitive operations, from reflexive unconscious reasoning to formal mathematics. The cognitive science of reasoning is dominated by two major methodologies: one is symbolic, propositional, or *linguistic,* and the other is nonpropositional or *connectionist.* The first methodology is predicated on the linguistic formalization of all knowledge and on the rule-based utilization of learned symbols. The second is predicated on the fast, expert, and spontaneous processing of information through preestablished cognitive networks. According to connectionist models, this processing takes place within each network mostly in parallel, along many channels at the same time.

The brain mechanisms of reasoning are not known, but it seems increasingly evident that both forms of processing, linguistic and connectionist, are compatible with each other and with the available facts of neuroscience. The human brain obviously uses both. Much as the construction of language relies on the interplay of lexical and cognitive networks (Chapter 7), reasoning probably does too. The linguistic–

connectionist polarity is another of those pairs of opposing positions in cognitive neuroscience that can be reconciled by the concept of neural transactions at several levels in a hierarchy of organized cortical cognits. Both the linguistic and the connectionist approaches have led to interesting models of the functional architecture of reasoning in the cortex. Some of these models have considerable neural plausibility, in that they accommodate a number of known facts of cortical anatomy, physiology and dysfunction.

Symbolic models of reasoning, as have been proposed in the field of AI, are usually characterized by an executive processing unit or *agent* of some sort. That agent contains a plan to control successive stages of the processing of symbols (words) and propositions, which are intelligible at every stage. All the processing takes place in accord with a preestablished set of rules. Connectionist models, on the other hand, postulate neither a central executive nor a set of rules. Knowledge is distributed among many units of the cognitive network. The process of reasoning occurs in parallel through nodes of those units connected to one another as a result of the prior operation of learning principles at synapses. In the reasoning process, numerical values are passed through the system from unit to unit in close dependence on synaptic weight or another such variable or variables of transmissibility between units.

The simplest form of reasoning is *reflexive reasoning*. It consists of the rapid, automatic, and effortless drawing of inferences from a given situation with the assistance of a large permanent store of knowledge. This kind of reasoning, akin to intuitive fast-acting common sense, pervades all intelligent living. Every day our brains process a huge amount of information in that manner. Our lives are in reality guided by innumerable inferences drawn instantly from current situations and prior experience, without our being conscious of either the antecedents or the consequents of that covert reasoning. Nothing is known about the cerebral mechanisms of reflexive reasoning, though several attempts have been made to explain it in neural terms. One of the most appealing attempts is the one by Shastri and Ajjanagadde (1993). Their model is essentially connectionist, but contains certain features that make it applicable to propositional, rule-guided, symbolic reasoning. Its architecture consists of a large network that encodes millions of facts in its patterns of connectivity. In that network, facts have units and nodes in common. Together with the facts, also encoded in patterns of connectivity, is a set of elementary rules of in-

ference, which make the system in effect capable of deductive reasoning. From that large conglomerate of facts and rules, inferences are
drawn in a few hundred milliseconds by a process of rapid propagation of dynamic bindings within the network. Such bindings consist
of the synchronous activation of groups of representational nodes.
Reasoning is the transient propagation of rhythmic patterns of activity through the system, each pattern representing an item of knowledge. The essence of the reasoning process is the matching of incoming temporal patterns to those patterns inherent in subnetworks
that represent specific long-term facts. That process of rapid matching is governed by the rules of contingency embedded in the system.

   A model such as the one just outlined is consonant not only with
our view of cortical cognits and of the operations between cognits,
but also with the matching of reality to cognits that we have seen at
the root of several of those operations (e.g., perception, recognition,
attentive search). Binding, in that model as in ours, refers to the selective activation of all the neural elements that by prior association
have come to represent an object, a fact, or a proposition. Further,
that activation is accompanied by certain regularities in the patterns
of discharge of those neural elements. There is a basic difference,
however, between the reflexive-reasoning model outlined and ours.
In that model, the information in process is encoded by hypothesized
regularities in unit firing. In our model, that information is encoded
by the architecture of the network, in other words, by a spatial (i.e.,
connective) pattern in brain space; the firing regularities derive from
the activation of that architecture, that is, from the characteristics of
its intrinsic circuitry.

   Almost without exception, computational models of cognitive
function, like the reasoning model above, become implausible at the
level of the specific neural mechanism and its algorithms. There are
two reasons for this. One is the sparcity, in those models, of empirically established assumptions of cortical biophysics. The second reason is the imposition on the models of assumptions that are based on
questionable interpretations of neural data. One example of a questionable interpretation leading to a questionable assumption is the
attribution of a temporal code to the periodic oscillations of cell firing observed in animals during cognitive performance. The significance of such oscillations was discussed in Chapters 4 and 6, where
they were considered unlikely to constitute that kind of code.

   Johnson-Laird (1995) has proposed a view of deductive reasoning similar in some respects to the one presented above with respect

to reflexive reasoning. His theory also incorporates an idea akin to that of matching cognits to reality. He postulates that deductive reasoning essentially consists of the construction of multiple *mental models* of reality. Model construction, which in his theory includes the formation of spatial relations, is nonverbal and nonpropositional, although propositional representations may enter the process as an ancillary means to the making of models. Thus, in the reasoning process, the human mind tests multiple alternative models, as well as the consequences of their assumptions, against reality. Because the process is largely nonverbal, the theory predicts that the construction and testing of models take place, for the most part, in nonverbal processing areas of the cortex. Some support for this prediction can be found in the evidence (Chapter 7) that lesions of right-hemisphere cortex lead to disorders of nonverbal—for example, spatial—aspects of reasoning (Caramazza et al., 1976; Zaidel et al., 1981).

Recent studies of functional imaging, however, uphold the linguistic and propositional nature of all *deductive reasoning* and the role in it of the language areas of the left hemisphere. The evidence from these studies is also in agreement with the neuropsychological findings of some lesion studies (Gazzaniga, 1985; Deglin and Kinsbourne, 1996). Goel et al. (1998) had their subjects perform three kinds of deductive reasoning tasks (syllogism, spatial relational inference, and nonspatial relational inference). In all three tasks, the subject had to inspect three propositions and decide (by pressing a button) if the third followed logically from the first two. Table 8.1 shows examples of the propositions used by the authors in the three tasks and presented to the subject on a computer monitor. Three baseline control tasks were used, each requiring judgments about the semantic content of the sentences, but without any logical requirement. While the subjects performed the tasks, cortical metabolic activity was assessed by means of PET with oxygen-labeled water. Activity in each baseline task was subtracted from activity in the corresponding reasoning task. The subtraction results revealed that the three conditions of deductive reasoning induced the relative activation of areas in the left hemisphere only (Fig. 8.3). Those areas included portions of the inferior and middle frontal gyri and portions of temporal and anterior cingulate cortex. No significant right-hemisphere or parietal activation was observed. These results are remarkable because they indicate (*1*) the intimate coexistence, if not identity, of the cortical substrates for language and deductive reasoning; (*2*) the activation of language areas, and not spatial-processing areas, in spatial reasoning; and (*3*) the

Table 8.1. Example Stimuli used by
Goel et al. (1998)

Syllogism

Some officers are generals.
No privates are generals.
Some officers are not privates.

Spatial Relational

Officers are standing next to generals.
Privates are standing behind generals.
Privates are standing behind officers.

Nonspatial Relational

Officers are heavier than generals.
Generals are heavier than privates.
Privates are lighter than officers.

sharing of the same cortical substrate by spatial and nonspatial reasoning. Exceptionally strong activation of dorsolateral prefrontal cortex during syllogistic reasoning indicates the heavy involvement of
this cortex in the integrative demands of this form of reasoning.

It is unlikely, nonetheless, that the language areas of the left
hemisphere are the only ones involved in deductive reasoning. Other
areas of either hemisphere may participate in it, albeit with more
subtle and time-limited contributions that escape detection by imaging methods. A more recent study (Houdé et al., 2000), while supporting some of the essential findings of the one just described, provides a more dynamic picture of cortical reasoning and of the
participation of those other areas in it. Above all, this study, which is
briefly described below, provides evidence of the critical role that *inhibition* plays in reasoning, as it does in every other cognitive function.
Earlier in this chapter, in the section on development, I mentioned
the putative function of the perception-action cycle at the summit of
the hierarchical organization of intelligence. As noted in Chapters 4
and 6, the feedback connections from frontal to posterior cortical regions serve that cycle by providing monitoring and inhibitory control
over the perceptual sector of cognition. The inhibitory control at the
top of the perception-action cycle would thus play in that sector of
cognition the exclusionary role of attention, suppressing the competing percepts and inferences that interfere with current reasoning.

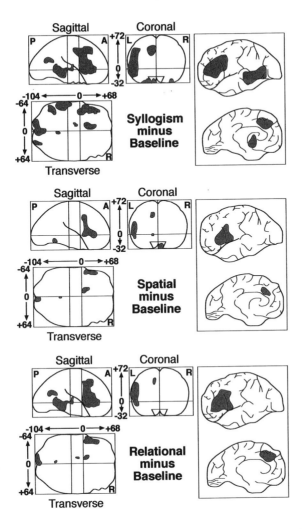

Figure 8.3. PET activation during the three reasoning tasks explained in the text and in Table 8.1. *In the left and middle columns,* relative increases in rCBF are shown in standard cross-sectional projections of statistically estimated activation. *In the right column,* the activations are shown in surface images of the left hemisphere (Talairach map). From Goel et al. (1998), modified, with permission.

That inhibitory control can be enhanced by training, and such training is the critical variable in the study by Houdé and his colleagues. Here the subject performs a reasoning task with colored geometrical forms arranged in pairs (left-right). The task is guided by a logical rule that prescribes certain color-form-position combinations (e.g., "if not the red square on the left, then the yellow circle on the right") and forbids others as illogical. Untrained subjects commit nu-

merous errors of matching due to incorrect perceptual bias from mis-
interpreting the rule (e.g., ignoring the negation). They strongly
tend to succumb to a systematic matching bias (Evans, 1998). With
appropriate training—to develop a *logical bias*—they overcome that
perceptual bias, and their performance rapidly improves. By functional imaging, Houdé et al. (2000) demonstrate that the logical
training of a subject induces marked displacement of the activation
of the cortex during performance of the task from posterior (i.e, perceptual) areas to frontal (i.e., executive) areas (Fig. 8.4). The authors

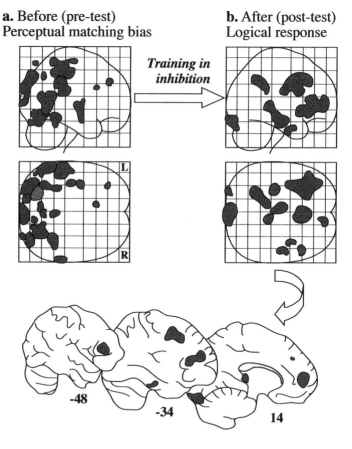

a. Before (pre-test)
Perceptual matching bias

b. After (post-test)
Logical response

*Training in
inhibition*

Figure 8.4. Regions activated (increased rCBF) during a rule falsification task (see
text) in two conditions: (*a*) before training in inhibition of perceptual bias and
(*b*) after training in inhibition of perceptual bias. *Top:* Statistical Z maps of activation. *Bottom:* Sagittal views of regional clusters of activation after training. Note
the logic-dependent (posttraining) shift of activation from posterior to frontal
regions. From Houdé et al. (2000), slightly modified, with permission.

interpret that shift as the result of the inhibition of the perceptual bias from posterior areas—inhibition brought about by the training. Thus, the exercise of logical reasoning seems to overcome the biasing influences from posterior cortex and to lend to the prefrontal cortex the effective control of the reasoning task.

In conclusion, reflexive reasoning consists of the rapid, parallel, and unconscious processing of neural information between permanent cognits at relatively low levels of the cortical organization. A key component of that process would be the expeditious matching of reality to existing cognits. Inferences would derive automatically (*reflexively*) from that matching, without intervention of inhibitory feedback or the mediation of contingencies across time. Deductive reasoning, on the other hand, can be conceived as an integrative process at the top of the perception-action cycle. Logical inferences are reached after sequential matching of alternative cognits against reality and against permanent cognits. Symbols and language intervene in the process; thus, so do the language areas of the left hemisphere. Inasmuch as it requires the integration of complex information and the rejection of alternatives, the process requires lateral prefrontal cortex, especially of the left hemisphere. The role of this cortex is especially critical in those forms of deductive reasoning (e.g., syllogistic reasoning) that tax the capacity for temporal integration and/or the inhibition of inferences that are logically nearly true.

Problem Solving

In everyday life, as in science, we use far more inductive than deductive reasoning. These two forms of reflective reasoning, however, are intimately entwined and, as we will see, appear to share the same cortical substrate. In the previous section we dealt mainly with deduction. In this one we deal with induction, for this kind of logical thinking plays a key role in the solution of problems, which is our next subject.

First, let us attempt to clarify in what ways induction differs from deduction. The aims of deductive reasoning are to draw and to verify logically valid inferences from premises. *Validity* in this context is defined as the logical consistency between inference and premises—regardless of the validity of the premises. The aims of inductive reasoning, on the other hand, are to draw *plausible* inferences from current observations and from preexisting knowledge and to estimate the probability of those inferences. J. Stuart Mill defined induction as "the process by which we conclude that what is true of certain individuals is true of a class, what is true of part is true of the whole class, or what is true at certain times will be true in similar circumstances at all times" (English and English, 1958). Induction, however, can at best only attain high probability, not truth. Absolute truth is barred to induction by the probabilistic, not deterministic, nature of observations and knowledge (sometime, somewhere, a black swan may yet be found!). The logic of scientific discovery (Popper, 1980) relies heavily on inductive reasoning, as natural science is a process of successive probabilistic approximations of our knowledge to the reality of the physical world.

Ordinary problem solving, which is also called *practical intelligence* (Sternberg, 1985), is essentially based on inductive arguments toward the goal of solving a problem. Often these arguments derive from similarities and lead to conclusions by similarity in a cognitive process that has been called *analogical reasoning*. In the inferential logic of this form of reasoning, similar stimuli are treated as equal; the strategy used in a solved problem will be applied again to a similar new problem. Analogical reasoning extends to the *relationships* between stimuli, between objects, and between events. Thus, the reasoner treats patterns of such relationships (associations) as analogous, and transfers them as such from one situation to another and from one problem to another. It is a process similar to what Gestalt psychology postulates the perceiver does in the making and recognition of percepts (Chapter 4). The reasoner, therefore, creates *analogical mappings* that represent in abstract form those patterns of relationship. The mappings are essentially abstract cognits. In analogical reasoning, they are used as cognitive units (gestalts). Their complexity varies as a function of the number of relationships they incorporate (Holyoak and Thagard, 1995). One of the tests now being used in neuroscience to challenge analogical reasoning and the intellectual ability to handle relational complexity is the RPM test. A variant of it is depicted in Figure 8.5.

The neuroscience of problem solving is the neuroscience of the cortical representations and operations that support reasoning toward the solution of problems. Thus, the cortical representations used in problem solving consist of cognits of established knowledge as well as of current or recent sensory information. The operations consist of neural transactions within and between those cognits. These transactions are the result of the excitatory and inhibitory mechanisms in

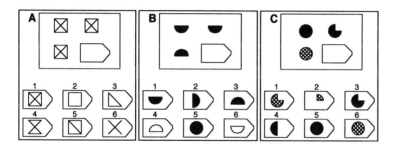

Figure 8.5. Variant of the RPM test. The subject has to choose the item from the bottom that completes the pattern at the top. In *A* (nonrelational problem), the correct choice is 1; in *B* (one-relation problem, vertical transformation), the correct choice is 3; in *C* (two-relation problem, vertical and horizontal transformation), the correct choice is 1. From Waltz et al. (1999), modified, with permission.

cortical networks by which the various cognitive functions lead reasoning to problem solution. The cognitive functions most important for problem solving are attention, perception, memory, and the integration of conditional contingencies ("if . . . then . . ."). As those contingencies become multiple and complex, the integration gains in temporal dimension; it becomes temporal integration. Then the temporal integrative aspects of attention and memory become critical, especially working memory and planning or *prospective memory*. Time and complexity become critical variables in the reasoning process, and thus in its supporting neural functions.

The ability of nonhuman primates to solve problems has been extensively tested, notably by the use of cross-temporal contingency tasks such as delay tasks. These tasks test some of the basic functions of temporal integration in problem solving, especially working memory and prospective set. The neural mechanisms by which cortical networks support these two functions, under the control of the prefrontal cortex, were discussed in Chapter 6. Here we will focus briefly on studies of functional neuroimaging conducted in humans performing problem solving. The data from these studies do not contribute substantially to our understanding of neural mechanisms, but they provide valuable insights into the cortical topography of cognits and of the neural operations behind the processes of reasoning that enable the solution of problems.

Almost without exception, functional neuroimaging during problem solving reveals the activation of large expanses of cortex of the left hemisphere and, in some cases, also the right. Generally, two groups of areas are activated, each with certain prominent foci of activation. One group of areas is in posterior cortex; the extent of their activation depends on the nature of the information that the subject has to deal with to solve the problem. The other group is in frontal cortex, often including the anterior cingulate cortex, Broca's area in the inferior frontal gyrus, and a portion of lateral prefrontal cortex. Because of the limitations of imaging methods and their difficulty in handling variability, the precise confines of the activated areas cannot be ascertained with confidence. Similarly, because of their insufficient temporal resolution, these methods cannot disclose the time course of the component neural processes that take place before the solution of a problem is reached. Thus, the tomographic activation of perceptual and executive areas in a problem-solving task does not necessarily imply that those activations are simultaneous. The all-important serial processing that presumably takes place in problem solving remains undisclosed by neuroimaging.

Spatial-reasoning problems, in which the subject must visually imagine the rotational transformation of bodies, are accompanied by the activation of areas in or around the junction of the occipital, parietal, and temporal lobes, especially on the left (Cohen et al., 1996; Zacks et al., 1999). Problems that require analogical reasoning, such as the RPM task (Fig. 8.5), induce the activation of posterior parietal areas (Wharton et al., 2000; Kroger et al., 2002). Text-processing problems activate Wernicke's area (Prabhakaran et al., 2001). Mental arithmetic activates inferior parietal cortex (Burbaud et al., 1999). All six studies referenced in this paragraph reveal, in addition to posterior cortical activation, the prominent activation of one or several lateral prefrontal areas.

Problem solving, therefore, seems to activate at least one region of posterior cortex that specializes in the representation and processing of the particular cognitive material that the subject must use for correct solution of the problem. In addition, problem solving activates prefrontal cortex. It is reasonable to conclude that a problem task is assisted by the activation of perceptual cognits representing the sensory or semantic content of the problem. Further, the performance of the task and the solution of the problem depend on the activation of executive networks of the prefrontal cortex.

The consistent activation of prefrontal cortex in problem solving is illustrated by the *meta-analysis* of neuroimaging studies conducted by Duncan and Owen (2000). Three prefrontal regions seem to be activated, sometimes in common, by the performance of many tasks (Fig. 8.6): the anterior cingulate region, the lateral region, and the orbital region. As we noted in Chapter 6, the anterior cingulate region seems activated by all tasks that require heightened attentive effort. The lateral prefrontal region, on the other hand, is active in tasks that require temporal integration, whatever the nature of the information essential to the task at hand or the solution of the problem. Accordingly, lateral prefrontal activation has been observed in tasks that load the two temporal integrative functions of the prefrontal cortex: working memory, as in delay tasks (Grasby et al., 1993; Jonides et al., 1993; Petrides et al., 1993b), and planning, as in chess playing (Nichelli et al., 1994). The activation of orbital and inferior prefrontal areas seems associated with the role that inhibition plays in exclusionary at-

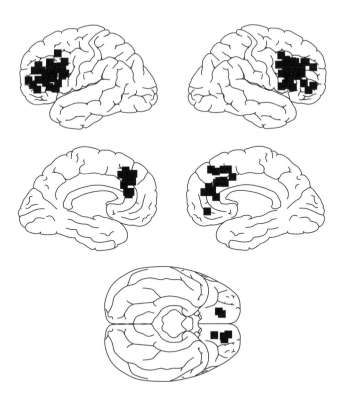

Figure 8.6. Peak prefrontal activations observed in assorted neuroimaging studies of problem solving. From Duncan et al. (2000), modified, with permission.

tention, that is, the inhibition of posterior cognits that interfere with the correct solution of the problem (see above, Reasoning).

The integrative role of the prefrontal cortex in problem solving is graded and adjusted to need. Three factors determine that need, with considerable trade-off between them: integration time, complexity, and novelty. (Their interactions and impact on delay-task performance are discussed in Fuster, 1997.) The three factors, singly or in combination, determine the degree of involvement of lateral frontal cortex in problem solving. In general, prefrontal cortical involvement correlates with the amount of effort that the subject must devote to solving the problem. Thus, the relational complexity—the number of relations to be integrated—in an analogical task (RPM) correlates with the level of lateral prefrontal activation (Kroger et al., 2002). Conversely, prefrontal damage affects adversely the performance of an analogical task as a function of relational complexity (Waltz et al., 1999). Problems of inductive reasoning that require probabilistic inferences have been seen to induce more activation of left prefrontal cortex than less demanding problems of deductive reasoning (Osherson et al., 1998). Finally, there seems to be a natural tendency toward *economy* of prefrontal resources, which is presumably correlated with economy of attentive effort. As they become automatic and effortless, numerical and verbal problems elicit less frontal activation (Jahanshahi et al., 2000; Reichle et al., 2000). Dehaene et al. (1998) postulate that, by regulating up or down the contribution of its neurons, the prefrontal cortex opens or closes, according to need, the "workspace" available for the solution of problems.

Decision Making

In ordinary language, the decision of a human to act at a certain time in a certain way carries the almost obligatory implication of reasoned free choice. Even in neuroscientific discourse, it is practically impossible to elude the phenomenological connotations of decision making. Yet we cannot usefully approach such a cardinal aspect of intelligence without studiously ignoring its implications of consciousness and free will. The failure to do it inevitably leads to the assumption of a free and conscious neural agent in the frontal lobe or elsewhere, which is an unnecessary and indefensible entity. Moreover, that spurious assumption takes the neuroscientist away from critical evidence for any argument on the neural basis of decision making. Such is the evidence that (*1*) the human is not the only organism capable of making decisions; (*2*) not all decisions are rational; (*3*) some decisions are unconscious; and (*4*) many decisions, indeed most, are in part the product of earlier experience of which we are not aware (implicit memory). Again we must descend to neurobiology to understand the roots of a cognitive function.

The decision to act, that is, the choice of an action between alternatives (including not to act), is inextricably and by definition tied to the *executive* functions of the organism. Therefore, it is reasonable to assume, a priori, that in primates decision making is a frontal lobe function. However, any role of frontal cortex in decision making must be viewed as the upward expansion of the role of hierarchically lower executive structures in action selection. Further, that role of frontal cortex must be construed within the framework of its input connections, which provide the antecedents to a decision, much as in reasoning those connections provide the antecedents to or premises of an inference. The following discussion of neural correlates of decision making takes place within those two broad theoretical constraints: executive frontal function and neural inputs to the frontal lobe.

William James (1890) wrote that any choice of adequate behavior requires, as a prerequisite, a choice of stimuli. That both choices may be conscious and guided by attention is here beside the point. The important point in James' remark is that the decision to behave in a certain manner depends on the prior processing of certain kinds of sensory information. A decision, then, would be a product of *perception*. Following this reasoning, it could be argued that the decision begins with perception. In a broader conceptual framework, there is decision in every sensory–motor act; therefore, there is decision at all levels of the neural substrate of sensory–motor integration. At low levels, the decision is made by a system of more or less direct pathways between sensory and motor structures. At higher levels, in the cortex, the decision rests on both sides of the perception-action cycle. Thus, it is reasonable to ask, first, if there are in posterior cortex neuronal populations that react to identical, uncertain, or ambiguous stimuli in accord with the behavioral choices that the animal makes in response to them. Electrophysiological evidence from the human and the monkey indicates that this is indeed the case.

Begleiter and Porjesz (1975) recorded evoked potentials at the vertex of human subjects given repeatedly an identical visual stimulus and the choice of responding to it by one motor act or one other. The potentials evoked by the stimulus differed significantly, depending on the motor response that the subject chose to produce on every trial. Thus, the evoked sensory signal contained information on the forth-coming decision of the subject. We might conclude that the decision was made, at least in part, on the perceptual side of the processing of the action.

In the middle temporal (MT) visual area of the monkey's poste-rior cortex, cells respond selectively to moving visual stimuli. Mon-keys were presented with patterns of moving dots and trained to re-port with eye movements the perceived direction of the dots (Britten et al., 1996). The dot patterns were then scrambled to some degree, such that some of the dots moved in the same direction while the oth-ers moved at random. By changing the ratio of same-direction dots to random-moving dots, the task could be made more or less difficult and the monkey's choices more or less accurate. Under these condi-tions, MT neurons were noted to fire in correlation with the monkey's perceived and reported direction of movement (Fig. 8.7), even when the aggregate physical motion of same-direction dots was weak and indistinguishable from random by human observers. Thus, the cells "decided" what the monkey decided and vice versa. Similarly, MT cells make decisions for the monkey on the direction of ambiguous moving gratings (Logothetis and Schall, 1989). Also, in the somatosensory cortex, cells discriminate frequencies of mechanical vibrations to fin-gertips in accord with the monkey's perceived and reported differ-ences (Hernández et al., 2000).

To sum up, the cognitive networks that represent and process sensory information appear to categorize stimuli—that is, to perceive them (see Chapter 4)—in accord with the behavioral decisions those stimuli determine, not only in accord with their physical properties. It can be concluded that some decisions are made or initiated on the perceptual side of the cortical perception-action cycle before the sig-nals from perception reach the executive cortex.

But perception is not the only source of decisions. Reasoning is another, most importantly in the human. Other sources of decisions can be found in a wide range of emotional and social influences. Such influences include those that derive from the *theory of mind*, the ability to assess the mental states and intentions of others. That abil-ity appears to be founded mostly on intuitive perceptions of speech and demeanor. Finally, a most important source of human decisions is a host of social, esthetic, and ethical *values* that may be viewed as the

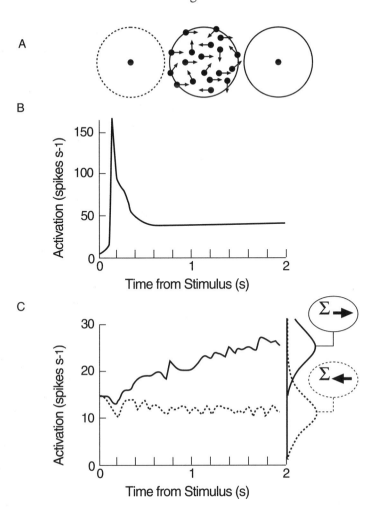

Figure 8.7. Neuronal discharge in MT cortex related to the direction of oculo-motor response to mixed patterns of dot movement (see text), as per experiments by Britten et al. (1996). *A:* Random moving dot pattern with a rightward bias. *B:* Firing of a neuron preferentially responding to rightward motion. *C:* Before the monkey's decision is made, the frequency of neuronal firing differs, depending on the animal's reported direction (firing is higher with a rightward decision than with a leftward decision). From Schall (2001), modified.

highest and most abstract cognits of perceptual and executive representation. Largely acquired by education and example, those values are part of the exclusive patrimony of our species.

Once a decision has been made, how is the consequent action initiated in the brain? This is one of the most challenging questions in cognitive neuroscience. Because it is a question highly relevant to philosophical issues, such as that of free will, it often invites speculation in favor of the existence of such quasi-phrenological concepts as a *center of will*. This would be a uniquely dedicated neural structure where decisions are made and carried out. Of course, the frontal lobe and its structures have been the most common targets of such speculation. The idea of a frontal center of voluntary action, however, like that of one for attention, is idle and misleading. For one thing, it leads to an infinite regress. If there is such a center, under which command is it? Is it under the command of another center somewhere else in the brain? And that one is located where, and under whose command is it? In any case, there is no evidence for a frontal neural commander of any kind. The empirical support for the speculation of a frontal center of conation consists of the following: (*1*) lesions of frontal cortex induce paralysis of voluntary movement or loss of spontaneity in speech and behavior; (*2*) stimulation of frontal cortex induces movements of the eyes, head, or limbs; and (*3*) surface potentials in the frontal lobe precede the initiation of voluntary action.

Both, however, the concept of a frontal center of conation and the interpretation of the evidence that appears to support it, ignore the evidence that every part of frontal cortex is embedded in a wealth of connections with other structures and subject to myriad inputs from them. The initiation of organized and goal-directed action is contingent on the activation of frontal networks by neural *inputs* that arrive at those networks from many sources. The nature of those inputs can be inferred from their sources (Fig. 8.8). Thus, from the internal milieu, through the limbic system, the frontal cortex receives information about the state of the visceral organs, about hormonal and chemical levels, and about the emotional and affective states of the organism. From the external environment, through the sensory organs and posterior cortex, the frontal cortex receives a constant flow of sensory information about the surrounding world. From other parts of the neocortex, the frontal cortex also receives a multitude of influences based on prior knowledge—in other words, influences from the cognitive spheres of perception, memory, reasoning, and language. Included among them are the influences from the domains of culture and values.

As we noted with regard to attention (Chapter 6) and earlier in this chapter with regard to reasoning and problem solving, the frontal cortex reciprocates the inputs from posterior cortex with critical *in-*

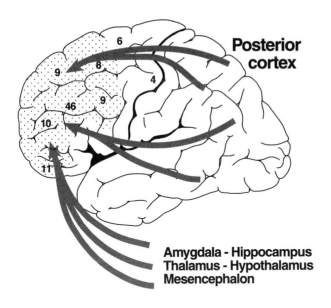

Figure 8.8. Inputs to prefrontal cortex.

hibitory outputs to that cortex that serve the exclusionary or gating role of attention. In addition, the frontal cortex sends inhibitory outputs to limbic structures to control the influx of impulses from those structures that serve drive and motivation. Those outputs originate mostly in orbitomedial areas of the prefrontal cortex. This is the reason that a lesion of orbitomedial cortex often results in clinical disorders characterized by poor impulse control, sociopathic behavior, intemperate risk-taking, and irrational decisions (Damasio, 1994; Adolphs et al., 1996; Fuster, 1997).

Essentially, then, the initiation of action, as well as its subsequent course, results from the *competition* of multiple influences arriving concomitantly in frontal cortex from assorted sectors of the organism. At any give time, by reason of their intensity or probability of occurrence, only a few of those influences prevail in that competition for executive attention. In humans, the influences may come from obscure sectors of the internal milieu that are the source of unconscious drives. Some of these may gain access to decision making unchecked by normal inhibitory control from frontal cortex. To the extent that we are unaware of those drives, we may feel free to execute the actions they determine. In any event, there is neither need nor evidence for a neural center of willed action. In terms of the brain, the old argument between determinism and free will may be theoretically resolved on intermediate probabilistic grounds. On the one hand, voluntary action is the result of competition between multiple input signals of varying strength and probability that arrive from many sources in the cortex of the frontal lobe. On the other, voluntary action is the result of competition between alternate executive cognits encoded in this cortex.

Creative Intelligence

Between the ages of 6 and 16, the intelligence of the child undergoes a tidal change from within. The essence of that change is the massive and progressive detachment of intelligence from the senses. In that decade, the sensory–motor modes of adaptation, which prevailed in early childhood, give way to ever more cognitive independence from the environment. The mind becomes less stimulus-bound and more the master of itself. Of course, the development of language promotes the transition. Some, like Vygotsky (1986), go even further, to claim that language is all there is to that transition at any age. Language is the indispensable key to the liberation of the child's intelligence from the sensory world. In the first section of this chapter we noted that in the last two Piagetian stages—the decade from 6 to 16—intellectual independence takes place in parallel and probably as a result of the maturation of the prefrontal cortex. Prefrontal cortical maturation essentially adds another hierarchical level to the perception-action cycle, a higher level of linguistic and behavioral integration. With it, the vocabulary of the child expands enormously, ever more symbols and imagination take the place of stimuli, time and deliberation intervene ever more often between stimuli and responses, and the associative cortex of the frontal lobe assumes its integrative role. Significantly, Luria—Vygotsky's disciple—postulated that the prefrontal cortex exerts that role by internalizing language within itself (Luria and Homskaya, 1964). Be that as it may, the maturation of higher association cortex sets the ground for creative intelligence.

It has been said that creative intelligence is the ability to invent goals, projects, and plans—in other words, we might say, to *invent the future*. It is also the ability to pursue those goals and to implement those projects and plans. Creative intelligence is an autonomous form of intelligence focused on the future. Its future aims, however, are firmly grounded in the past and in the present. Like all forms of intelligence, creative intelligence develops from all other cognitive functions. It develops from a broad base of knowledge, implicit and explicit, that was acquired in the past by attention and perception and symbolized by language. With the advent of creative intelligence, however, those functions that helped build it become its servants. They turn inside out and become part of the intelligent executive. Whereas beforehand there were the perceptual, mnemonic, attentional, and linguistic foundations of intelligence, now there is also intelligent perception, intelligent memory, intelligent attention, and intelligent language (Marina, 1993). Those slave functions become the agents for the intelligent executive in the cortex and help it devise new forms of perception as well as new forms of action.

As mentioned in Chapter 7, some neuropsychologists, on the basis of lesion data, have argued for a special role of the *right hemisphere* in certain aspects of language and in visuospatial perception. Similarly, a special role of the right hemisphere has been claimed for creative intelligence, in particular spatial creativity. Such specialization of the right hemicortex, however, has not been conclusively shown by lesion studies. Nonetheless, many such studies make it evident that the right hemisphere contributes creative power to the brain (Luria and Simernitskaya, 1977; Cook, 1986; Lezak, 1995). The logical and linguistic capabilities of the left hemisphere have been shown to be considerably assisted by the functional integrity of the right hemisphere, even though the functions of the latter have not been entirely clarified. What seems beyond dispute, however, is the important role of the cortex of the frontal lobe, dorsolateral prefrontal cortex in particular, in several crucial aspects of creativity. On neuropsychological grounds, the critical functional position of this cortex in reasoning and problem solving, discussed in the previous two sections, seems to extend to creative intelligence as well. It could not be otherwise if we consider the proven role of the prefrontal cortex in the integration of new and complex structures of reason, language, and behavior (brief review in Fuster, 2001).

There are few reliable and directly pertinent studies of brain function in creative intelligence. Thus, our knowledge of the subject is very limited. In one study (Martindale and Hines, 1975), the amount of EEG alpha frequency was found to be positively correlated with creativity in tests of remote association and alternate uses. This finding is suggestive of synchrony and coherence of activity in large cortical networks during creative performance—as in previously referenced studies of general intelligence. The increase in alpha frequency related to creativity appears greater in the right hemisphere than in the left.

Carlsson et al. (2000) investigate differences in the regional cerebral blood flow (rCBF) of the prefrontal cortex as a function of creative ability. Using a test of creativity developed by one of those researchers, they divide subjects into two groups, a high creative group and a low creative group. Creativity, as measured by that test, is composed of such intellectual qualities as the capacity to express ideas, their originality, the breadth of creative interests, and the predictability of creative achievement. In their search for brain correlates of creativity, the investigators obtain measures of rCBF during rest and during performance of three tasks: automatic speech (counting numbers), verbal fluency (verbalizing words that begin with a certain letter), and an object-use test (*Brick*) that requires the naming of as many uses of bricks as the subject can think of. At rest, the high creative group has higher rCBF activity than the low creative group. The high creative group also shows a bilateral frontal increase in activity from rest to Brick performance, while the low creative group shows only a left frontal increase. The subtraction of Brick activity from verbal-fluency activity reveals relative increases of object-use activity in anterior and superior prefrontal areas of the high creative group (Fig. 8.9). Conversely, the low creative group shows relative decreases of that activity, especially in the right hemisphere. In sum, the study indicates that creativity, as measured by the ability to conceptualize the uses of construction objects, correlates with basal metabolic activity in the dorsolateral prefrontal cortex; further, in creative subjects engaged in creative performance, prefrontal activation increases beyond basal levels. Both hemispheres contribute resources to creativity in highly creative subjects, whereas only the left hemisphere seems to do it in less creative subjects.

However, the study just described also yields a couple of apparently paradoxical results of remarkable significance in the light of our previous discussion in this chapter. The first is the observation that the *level* of performance of Brick does not correlate with prefrontal activity. In some highly creative subjects, good performance is in fact negatively correlated with prefrontal activation. This finding again points to the economy of neural resources in intellectual performance (Parks et al., 1988; Boivin et al., 1992). Perhaps proficiency ob-

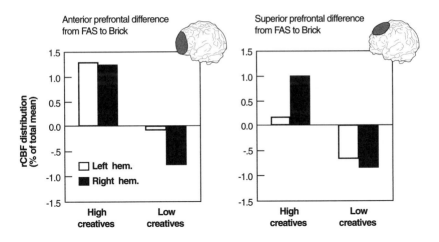

Figure 8.9. Relative activation of two prefrontal regions during object-use performance in high-creative and low-creative subjects. CBF in a word-fluency task (FAS) is subtracted from CBF in an object-use task (Brick). From Carlsson et al. (2000), modified, with permission.

viates the need for all of the resources available. The other finding is that the low creative group is superior to the high creative group in conventional intelligence tests. This points to the frequently noted dissociation between creativity and logical thinking (Guilford, 1967). Some have suspected a degree of incompatibility between the two. Logical and analytical thinking is deemed an impediment to creativeness (Reddy and Reddy, 1983).

What do the reported cortical increases in cerebral blood flow or EEG synchrony signify in terms of the neural mechanisms of creative achievement? We do not know. The reason is that imaging and electrophysiology cannot answer the question and no other appropriate methodology is currently available. Nevertheless, we can venture a reasonable (not creative!) answer on the basis of what we know about the cognitive physiology of the cortex, the prefrontal cortex in particular. A reasonable assumption is that the creative process consists of the formation of new cognits, that is, new network representations in the cortex. These representations result mostly from divergent thinking as opposed to convergent thinking. Convergent thinking consists of inductive and deductive reasoning, which converge toward logical inferences and the solution of problems (Guilford, 1967). Divergent thinking, on the other hand, is free of logical constraints, autonomous

and to some extent free-floating, reliant on imagination, and mini-
mally anchored in immediate reality. Creative cognits emerge mainly
from *divergent* thinking.

To create, in the present context, is to make new cognits out of
old ones. At the root of this process is the formation of new *associations* between old cognits. Thus, to invent the future is to reinvent the
past by making new associations in it. The new cognits are potentially
infinite, much as the old ones were, because the range of either is determined by the practically infinite combinatorial power of some 10
billion cells or subgroups (e.g., modules, assemblies) of them. Therefore, the spread and configuration of created cortical cognits and
their supporting networks are extremely variable. Inasmuch as they
contain perceptual components, they occupy postrolandic and post-
sylvian cortex; inasmuch as they contain executive components (all
do, by definition, for creation is an active process), they occupy prefrontal cortex.

Three major categories of neural inputs activate cortical networks in the creative process: inputs from mesencephalic and limbic
formations, from other cortical networks, and from sensory systems.
These categories of inputs, it will be noted, are the same ones that
converge on frontal cortex in decision making (previous section).
Now they contribute to the making of decisions, of sorts, that consist
in the creation of new perceptual and executive cognits. Like all
forms of decision making, the cortical creation of new cognits necessitates the inputs from subcortical structures. These structures, notably in the limbic system and the brain stem, provide to the creative
process inputs from drive, motivation, and attention. As will be recalled (Chapter 6), these influences from the internal milieu and the
world of affect enter the executive cortex mainly through afferent
connections to dorsolateral and cingulate prefrontal cortices. They
bring to the creative process the indispensable energizing tone from
biological sources. Probably those influences communicate that tone
to the neocortex through monoaminergic neurotransmitter systems
of subcortical origin (reviewed in Fuster, 1997). Not only is creativity
energized by influences from affect, but then also creativity, possibly
by feedback through reward systems of the basal brain, induces predictable changes of affect. Rather well known are the effects of creativity in allaying anxiety and uplifting mood.

From the limbic system and neocortex itself come also to cortical
cognits the excitatory inputs from value systems that facilitate and

maintain the process of creative intelligence. Included in those systems are the neural networks that represent a wealth of social, esthetic, and ethical values, which can be reasonably assumed to be partly innate and partly acquired.

The biophysical essence of creativity is the dynamic process of formation of new associative contacts between cognits. That process can begin with the activation of any cognit or group of cognits anywhere in the cortex. Networks that share neurons and associations activate one another, thus strengthening those associations and forming new ones between them. The *ignition* (Braitenberg's term) of neuronal assemblies can thus shift in succession from one network to another, leaving a trail of synaptic facilitation in wide expanses of cortex. Some of this serial recruitment of cognits is divergent and open-ended. It takes place in chain-like fashion mostly in associative networks of posterior cortex, presumably in the same manner as in the free association of ideas. The creative recruitment of cognits, however, takes place under prefrontal control and has the objective of organizing, that is, integrating, new executive cognits. Those cognits are what, in the form of goal-directed structures of action, will find their expression in the hands of the composer, the architect, or the novelist or in the words of the public speaker or the entertainer. At any point, the process can be prompted or assisted by sensory inputs. Such inputs, in fact, provide the essential feedback for the prefrontal cortex to be able to steer the perception-action cycle to the completion of the work. The prefrontal cortex of the creative genius imparts unparalleled richness, complexity, and harmony, as well as a worthy goal, to the spatial and temporal structure of that work.

9

Epilogue on Consciousness

Consciousness is the subjective experience of cognitive function. Because it is not itself a cognitive function, no special chapter has been dedicated to its neural substrate. Yet consciousness is not only a concomitant phenomenon of cognition, but also a valuable aid to study it. Therefore, as some have forcefully advocated (e.g., Searle, 1990), phenomenology—the analysis of consciousness—is increasingly recognized as a useful method in cognitive science and, accordingly, in cognitive neuroscience. Conscious experience can emerge from the operation of any cognitive function, whereby phenomenology can lead to new knowledge of that function. Indeed, phenomenology has helped us draw valuable inferences in every one of the five preceding chapters. Ordinarily, however, conscious experience results from the operation and interaction of several functions in complex assemblies of cortical networks. Thus, the cortical architecture of consciousness is the architecture of the five functions discussed in previous chapters. In neural terms, what James (1890) called the *stream of consciousness* appears to consist of the sequential activation, above a certain level or threshold, of the cortical networks (cognits) that support those functions. This is the central idea of this concluding chapter.

For a long time, neuroscience, under the influence of behaviorism, treated consciousness as an illegitimate scientific subject, an intrusive vestige of dualistic thinking. In recent decades, however, for reasons that are easy to understand, the neuroscience of consciousness has had a powerful surge. One reason for this surge is the discovery of certain cortical correlates of psychophysical function, namely, of the relationships between conscious experience and the physical parameters of sensory stimulation. Some of these cortical correlates have been discovered in the nonhuman primate by the use of indirect behavioral measures of consciousness. Another reason, in my view more profound and consequential, is the growing acceptance of the network model of cognition, which holds that *relations* are the essence of meaning. Meaning is the phenomenal experience of relations and of the integrated unity they form, in space and time. That unity in space and time, which can derive from any cognitive operation, is one of the basic qualities of consciousness.

It is that quality of integration, as it pertains to *perception,* that makes Gestalt phenomenology such an appealing method for the cognitive neuroscientist (Chapter 4). We are conscious of our percepts because these are the result of the integration of elementary sensations into categorical perceptual wholes. Conventionally, such categorical wholes or gestalts have been explored in the spatial domain. They constitute the central topic of the Gestalt psychology of visual perception. The associations that make a visual percept, essentially a segregated figure against a background, are considered the basis of *binding.* As we saw, certain patterns of electrocortical oscillation, especially prominent in the cat, have been assumed to be manifestations of the binding of the components of a visual percept in the cortex. From the observation of those patterns in visual perception, and from the phenomenology of the latter, some have concluded that fast-frequency oscillations are the physiological foundation of conscious experience. This argument is weakened by the evidence that the oscillations are found most conspicuously in anesthetized animals. Nonetheless, binding can be explained as a pattern of persistent reentry in cortical and thalamocortical circuits. Binding would be the tying together, by neural reentry, of the component cortical representations of the percept.

Whereas spatial gestalts are easy to demonstrate and amenable to study by neurophysiological methods, it is the temporal dimension that provides the phenomenal presence to a perceptual gestalt, whether spatial or nonspatial. In other words, temporal continuity is a necessary condition for the consciousness of a percept. That temporal continuity has two possible sources. One is the continuance in the environment of the sensory elements that, in the cortex, constitute the cognit of the percept. The other is the mental and neural trace of the percept after its sensory constituents have disappeared from the environment. That trace may simply consist of the iconic afterimage of the percept. When the percept, however, is to be integrated with later percepts for the organization of an action, the trace of the percept enters the focus of internalized attention and becomes working memory. Working memory (Chapter 6) is the internalized attention on a recent percept for prospective action, and thus the persistent activation of the cognitive network that represents that percept.

Memory can enter consciousness in a multitude of forms and states. The recall of any memory is conscious by definition. Imagining is also conscious in that it consists essentially of the conscious retrieval of long-term memories and established cognits, assembled and reconfigured in a variety of ways. Creative intelligence is served by the conscious interaction of memory and imagination. In all likelihood, that interaction rests on sequences of reentrant functional linkages between posterior and frontal cortices. Any such sequence may commence in structures that represent affective states or states of the internal milieu. Thus, for example, impulses of limbic origin related to affect or motivation can activate cognits in posterior cortical areas, which in turn feed inputs into the prefrontal cortex. Then, by way of top-down feedback, the temporal integrative and planning functions of the prefrontal cortex arrange those cognits in new ways, creating new structures of action of esthetic or social value.

While we deal in daily life with the world around us, recognition is by and large a more prevalent form of memory retrieval than recall. The reason for that dominant role of recognition lies in the interactions between memory and perception. As we saw in Chapter 4, the essence of all perception is recognition. Perception is the recognition of categories of sensory stimuli, whether that recognition is conscious or not. As perception enters the focus of attention, it becomes conscious. Thus, at the phenomenal level, consciousness emerges from complex interactions between three cognitive functions: perception, memory, and attention. It is the last, however, that contributes most to consciousness. We are consciously aware of what we attend to, whether it is an object, its place and time, a trend of thought, an old

memory, a fantasy, or a future plan. Therein lies the reason that attention is commonly treated as synonymous with consciousness.
Therein also lies the reason that the neural correlates of attention are
frequently interpreted as the neural correlates of consciousness.
However, whereas manipulating attention may be useful for the study
of consciousness in the human brain, or even the animal brain, equat-
ing consciousness with attention is an oversimplification at both the
phenomenal and physiological levels. The content of attention is the
content of consciousness, though not all the content of consciousness
necessarily falls within the focus of attention. Nevertheless, *attention* is
the cognitive function that relates consciousness most directly to cortical physiology.

All attentive phenomena have the essential property of consciousness: integrated unity. Any content of attention possesses the
phenomenal attribute of spatial and temporal unity. Even the most elementary sensation, if and when it enters the focus of attention, constitutes an act of integration, for it unifies the associated qualia that
derive from prior experience with similar sensations. Every attended
percept unifies the associated properties of the members of its class.
At the same time, that percept is associated with its context and dis-
sociated from—that is, negatively associated with—its background.
The integration of an attended percept, therefore, derives from the
associative properties of the cognit that represents it, which is to say,
from the associative structure of its cortical network. It is the concomitant activation of the associated elements of that network that
confers unity on the conscious experience of the attentive act. That
unity applies to the experience of perceptual attention as well as to
that of motor attention. The performance of a goal-directed task, especially if the task is new and deliberate, confers on the performer
the conscious experience of unity, much as an attended percept does
on the perceiver. Thus, through attention, all perceptual and motor
aspects of language and intellectual performance have access to consciousness.

In principle, then, to follow that line of reasoning, the cortical
distribution of an integrated conscious experience coincides with the
distribution of the cognitively activated cortical network that gives
rise to it. Attention is the cognitive function that most discretely and
intensely activates a network from which consciousness emerges. In
these final pages, I wish to discuss briefly the properties of that net-

work and the physiological conditions under which its activation gains access to consciousness.

In the broadest topographical terms, the cortical networks activated by the performance of a sensory–motor task may extend across both hemispheres. This is in part determined by the dual-hemispheric distribution of sensory and motor cortices and their inputs and outputs. It is also in part determined by the connectivity of those cortices with associative areas of both hemispheres. Thus, the attention to the successive components of a task may activate a succession of interconnected networks in the two hemispheres. Under certain conditions, however, a task can be shown to engage networks confined to one hemisphere. Patients with split brain from section of the corpus callosum can be taught to perform concomitantly two visuomotor memory tasks, each under full control of one hemisphere or the other (Holtzman and Gazzaniga, 1985). In such patients, who can perform both tasks considerably better than normal subjects, it can be ascertained that both visuomotor attention and consciousness are split between the two tasks. The cognits of each task are limited to one hemisphere, and as they become active, they give rise to a series of unitary conscious experiences.

In a serial task, attention shifts fluidly from one cognit to another and thus from one network to another until the task is completed. Accordingly, consciousness shifts from one content to another, and its flow follows the performance as if it were its phenomenal shadow. Each successive experience derives its conscious unity from the integration of the corresponding cognit in the series. That cognit, however, is embedded in the more general cognit of the task, which includes associations with its origin, context, and goals. Therefore, the unity of the experience is part of the larger unity of the task as a whole, which at any given time may not be entirely conscious or fall within the focus of attention. Similar considerations apply to the performance of the innumerable cognitive tasks required by language and intellectual activity. At a given time, we may be aware of a word, a sentence, or a premise, but not necessarily of the thrust of our discourse or of our line of reasoning.

When a task imposes demands on the brain's capacity to integrate information across time, attention becomes arrested in the activation and retention of time-integrating cognits, as these become the content of *working memory*. With the need to integrate information temporally, the flow of consciousness becomes less fluid in that the focus of attention remains temporarily on those cognits. Thus, during the intervals of cross-temporal transfer of information, working memory can be best characterized as a critical part of the *remembered present,* which Edelman (1989) identifies with consciousness. Consequently, working memory provides a unique methodological opportunity for investigating the neural correlates of consciousness in a temporarily steady state.

It is reasonable to assume that the conscious awareness of a cognit coincides with the temporary activation of its cortical network while it is being retained in working memory. As discussed in Chapter 6, the electrophysiological and neuroimaging literatures indicate that the cortical topography of working memory coincides with the topography of the cognit retained in working memory. The distribution of that cognit depends on the architecture of the cortical network that represents its associated components. In a monkey performing a delay task, working-memory cells are found in widely dispersed cortical areas containing assemblies of cells that represent assorted sensory or motor attributes of the memorandum. Thus, for example, while the animal must retain temporarily a visual stimulus in working memory, as in a visual delayed matching-to-sample task, active memory cells can be found in inferotemporal as well as dorsolateral prefrontal cortex. In the human performing a spatial delay task, activated areas can be found in parietal as well as prefrontal cortex.

Two questions remain unanswered: What degree of activation must a cognit reach in order to enter consciousness? What is the mechanism underlying the sustained activation of a cognitive network in working memory and thereby in consciousness? With regard to the first question, we can only speculate. As the focus of attention shifts from one item to another, activation probably shifts from one cognit or network to another. As the activation of a cognit or network rises above a certain level, it is likely to give rise to the conscious experience of it. It has been suggested that a percept must be in focus for a minimum of 200 ms to enter consciousness (Tononi and Edelman, 1998). Thus, the stream of consciousness would consist of an uninterrupted succession of those temporary activations of cognits and their networks.

The processing of information in cortical networks can take place, however, without giving rise to conscious experience. As we have seen in previous chapters with regard to each of the cognitive functions, much of that processing may be unconscious. Evidently, therefore, the activation of a cortical network in the processing of information may not reach a high enough level or persist long enough to yield conscious experience. Thus, it is reasonable to hypothesize that the activation of that network has two thresholds (Fig. 9.1): a threshold for the processing of information and a threshold for the consciousness of it. The activation of the network above the threshold for consciousness would serve the focus of attention and coincide with what Tononi and Edelman (1998) call the *dynamic core*.

When the focus of attention or the dynamic core of consciousness resides in a given network to maintain the cognit it represents in working memory, there must be cortical and corticothalamic mechanisms that keep the network persistently active. The most plausible of such mechanisms is reentry. Hebb (1949) was the first to postulate a role of reverberating reentry in recurrent circuits for sustaining visual short-term memory in occipital areas. As noted in Chapter 6, reentry is emerging as the key mechanism in working memory. The most plausible computational models of working memory have recurrent network architecture. Working memory, according to some of these models (e.g., Zipser et al., 1993), would consist of the sustained reentry of excitation between the associated components of the cognitive network that represents the mnemonic content in the cortex.

The prefrontal cortex, because of its substantiated role in the top-down control of other structures for attention and working mem-

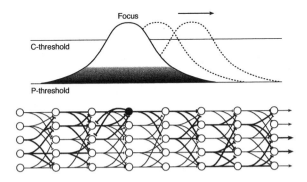

Figure 9.1. Hypothetical displacement of cortical-network activation with changes in the focus of attention. At a given time, the activation of a given part of the network may reach the P-threshold for processing and, at a higher level, the C-threshold for consciousness.

ory, has been considered a putative neural *seat of consciousness*. That cortex, however, does not appear to contribute to consciousness any more than any other cortical region. Any portion of neocortex can generate conscious phenomena as a participant in cognitive function. Thus, the neocortical contribution to consciousness varies from one time to another and from one area to another. The conscious experience can change accordingly in a wide variety of ways as neural activity migrates within and between the many potential cortical networks that we call cognits.

In conclusion, the seat of consciousness has eluded several generations of neuroscientists because consciousness is an epiphenomenon of activity in a shifting neural substrate. In earlier times, that "seat" was identified with certain reticular and neurotransmitter systems of the brain stem on account of their critical importance for the transition from sleep to wakefulness and for attentive vigilance. Now it is generally accepted that the role of those brain-stem systems in consciousness and vigilance lies in the global excitatory influences that those systems have over the cerebral cortex. In sleep, those influences cease or diminish.

Even during sleep, however, the cortex may be subject to influences from other brain structures. That may be the case in dreaming, for example. It seems possible that *dreams* result from the patchy activation of cortical regions during rapid eye movement (REM) sleep (Hobson, 1988). The source of that cortical activation may lie in limbic structures. During REM sleep, inputs from these structures, especially the amygdala, which provide emotional associations to neocortical networks (Chapter 3), can have associative access to those networks. Thus, the manifestations of the unconscious in the dream would essentially result from the limbic activation of fragmentary cortical cognits linked to emotion. Without inputs from other cortical regions to provide the integration with reality that characterizes consciousness, those activated fragments of cognition would fill the oneiric experience with distorted representations devoid of real context in space or time. *Delusions* may have an origin similar to that of dreams. Presumably as a result of functional disconnection in the cortex, emotion-laden and distorted cognits of reality erupt uncontrollably in the consciousness of the psychotic patient. In any case, further speculation about the neural basis of altered states of consciousness must await a better understanding than we now have of the cortical physiology in normal states.

References

....

Abeles, M. *Local Cortical Circuits: An Electrophysiological Study* (New York: Springer, 1982).

Aboitiz, F. Comparative development of the mammalian isocortex and the reptilian dorsal ventricular ridge. Evolutionary considerations. *Cerebral Cortex* 9: 783–791, 1999.

Aboitiz, F. and Ide, A. Anatomical asymmetries in language-related cortex and their relation to callosal function. In: *Handbook of Neurolinguistics*, ed. B. Stemmer and H. A. Whitaker (San Diego: Academic Press, 1998), 393–404.

Adolphs, R., Tranel, D., Bechara, A., Damasio, H., and Damasio, A. R. Neuropsychological approaches to reasoning and decision-making. In: *Neurobiology of Decision-Making*, ed. A. R. Damasio, A. R. Damasio, and Y. Christen (Berlin: Springer, 1996), 157–179.

Alexander, G. E., Delong, M. R., and Crutcher, M. D. Do cortical and basal ganglia motor areas use 'motor programs' to control movement? *Behav. Brain Sci.* 15: 656–665, 1992.

Allman, J. Evolution of neocortex. In: *Cerebral Cortex*, ed. E. G. Jones and A. Peters (New York and London: Plenum Press, 1984), 269–283.

Allman, J. K. and Kaas, J. H. A representation of visual field in the caudal third of the middle temporal gyrus of the owl monkey. *Brain Res.* 31: 84–105, 1971.

Allport, D. A. Distributed memory, modular subsystems and dysphasia. In: *Current Perspectives in Dysphasia,* ed. S. Newman (Edinburgh: Churchill Livingston, 1985), 32–60.

Andersen, R. A. Bracewell, R. M., Barash, S., Gnadt, J. W., and Fogassi, L. Eye position effects on visual, memory, and saccade-related activity in areas LIP and 7a of macaque. *J. Neuroscience* 10: 1176–1196, 1990.

Anderson, J. R. *Cognitive Psychology and Its Implications* (New York: W. H. Freeman, 1995).

Anokhin, A., Lutzenberger, W., and Birbaumer, N. Spatiotemporal organization of brain dynamics and intelligence: An EEG study in adolescents. *Int. J. Psychophysiol.* 33: 259–273, 1999.

Arbib, M. A, Érdi, P., and Szentágothai, J. *Neural Organization* (Cambridge, MA: MIT Press, 1998).

Asanuma, H. Recent developments in the study of the columnar arrangement of neurons within the motor cortex. *Physiol. Rev.* 55: 143–156, 1975.

Ashby, W. R. Design for a brain. *Engineering* 20: 379–383, 1948.

Atkinson, R. C. and Shiffrin, R. M. Human memory: A proposed system and its control processes. In: *The Psychology of Learning and Motivation: Advances in Research and Theory. Vol. 2,* ed. K. W. Spence and J. T. Spence (New York: Academic Press, 1968), 89–195.

Attneave, F. Some informal aspects of visual perception. *Psychol. Rev.* 61: 183–193, 1954.

Bach-y-Rita, P. Neurotransmission in the brain by diffusion through the extracellular fluid: a review. *NeuroReport* 4: 343–350, 1993.

Baddeley, A. *Working Memory* (Oxford: Clarendon Press, 1986).

Baker, S. C., Rogers, R. D., Owen, A. M., Frith, C. D., Dolan, R. J., Frackowiak, R. S. J., and Robbins, T. W. Neural systems engaged by planning: A PET study of the Tower of London task. *Neuropsychologia* 34: 515–526, 1996.

Barbizet, J., Duizabo, P., and Flavigny, R. Rôle des lobes frontaux dans le langage. *Rev. Neurol.* 131: 525–544, 1975.

Barkovich, A. J. *Pediatric Neuroimaging.* New York: Raven Press, 1995.

Barnes, C. A. Memory deficits associated with senescence: A neurophysiological and behavioral study in the rat. *J. Comp. Physiol. Psychol.* 93: 74–104, 1979.

Barris, R. W. and Schuman, H. R. Bilateral anterior cingulate gyrus lesions: Syndrome of the anterior cingulate gyri. *Neurology* 3: 44–52, 1953.

Barsalou, L. W. Perceptual symbol systems. *Behav. Brain Sci.* 22: 577–660, 1999.

Baxter, L. R., Phelps, M. E., Mazziotta, J. C., Guze, B. H., Schwartz, J. M., and Selin, C. E. Local cerebral glucose metabolic rates in obsessive-compulsive disorder. *Arch. Gen. Psychiatry* 44: 211–218, 1987.

Becker, L. E., Armstrong, D. L., Chan, F., and Wood, M. M. Dendritic development in human occipital cortical neurons. *Dev. Brain Res.* 13: 117–124, 1984.

Begleiter, H. and Porjesz, B. Evoked brain potentials as indicators of decision making. *Science* 187: 754–755, 1975.

Belin, P., Zilbovicius, M., Crozier, S., Thivard, L., and Fontaine, A. Lateralization of speech and auditory temporal processing. *J. Cognit. Neurosci.* 10: 536–540, 1998.

Benson, F. D. and Geschwind, N. Aphasia and related disorders: A clinical approach. In: *Principles of Behavioral Neurology*, ed. M.-M. Mesulam (Philadelphia: F. A. Davis, 1985), 193–238.

Berger, H. Über das Elektroenzephalogramm des Menschen. *Arch. Psychiatr. Nervenkr.* 87: 527–528, 1929.

Berkeley, G. An essay toward a new theory of vision (1709). In: *Berkeley's Work on Vision*, ed. C. M. Turbnyne (New York: Bobbs-Merrill, 1963), 7–102.

Berthier, M. L., Starkstein, S. E., Lylyk, P., and Leiguarda, R. Differential recovery of languages in a bilingual patient: A case study using selective amytal test. *Brain Lang.* 38: 449–453, 1990.

Best, C. T. The emergence of cerebral asymmetries in early human development: A literature review and a neuroembryological model. In: *Brain Lateralization in Children: Developmental Implications*, ed. D. L. Molfese and S. J. Segalowitz (New York: Guilford Press, 1988), 5–34.

Betz, W. Anatomischer Nachweis zweier Gehirncentra. *Cent. Med. Wissensch.* 12: 578–580; 595–59, 1874.

Binder, J. R., Frost, J. A., Hammeke, T. A., Cox, R. W., Rao, S. M., and Prieto, T. Human brain language areas identified by functional magnetic resonance imaging. *J. Neurosci.* 17: 353–362, 1997.

Black, J. E. and Greenough, W. T. Induction of pattern in neural structure by experience: Implications for congnitive development. In: *Advances in Developmental Psychology*, ed. M. E. Lamb, A. L. Brown, and B. Rogoff (Hillsdale, NJ: Erlbaum, 1986), 1–50.

Blakemore, C., Garey, L. J., and Vital-Durand, F. The physiological effects of monocular deprivation and their reversal in the monkey's visual cortex. *J. Physiol.* 283: 223–262, 1978.

Bliss, T. V. P. and Lømo, T. Long-lasting potentiation of synaptic transmission in the dentate area of the anaesthetized rabbit following stimulation of the perforant path. *J. Physiol.* 232: 331–356, 1973.

Bodner, M., Kroger, J., and Fuster, J. M. Auditory memory cells in dorsolateral prefrontal cortex. *NeuroReport* 7: 1905–1908, 1996.

Bodner, M., Zhou, Y. -D., and Fuster, J. M. High-frequency transitions in cortical spike trains related to short-term memory. *Neuroscience* 86: 1083–1087, 1998.

Bogen, J. E. and Gordon, H. W. Musical tests for functional lateralisation with intracaratoid amobarbital. *Nature* 230: 524–525, 1971.

Boivin, M., Giordani, B., Beret, S., Amato, D., Lehtinen, S., Koeppe, R., Buchtel, H. A., Foster, N., and Kuhl, D. E. Verbal fluency and positron emission tomographic mapping of regional cerebral glucose metabolism. *Cortex* 2: 231–239, 1992.

Bonin, G. V. *Essay on the Cerebral Cortex* (Springfield, IL.: Charles C. Thomas, 1950).

Boring, E. G. *The Physical Dimensions of Consciousness* (New York: The Century Co., 1933).

Boring, E. G. *A History of Experimental Psychology* (New York: Appleton-Century-Crofts, 1942).

Bourgeois, J. P., Goldman-Rakic, P. S., and Rakic, P. Synaptogenesis in the prefrontal cortex of rhesus monkeys. *Cerebral Cortex* 4: 78–96, 1994.

Bower, G. H., Clark, M. C., Lesgold, A. M., and Winzenz, D. Hierarchical retrieval schemes in recall of categorized word lists. *J. Verbal Learning Verbal Behav.* 8: 323–343, 1969.

Braitenberg, V. *Vehicles* (Cambridge, MA: MIT Press, 1996).

Bressler, S. L. The gamma wave: A cortical information carrier? *Trends NeuroSci.* 13: 161–162, 1990.

Britten, K., Newsome, W., Shadlen, M., Celebrini, S., and Movshon, J. A relationship between behavioral choice and the visual responses in macaque MT. *Visual Neurosci.* 13: 87–100, 1996.

Broca, P. Rémarques sur la siège de la faculté du langage articulé, suivi d'une observation d'aphemié. *Bull. Anat. Soc. (Paris)* 2: 330–357, 1861.

Brody, B. A., Kinney, H. C., Kloman, A. S., and Gilles, F. H. Sequence of central nervous system myelination in human infancy. I. An autopsy study of myelination. *J. Neuropathol. Exp. Neurol.* 46: 283–301, 1987.

Brown, J. W. *Aphasia, Apraxia and Agnosia.* (Springfield, IL: Charles C. Thomas, 1972).

Brown, T. H., Kairiss, E. W., and Keenan, C. L. Hebbian synapses: Biophysical mechanisms and algorithms. *Annu. Rev. Neurosci.* 13: 475–511, 1990.

Brunia, C. H. M., Haagh, S. A. V. M., and Scheirs, J. G. M. Waiting to respond: Electrophysiological measurements in man during preparation for a voluntary movement. In: *Motor Behavior,* ed. H. Heuer, U. Kleinbeck, and K.-H. Schmidt (New York: Springer, 1985), 35–78.

Brust, J. C. Music and language: Musical alexia and agraphia. *Brain* 103: 367–392, 1980.

Buonomano, D. V. and Byrne, J. H. Long-term synaptic changes produced by a cellular analog of classical conditioning in Aplysia. *Science* 249: 420–423, 1990.

Burbaud, P., Camus, O., Guehl, D., Bioulac, B., Caillé, J., and Allard, M. A functional magnetic resonance imaging study of mental subtraction in human subjects. *Neurosci. Lett.* 273: 195–199, 1999.

Butler, A. B. The evolution of the dorsal pallium in the telencephalon of amniotes: Cladistic analysis and a new hypothesis. *Brain Res. Rev.* 19: 66–101, 1994.

Cabeza, R. and Nyberg, L. Imaging cognition II: An empirical review of 275 PET and MRI studies. *J. Cognit. Neurosci.* 12: 1–47, 2000.

Cajal, S. R. La fine structure des centres nerveux. *Proc. R. Soc. Lond.* 55: 444–468, 1894.

Caramazza, A., Gordon, J., Zurif, E. B., and DeLuca, D. Right-hemispheric damage and verbal problem solving behavior. *Brain Lang.* 3: 41–46, 1976.

Caramazza, A. and Hillis, A. E. Lexical organization of nouns and verbs in the brain. *Nature* 349: 788–790, 1991.

Caramazza, A. and Shelton, J. R. Domain specific knowledge systems in the brain: The animate–inanimate distinction. *J. Cognit. Neurosci.* 10: 1–34, 1998.

Carew, T. J., Hawkins, R. D., Abrams, T. W., and Kandel, E. A test of Hebb's postulate at identified synapses which mediate classical conditioning in Aplysia. *J. Neurosci.* 4: 1217–1224, 1984.

Carlsson, I., Wendt, P., and Risberg, J. On the neurobiology of creativity. Differences in frontal activity between high and low creativity subjects. *Neuropsychologia* 38: 873–885, 2000.

Carroll, R. *Vertebrate Paleontology and Evolution* (New York: Freeman, 1988).

Cavada, C. and Goldman-Rakic, P. S. Posterior parietal cortex in rhesus monkey: I. Parcellation of areas based on distinctive limbic and sensory corticocortical connections. *J. Comp. Neurol.* 287: 393–421, 1989a.

Cavada, C. and Goldman-Rakic, P. S. Posterior parietal cortex in rhesus monkey: II. Evidence for segregated corticocortical networks linking sensory and limbic areas with the frontal lobe. *J. Comp. Neurol.* 287: 422–445, 1989b.

Changeux, J.-P. and Danchin, A. Selective stabilisation of developing synapses as a mechanism for the specification of neuronal networks. *Nature* 264: 705–712, 1976.

Chelazzi, L., Miller, E. K., Duncan, J., and Desimone, R. A neural basis for visual search in inferior temporal cortex. *Nature* 363: 345–347, 1993.

Chomsky, N. *Reflections on Language* (New York: Pantheon Books, 1975).

Chomsky, N. *Knowledge of Language* (New York: Praeger, 1986).

Cohen, M. S., Kosslyn, S. M., Breiter, H., DiGirolamo, G., Thompson, W. L., Anderson, A., Brookheimer, S., Rosen, B. R., and Belliveau, J. W. Changes in cortical activity during mental rotation. A mapping study using functional MRI. *Brain* 119: 89–100, 1996.

Cohen, N. J. and Eichenbaum, H. *Memory, Amnesia, and the Hippocampal System* (Cambridge, MA: MIT Press, 1993).

Cohen, N. J. and Squire, L. R. Preserved learning and retention of pattern-analyzing skill in amnesia: Dissociation of knowing how and knowing that. *Science* 210: 207–210, 1980.

Colebatch, J. G., Deiber, M.-P., Passingham, R. E., Friston, K. J., and Frackowiak, S. J. Regional cerebral blood flow during voluntary arm and hand movements in human subjects. *J. Neurophysiol.* 65: 1392–1401, 1991.

Collins, A. M. and Loftus, E. F. A spreading-activation theory of semantic processing. *Psychol. Rev.* 82: 407–428, 1975.

Conel, J. L. *The Postnatal Development of the Human Cerebral Cortex*, Vols. 1–6 (Cambridge, MA: Harvard University Press, 1963).

Cook, N. *The Brain Code: Mechanisms of Information Transfer and the Role of the Corpus Callosum* (London: Methuen, 1986).

Corbetta, M., Miezin, F. M., Shulman, G. L., and Petersen, S. E. A PET study of visuospatial attention. *J. Neurosci.* 13: 1202–1226, 1993.

Corbin, J., Nery, S., and Fishell, G. Telencephalic cells take a tangent: non-radial migration in the mammalian forebrain. *Nature Neurosci. Suppl.* 4: 1177–1182, 2001.

Coryell, J. Infant rightward asymmetries predict right-handedness in childhood. *Neuropsychologia* 23: 269–271, 1985.

Cotman, C. W., Monaghan, D. T., Ottersen, O. P., and Storm-Mathisen, J. Anatomical organization of excitatory amino acid receptors and their pathways. *Trends NeuroSci.* 10: 273–280, 1987.

Cragg, B. G. The development of synapses in kitten visual cortex during visual deprivation. *Exp. Neurol.* 46: 445–451, 1975.

Creutzfeldt, O. D. *Cortex Cerebri.* Oxford: Oxford University Press, 1995.

Crewther, D. P., Crewther, G. S., and Sanderson, K. J. Primary visual cortex in the brushtailed possum: Receptive field properties and corticocortical connections. *Brain Behav. Evol.* 24: 184–197, 1984.

Critchley, M. and Henson, R. A. *Music and the Brain.* (London: Heinemann Medical Books, 1977).

Crutcher, M. D. and Alexander, G. E. Movement-related neuronal activity selectively coding either direction or muscle pattern in three motor areas of the monkey. *J. Neurophysiol.* 64: 151–163, 1990.

Cummings, J. L., Benson, D. F., Walsh, M. J., and Levine, H. L. Left-to-right transfer of language dominance: A case study. *Neurology* 29: 1547–1550, 1979.

Daffner, K. R., Mesulam, M.-M., Scinto, L. F. M., Acar, D., Calvo, V., Faust, R., Chabrerie, A., Kennedy, B., and Holcomb, P. The central role of the prefrontal cortex in directing attention to novel events. *Brain* 123: 927–939, 2000.

Damasio, A. R. The brain binds entities and events by multiregional activation from convergence zones. *Neural Comput.* 1: 123–132, 1989a.

Damasio, H. Neuroimaging contributions to the understanding of aphasia. In: *Handbook of Neuropsychology,* ed. F. Boller and J. Grafman (Amsterdam: Elsevier, 1989b), 3–46.

Damasio, A. R. *Descartes' Error: Emotion, Reason and the Human Brain* (New York: Grosset Putnam, 1994).

Damasio, H., Grabowski, T., Tranel, D., Hichwa, R. D., and Damasio, A. R. A neural basis for lexical retrieval. *Nature* 380: 499–505, 1996.

Damasio, A. R. and Tranel, D. Nouns and verbs are retrieved with differently distributed neural systems. *Proc. Natl. Acad. Sci. USA* 90: 4957–4960, 1993.

Darwin, C. *The Expression of the Emotions in Man and Animals.* (Oxford: Oxford University Press, 1998).

Davidoff, J. B. and Ostergaard, A. L. Colour anomia resulting from weakened short-term colour memory. *Brain* 107: 415–431, 1984.

Deacon, T. W. Rethinking mammalian brain evolution. *Am. Zool.* 30: 629–705, 1990.

Deacon, T. W. *The Symbolic Species* (New York: Norton, 1998).

Decker, M. W. and McGaugh, J. L. The role of interactions between the cholinergic system and other neuromodulatory systems in learning and memory. *Synapse* 7: 151–168, 1991.

Deglin, V. and Kinsbourne, M. Divergent thinking styles of the hemispheres: How syllogisms are solved during transitory hemisphere suppression. *Brain Cognition* 31: 285–307, 1996.

Dehaene, S. and Changeux, J.-P. Development of elementary numerical abilities: A neuronal model. *J. Cognit. Neurosci.* 5: 390–407, 1993.

Dehaene, S., Kerszberg, M., and Changeux, J.-P. A neuronal model of a global workspace in effortful cognitive tasks. *Proc. Natl. Acad. Sci. USA* 95: 14529–14534, 1998.

Desimone, R. Face-selective cells in the temporal cortex of monkeys. *J. Cognit. Neurosci.* 3: 1–8, 1991.

Desimone, R., Albright, T. D., Gross, C. G., and Bruce, C. Stimulus-selective properties of inferior temporal neurons in the macaque. *J. Neurosci.* 4: 2051–2062, 1984.

Desimone, R. and Duncan, J. Neural mechanisms of selective visual attention. *Annu. Rev. Neurosci.* 18: 193–222, 1995.

Di Pellegrino, G., Fadiga, L., Fogassi, L., Gallese, V., and Rizzolatti, G. Understanding motor events: A neurophysiological study. *Exp. Brain Res.* 91: 176–180, 1992.

Diamond, M. C. *Enriching Heredity* (New York: Free Press, 1988).

Diamond, M. C., Law, F., Rhodes, H., Lindner, B., Rosenzweig, M. R., Krech, D., and Bennett, E. L. Increases in cortical depth and glia numbers in rats subjected to enriched environment. *J. Comp. Neurol.* 128: 117–126, 1966.

Dobbs, A. R. and Rule, B. G. Prospective memory and self-reports of memory abilities in older adults. *Can. J. Psychol.* 41: 209–222, 1987.

Duncan, J., Burgess, P., and Emslie, H. Fluid intelligence after frontal lobe lesions. *Neuropsychologia* 33: 261–268, 1995.

Duncan, J., Emslie, H., Williams, P., Johnson, R., and Freer, C. Intelligence and the frontal lobe: The organization of goal-directed behavior. *Cognit. Psychol.* 30: 257–303, 1996.

Duncan, J. and Owen, A. M. Common regions of the human frontal lobe recruited by diverse cognitive demands. *Trends NeuroSci.* 23: 475–483, 2000.

Duncan, J., Seitz, R. J., Kolodny, J., Bor, D., Herzog, H., Ahmed, A., Newell, F., and Emslie, H. A neural basis for general intelligence. *Science* 289: 457–460, 2000.

Earle, J. Task difficulty and EEG alpha asymmetry: An amplitude and frequency analysis. *Neuropsychology* 20: 95–112, 1988.

Eayrs, J. T. Influence of the thyroid on the central nervous system. *Br. Med. Bull.* 16: 122–127, 1960.

Ebbinghaus, H. *Memory: A Contribution to Experimental Psychology* (New York: Columbia University Press, 1885).

Eccles, J. C. The initiation of voluntary movements by the supplementary motor area. *Arch. Psychiatr. Nervenkr.* 231: 423–441, 1982.

Edelman, G. and Gally, J. A. Degeneracy and complexity in biological systems. Proc. Natl. Acad. Sci. USA 98: 13763–13768, 2001.

Edelman, G. M. *Neural Darwinism* (New York: Basic Books, 1987).

Edelman, G. M. *The Remembered Present* (New York: Basic Books, 1989).

Edelman, G. M. and Mountcastle, V. B. *The Mindful Brain* (New York: Plenum Press, 1978).

Elman, J. L., Bates, E. A., Johnson, M. H., Karmiloff-Smith, A., Parisi, D., and Plunkett, K. *Rethinking Innateness. A Connectionist Perspective on Development* (Cambridge, MA: MIT Press, 1996).

Engel, A. K., König, P., Kreiter, A. K., and Singer, W. Interhemispheric synchronization of oscillatory neuronal responses in cat visual cortex. *Science* 252: 1177–1179, 1991.

English, H. B. and English, A. C. *A Comprehensive Dictionary of Psychological and Psychoanalytic Terms* (New York: Longmans, Green, 1958).

Entus, A. K. Hemispheric asymmetry in processing of dichotically presented speech and nonspeech stimuli by infants. In: *Language Development and Neurological Theory*, ed. S. J. Segalowitz and F. A. Gruber (New York: Academic Press, 1977), 63–73.

Eulitz, C., Maess, B., Pantev, C., Friederici, A. D., Feige, B., and Elbert, T. Oscillatory neuromagnetic activity induced by language and non-language stimuli. *Cognit. Brain Res.* 4: 121–132, 1996.

Evans, J. Matching bias in conditional reasoning. *Thinking Reasoning* 4: 45–82, 1998.

Feigl, H. *The "Mental" and the "Physical"* (Minneapolis: University of Minnesota Press, 1967).

Felleman, D. J. and Van Essen, D. C. Distributed hierarchical processing in the primate cerebral cortex. *Cerebral Cortex* 1:1–47, 1991.

Fiez, J. A. and Petersen, S. E. Neuroimaging studies of word reading. *Proc. Natl. Acad. Sci. USA* 95: 914–921, 1998.

Finlay, B. L. and Darlington, R. B. Linked regularities in the development and evolution of mammalian brains. *Science* 268: 1578–1584, 1995.

Flechsig, P. Developmental (myelogenetic) localisation of the cerebral cortex in the human subject. *Lancet* 2: 1027–1029, 1901.

Flechsig, P. *Anatomie des Menschlichen Gehirns und Rückenmarks auf Myelogenetischer Grundlage* (Leipzig: Thieme, 1920).

Fletcher, P. C., Shallice, T., and Dolan, R. J. The functional roles of prefrontal cortex in episodic memory. I. Encoding. *Brain* 121: 1239–1248, 1998a.

Fletcher, P. C., Shallice, T., Frith, C. D., Frackowiak, R. S. J., and Dolan, R. J. The functional roles of prefrontal cortex in episodic memory. II. Retrieval. *Brain* 121: 1249–1256, 1998b.

Fodor, J. A. *The Modularity of Mind* (Cambridge, MA: MIT Press, 1983).

Foundas, A. L., Leonard, C. M., and Heilman, K. M. Morphologic cerebral asymmetries and handedness: The pars triangularis and planum temporale. *Arch. Neurol.* 52: 501–508, 1995.

Frahm, H. D., Stephan, H., and Stephan, M. Comparison of brain structure volumes in insectivora and primates. I. Neocortex. *J. Hirnforsch.* 23: 375–389, 1982.

Freeman, W. J. *Mass Action in the Nervous System* (New York: Academic Press, 1975).

Freud, S. *On Aphasia* (English translation from German *Zur Auffassung der Aphasien, 1891*) (London: Imago, 1953).

Friedlander, M. J., Martin, K. A. C., and Wassenhove-McCarthy, D. Effects of monocular visual deprivation on geniculocortical innervation of area 18 in cat. *J. Neurosci.* 11: 3268–3288, 1991.

Frith, C. D., Friston, K. J., Liddle, P. F., and Frackowiak, R. S. J. A PET study of word finding. *Neuropsychologia* 29: 1137–1148, 1991.

Frost, D. O. and Metin, C. Induction of functional retinal projections to the somatosensory system. *Nature* 317: 162–164, 1985.

Fujita, I., Tanaka, K., Ito, M., and Cheng, K. Columns for visual features of objects in monkey inferotemporal cortex. *Nature* 360: 343–346, 1992.

Fukuchi-Shimogori, T. and Grove, E. Neocortex patterning by the secreted signaling molecule FGF8. *Science* 294: 1071–1074, 2001.

Funahashi, S., Bruce, C. J., and Goldman-Rakic, P. S. Mnemonic coding of visual space in the monkey's dorsolateral prefrontal cortex. *J. Neurophysiol.* 61: 331–349, 1989.

Fuster, J. M. Effects of stimulation of brain stem on tachistoscopic perception. *Science* 127: 150, 1958.

Fuster, J. M. Unit activity in prefrontal cortex during delayed-response performance: Neuronal correlates of transient memory. *J. Neurophysiol.* 36: 61–78, 1973.

Fuster, J. M. Inferotemporal units in selective visual attention and short-term memory. *J. Neurophysiol.* 64: 681–697, 1990.

Fuster, J. M. *Memory in the Cerebral Cortex: An Empirical Approach to Neural Networks in the Human and Nonhuman Primate* (Cambridge, MA: MIT Press, 1995).

Fuster, J. M. *The Prefrontal Cortex: Anatomy, Physiology, and Neuropsychology of the Frontal Lobe* (Philadelphia: Lippincott-Raven, 1997).

Fuster, J. M. The prefrontal cortex—an update: time is of the essence. *Neuron* 30: 319–333, 2001.

Fuster, J. M. and Alexander, G. E. Neuron activity related to short-term memory. *Science* 173: 652–654, 1971.

Fuster, J. M., Bauer, R. H., and Jervey, J. P. Cellular discharge in the dorsolateral prefrontal cortex of the monkey in cognitive tasks. *Exp. Neurol.* 77: 679–694, 1982.

Fuster, J. M., Bauer, R. H., and Jervey, J. P. Functional interactions between inferotemporal and prefrontal cortex in a cognitive task. *Brain Res.* 330: 299–307, 1985.

Fuster, J. M., Bodner, M., and Kroger, J. Cross-modal and cross-temporal association in neurons of frontal cortex. *Nature* 405: 347–351, 2000.

Fuster, J. M. and Jervey, J. Inferotemporal neurons distinguish and retain behaviorally relevant features of visual stimuli. *Science* 212: 952–955, 1981.

Fuster, J. M. and Jervey, J. P. Neuronal firing in the inferotemporal cortex of the monkey in a visual memory task. *J. Neurosci.* 2: 361–375, 1982.

Gabor, D. Improved holographic model of temporal recall. *Nature* 217: 1288–1289, 1968.

Gainotti, G. Neuroanatomical correlates of category-specific semantic disorders: A critical survey. *Memory* 3: 247–264, 2001.

Gainotti, G., Silveri, M. C., Daniele, A., and Giustolisi, L. Neuroanatomical correlates of category-specific semantic disorders: A critical survey. *Memory* 3: 247–264, 1995.

Galaburda, A. M., Anatomic basis of cerebral dominance. In: *Brain Asymmetry*, ed. R. J. Davidson and K. Hugdahl (Cambridge, MA: MIT Press, 1995), 51–73.

Gall, F. I. *Sur les Fonctions du Cerveau et sur Celles de Chacune de ses Parties* (Paris: Bailliere, 1825).

Gazzaniga, M. S. *The Social Brain* (New York: Basic Book, 1985).

Georgopoulos, A. P., Kalaska, J. F., Caminiti, R., and Massey, J. T. On the relations between the direction of two-dimensional arm movements and cell discharge in primate motor cortex. *J. Neurosci.* 2: 1527–1537, 1982.

Georgopoulos, A. P., Schwartz, A. B., and Kettner, R. E. Neuronal population coding of movement direction. *Science* 233: 1416–1419, 1986.

Geschwind, N. Alexia and colour-naming disturbance. In: *Functions of the Corpus Callosum*, ed. G. Ettlinger (London: Churchill, 1965a), 95–114.

Geschwind, N. Disconnexion syndromes in animals and man. *Brain* 88: 237–274, 585, 1965b.

Geschwind, N. The varieties of naming errors. *Cortex* 3: 97–112, 1967.

Geschwind, N. The organization of language and the brain. *Science* 170: 940–944, 1970.

Geschwind, N. and Levitsky, W. Human brain: Left–right asymmetries in temporal speech region. *Science* 161: 186–187, 1968.

Gibson, K. R. Myelination and behavioral development: A comparative perspective on questions of neoteny, altriciality and intelligence. In: *Brain Maturation and Cognitive Development*, ed. K. R. Gibson and A. C. Petersen (New York: Aldine de Gruyter, 1991), 29–63.

Gilbert, C. D. Adult cortical dynamics. *Physiol. Rev.* 78: 467–485, 1998.

Glickman, S. E. Perseverative neural processes and consolidation of the memory trace. *Psychol. Bull.* 58: 218–233, 1961.

Globus, A., Rosenzweig, M. R., Bennett, E. L., and Diamond, M. C. Effects of differential experience on dendritic spine counts in rat cerebral cortex. *J. Comp. Physiol. Psychol.* 82: 175–181, 1973.

Globus, A. and Scheibel, A. B. Synaptic loci on visual cortical neurons of the rabbit: The specific afferent radiation. *Exp. Neurol.* 18: 116–131, 1967.

Gloor, P. Amygdala. In: *Handbook of Physiology. Neurophysiology*, ed. J. Field and

H. W. Magoun (Washington, DC: American Physiological Society, 1960), 1395–1420.

Goel, V., Gold, B., Kapur, S., and Houle, S. Neuroanatomical correlates of human reasoning. *J. Cognit. Neurosci.* 10: 293–302, 1998.

Goldberg, E., Antin, S. P., Bilder, R. M., Gerstman, L. J., Hughes, J. E. O., and Mattis, S. Retrograde amnesia: Possible role of mesencephalic reticular activation in long-term memory. *Science* 213: 1392–1394, 1981.

Goldman-Rakic, P. S. Development and plasticity of primate frontal association cortex. In: *The Organization of the Cerebral Cortex,* ed. E. O. Schmitt (Cambridge, MA: MIT Press, 1981), 69–97.

Goldman-Rakic, P. S. Circuitry of primate prefrontal cortex and regulation of behavior by representational memory. In: *Handbook of Physiology; Nervous System, Vol. V: Higher Functions of the Brain, Part 1,* ed. F. Plum (Bethesda, MD: American Physiological Society, 1987), 373–417.

Goldman-Rakic, P. S. Topography of cognition: Parallel distributed networks in primate association cortex. *Annu. Rev. Neurosci.* 11: 137–156, 1988.

Goldman-Rakic, P. S. Architecture of the prefrontal cortex and the central executive. *Proc. Natl. Acad. Sci. USA* 769: 71–83, 1995.

Goldman-Rakic, P. S., Bourgeois, J. P., and Rakic, P. Synaptic substrate of cognitive development: Lifespan analysis of synaptogenesis in the prefrontal cortex of the nonhuman primate. In: *Development of Prefrontal Cortex. Evolution, Neurobiology and Behavior,* ed. N. A. Krasnogor, G. R. Lyon, and P. Goldman-Rakic (Baltimore: P. H. Brukes, 1997), 27–47.

Goldman-Rakic, P. S. and Brown, R. M. Postnatal development of monoamine content and synthesis in the cerebral cortex of rhesus monkeys. *Dev. Brain Res.* 4: 339–349, 1982.

Goldstein, K. *Language and Language Disturbances* (New York: Grune & Stratton, 1948).

Goldstein, K. Functional disturbances in brain damage. In: *American Handbook of Psychiatry, Vol. I,* ed. S. Arieti (New York: Basic Books, 1959), 770–794.

Goodglass, H., Klein, B., Carey, P., and Jones, K. Specific semantic word categories in aphasia. *Cortex* 2: 74–89, 1966.

Grafton, S. T., Mazziotta, J. C., Woods, R. P., and Phelps, M. E. Human functional anatomy of visually guided finger movements. *Brain* 115: 565–587, 1992.

Grasby, P. M., Frith, C. D., Friston, K. J., Bench, C., Frackowiak, R. S. J., and Dolan, R. J. Functional mapping of brain areas implicated in auditory–verbal memory function. *Brain* 116: 1–20, 1993.

Greenfield, P. M. Language, tools and brain: The ontogeny and phylogeny of hierarchically organized sequential behavior. *Behav. Brain Sci.* 14: 531–595, 1991.

Grossberg, S. How does a brain build a cognitive code? *Psychol. Rev.* 87: 1–42, 1980.

Grossberg, S. The link between brain learning, attention, and consciousness. *Consciousness Cognition* 8: 1–44, 1999.

Guilford, J. *The Nature of Human Intelligence* (New York: McGraw-Hill, 1967).

Gustavson, C. R., Garcia, J., Hankins, W. G., and Rusiniak, K. W. Coyote predation control by aversive conditioning. *Science* 184: 581–583, 1974.

Hagoort, P. The shadows of lexical meaning in patients with semantic impairments. In: *Handbook of Neurolinguistics.*, ed. B. Stemmer and H. A. Whitaker (San Diego, CA: Academic Press, 1998), 235–248.

Halford, G. S. *Children's Undestanding: The Development of Mental Models* (Hillsdale, NJ: Erlbaum, 1993).

Halsband, U., Ito, N., Tanji, J., and Freund, H.-J. The role of premotor cortex and the supplementary motor area in the temporal control of movement in man. *Brain* 116: 243–266, 1993.

Hamlyn, L. H. An electron microscope study of pyramidal neurons in the Ammon's horn of the rabbit. *J. Anat.* 97: 189–201, 1962.

Hart, J. and Gordon, B. Neural subsystems for object knowledge. *Nature* 359: 60–64, 1992.

Hasegawa, I., Fukushima, T., Ihara, T., and Miyashita, Y. Callosal window between prefrontal cortices: Cognitive interaction to retrieve long-term memory. *Science* 281: 814–818, 1998.

Hayek, F. A. *The Road to Serfdom.* Chicago: University of Chicago Press, 1944.

Hayek, F. A. *The Sensory Order* (Chicago: University of Chicago Press, 1952).

Hayes, T. L. and Lewis, D. A. Anatomical specialization of the anterior motor speech area: Hemispheric differences in magnopyramidal neurons. *Brain Lang.* 49: 289–308, 1995.

Hebb, D. O. *The Organization of Behavior* (New York: Wiley, 1949).

Helmholtz, H. v. Helmholtz's Treatise on Physiological Optics (translated from German by J.P.C. Southall) (Banta, Menasha, WI: Optical Society of America, 1925).

Hernández, A., Zainos, A., and Romo, R. Neuronal correlates of sensory discrimination in the somatosensory cortex. *Proc. Natl. Acad. Sci. USA* 97: 6191–6196, 2000.

Herrick, C. J. *The Brain of the Tiger Salamander* (Chicago: University of Chicago Press, 1948).

Herrick, C. J. *The Evolution of Human Nature* (Austin: University of Texas Press, 1956).

Hikosaka, O., Nakahara, H., Rand, M. K., Sakai, K., Lu, X., Nakamura, K., Miyachi, S., and Doya, K. Parallel neural networks for learning sequential procedures. *Trends NeuroSci.* 22: 464–471, 1999.

Hiscock, M. Brain lateralization across the life span. In: *Handbook of Neurolinguistics*, ed. B. Stemmer and H. A. Whitaker (San Diego, CA: Academic Press, 1998), 357–368.

Hobson, J. A. *The Dreaming Brain* (New York: Basic Books, 1988).

Holloway, R. L. Human brain evolution: A search for units, models and synthesis. *Can. J. Anthropol.* 3: 215–230, 1983.

Holtzman, J. and Gazzaniga, M. S. Enhanced dual task performance following corpus commissurotomy in humans. *Neuropsychologia* 23: 315–321, 1985.

Holyoak, K. J. and Thagard, P. *Mental Leaps: Analogy in Creative Thought* (Cambridge, MA: MIT Press, 1995).

Homan, R. W., Criswell, E., Wada, J. A., and Ross, E. D. Hemispheric contributions to manual communication (signing and finger spelling). *Neurology* 32: 1020–1023, 1982.

Houdé, O. Inhibition and cognitive development: Object, number, categorization, and reasoning. *Cognit. Dev.* 15: 63–73, 2000.

Houdé, O., Zago, L., Mellet, E., Moutier, S., Pineau, A., Mazoyer, B., and Tzourio-Mazoyer, N. Shifting from the perceptual brain to the logical brain: The neural impact of cognitive inhibition training. *J. Cognit. Neurosci.* 12: 721–728, 2000.

Hubel, D. H. and Wiesel, T. N. Receptive fields and functional architecture of monkey striate cortex. *J. Physiol.(Lond.)* 195: 215–243, 1968.

Hutsler, J. J. and Gazzaniga, M. S. The organization of human language cortex: Special adaptation or common cortical design? *Neuroscientist* 3: 61–72, 1997.

Huttenlocher, P. R. Morphometric study of human cerebral cortex development. *Neuropsychologia* 28: 517–527, 1990.

Huttenlocher, P. R. and Dabholkar, A. S. Regional differences in synaptogenesis in human cerebral cortex. *J. Comp. Neurol.* 387: 167–178, 1997.

Igarashi, S. and Kamiya, T. *Atlas of the Vertebrate Brain* (Baltimore: University Park Press, 1972).

Ingvar, D. H. "Memory of the future": An essay on the temporal organization of conscious awareness. *Human Neurobiol.* 4: 127–136, 1985.

Ingvar, D. H. Serial aspects of language and speech related to prefrontal cortical activity. *Hum. Neurobiol.* 2: 177–189, 1983.

Inhelder, B. and Piaget, J. *The Growth of Logical Thinking from Childhood to Adolescence* (New York: Basic Books, 1958).

Iriki, A., Pavlides, C., Keller, A., and Asanuma, H. Long-term potentiation in the motor cortex. *Science* 245: 1385–1387, 1989.

Jackson, J. H. *Selected Writings* (New York: Basic Books, 1958).

Jacobs, B. and Scheibel, A. B. A quantitative dendritic analysis of Wernicke's area in humans. I. Lifespan changes. *J. Comp. Neurol.* 327: 83–96, 1993.

Jacobson, S. and Trojanowski, J. Q. Prefrontal granular cortex of the rhesus monkey. I. Intrahemispheric cortical afferents. *Brain Res.* 132: 209–233, 1977.

Jahanshahi, M., Dirnberger, G., Fuller, R., and Frith, C. D. The role of the dorsolateral prefrontal cortex in random number generation: A study with positron emission tomography. *NeuroImage* 12: 713–725, 2000.

James, W. *Principles of Psychology* (New York: Holt, 1890).

Janet, P. *Les Débuts de L'Intelligence* (Paris: Flammarion, 1935).

Jenkins, I. H., Brooks, D. J., Nixon, P. D., Frackowiak, R. S. J., and Passingham, R. E. Motor sequence learning: A study with positron emission tomography. *J. Neurosci.* 14: 3775–3790, 1994.

Jerison, H. J. *Evolution of the Brain and Intelligence* (New York: Academic Press, 1973).

Jerison, H. J. Fossil brains and the evolution of the neorcortex. In: *The Neocortex: Ontogeny and Phylogeny,* ed. B. L. Finlay, G. Innocenti, and H. Scheich (New York: Plenum Press, 1990), 5–19.

Johnson-Laird, P. Mental models, deductive reasoning, and the brain. In: *The Cognitive Neurosciences,* ed. M. S. Gazzaniga (Cambridge, MA: MIT Press, 1995), 999–1008.

Joliot, M., Ribary, U., and Llinás, R. Human oscillatory brain activity near 40 Hz coexists with cognitive temporal binding. *Proc. Natl. Acad. Sci. USA* 91: 11748–11751, 1994.

Jones, E. G. Cellular organization in the primate postcentral gyrus. In: *Information Processing in the Somatosensory System,* eds. O. Franzen and J. Westman (New York: Macmillan, 1991), 95–107.

Jones, E. G. Laminar distribution of cortical efferent cells. In: *Cerebral Cortex,* ed. A. Peters and E. G. Jones (New York and London: Plenum Press, 1984), 521–553.

Jonides, J., Smith, E. E., Koeppe, R. A., Awh, E., Minoshima, S., and Mintun, M. A. Spatial working memory in humans as revealed by PET. *Nature* 363: 623–625, 1993.

Julesz, B. A brief outline of the texton theory of human vision. *Trends Neuro-Sci.* 7: 41–48, 1984.

Junqué, C., Vendrell, P., and Vendrell, J. Differential impairments and specific phenomena in 50 Catalan-Spanish bilingual aphasic patients. In: *Aspects of Bilingual Aphasia,* ed. M. Paradis (Oxford: Pergamon Press, 1995), 177–209.

Kaas, J. H., Merzenich, M. M., and Killackey, H. P. The reorganization of somatosensory cortex following peripheral nerve damage in adult and developing mammals. *Annu. Rev. Neurosci.* 6: 325–356, 1983.

Kaes, T. *Die Grosshirnrinde des Menschen in ihren Massen und in ihrem Fasengehalt* (Jena: Fischer, 1907).

Kalaska, J. F., Sergio, L. E., and Cisek, P. Cortical control of whole-arm motor tasks. *Novartis Foundation Symp.* 218: 176–190, 1998.

Kandel, E. R. *Cellular Basis of Behavior* (San Francisco: W. H. Freeman, 1976).

Kandel, E. R. Cellular mechanisms of learning and the biological basis of individuality. In: *Principles of Neural Science,* ed. E. R. Kandel, J. H. Schwartz, and T. M. Jessell (Norwalk, CT: Appleton & Lange, 1991), 1009–1031.

Karten, H. J. The organization of the avian telencephalon and some speculations on the phylogeny of the amniote telecephalon. *Ann. N.Y. Acad. Sci.* 167: 164–179, 1969.

Kastner, S., Pinsk, M. A., De Weerd, P., Desimone, R., and Ungerleider, L. G. Increased activity in human visual cortex during directed attention in the absence of visual stimulation. *Neuron* 22: 751–761, 1999.

Katz, L. C. and Shatz, C. J. Synaptic activity and the construction of cortical circuits. *Science* 274: 1133–1138, 1996.

Kemali, M. and Braitenberg, V. *Atlas of the Frog's Brain* (Berlin: Springer-Verlag, 1969).

Kertesz, A., Polk, M., Black, S. E., and Howell, J. Anatomical asymmetries and functional laterality. *Brain* 115: 589–605, 1992.

Kim, J. J. and Fanselow, M. S. Modality specific retrograde amnesia of fear following hippocampal lesions. *Science* 256: 675–677, 1992.

Kimura, D. Left–right differences in the perception of melodies. *J. Exp. Psychol.* (*Gen.*) 16: 355–358, 1964.

Kimura, D. Neuromotor mechanisms in the evolution of human communication. In: *Neurobiology of Social Communication in Primates: An Evolutionary Perspective,* ed. H. D. Steklis and M. J. Raleigh (New York: Academic Press, 1979), 197–219.

Kimura, D. *Neuromotor Mechanisms in Human Communication* (Oxford: Oxford University Press, 1993).

Kinsbourne, M. The right hemisphere and recovery from aphasia. In: *Handbook of Neurolinguistics,* ed. B. Stemmer and H. A. Whitaker (San Diego, CA: Academic Press, 1998), 385–392.

Klein, D., Zatorre, R. T., Milner, B., Meyer, E., and Evans, A. C. The neural substrates of bilingual language processing: Evidence from positron emission tomography. In: *Aspects of Aphasia,* ed. M. Paradis (Oxford: Pergamon Press, 1995), 23–36.

Knight, R. T. Decreased response to novel stimuli after prefrontal lesions in man. *Electroencephalogr. Clin. Neurophysiol.* 59: 9–20, 1984.

Koffka, K. *Principles of Gestalt Psychology* (New York: Harcourt, Brace, 1935).

Köhler, W. *The Mentality of Apes* (New York: Harcourt, 1925).

Köhler, W. *Gestalt Psychology* (New York: Liveright, 1929).

Kohonen, T. *Associative Memory: A System-Theoretical Approach* (Berlin: Springer-Verlag, 1977).

Kohonen, T. *Self-Organization and Associative Memory* (Berlin: Springer, 1984).

Kornhuber, H. H. and Deecke, L. Hirnpotentialänderungen bei Willkürbewegungen und passiven Bewegungen des Menschen: Bereitschaftspotential und reafferent Potentiale. *Pfluegers Arch. Gesamte Physiol.* 284: 1–17, 1965.

Kosslyn, S. M. and Thompson, W. L. Shared mechanisms in visual imagery and visual perception: Insights from cognitive neuroscience. In: *The New Cognitive Neurosciences,* ed. M. S. Gazzaniga (Cambridge, MA: MIT Press, 2000), 975–985.

Krasne, F. B. Extrinsic control of intrinsic neuronal plasticity: An hypothesis from work on simple systems. *Brain Res.* 140: 197–216, 1978.

Kreiman, G., Koch, C., and Fried, I. Category-specific visual responses of single neurons in the human medial temporal lobe. *Nature Neurosci.* 3: 946–953, 2000.

Kroger, J. K., Sabb, F., Fales, C., Bookheimer, S. Y., Cohen, M. S., and Holyoak,

K. J. Recruitment of anterior dorsolateral prefrontal cortex in human reasoning: A parametric study of relational complexity. *Cerebral Cortex* 12: 477–485, 2002.

Krubitzer, L. The organization of neocortex in mammals: Are species differences really so different? *Trends NeuroSci.* 18: 408–417, 1995.

Krubitzer, L., Manger, P., Pettigrew, J., and Calford, M. Organization of somatosensory cortex in monotremes: In search of the prototypical plan. *J. Comp. Neurol.* 351: 261–306, 1995.

Kuffler, S. W. and Nicholls, J. *From Neuron to Brain* (Sunderland, MA: Sinauer, 1976).

Kuhn, T. S. *The Structure of Scientific Revolutions* (Chicago: University of Chicago Press, 1996).

Kutas, M. and Hillyard, S. A. Event-related brain potentials to grammatical errors and semantic anomalies. *Memory Cognition* 11: 539–550, 1983.

Lamberts, K. Information-accumulation theory of speeded categorization. *Psychol. Rev.* 107: 227–260, 2000.

Lashley, K. S. In search of the engram. *Symp. Soc. Exp. Biol.* 4: 454–482, 1950.

Lashley, K. S. The problem of serial order in behavior. In: *Cerebral Mechanisms in Behavior*, ed. L. A. Jeffress (New York: Wiley, 1951), 112–146.

LeDoux, J. E. Emotional memory systems in the brain. *Behav. Brain Res.* 58: 69–79, 1993.

Levi-Montalcini, R. The nerve growth factor 35 years later. *Science* 237: 1154–1162, 1987.

Lezak, M. D. *Neuropsychological Assessment* (New York: Oxford University Press, 1995).

Lhermitte, F., Deroulsne, J., and Signoret, J. L. Analyse neuropsychologique du syndrome frontal. *Rev. Neurol.* 127: 415–440, 1972.

Lichtheim, L. On aphasia. *Brain* 7: 433–484, 1885.

Lidow, M. S. and Rakic, P. Scheduling of monoaminergic neurotransmitter receptor expression in the primate neocortex during postnatal development. *Cerebral Cortex* 2: 401–416, 1992.

Liederman, J. Neonates show an asymmetric degree of head rotation but lack an asymmetric tonic neck reflex asymmetry: Neuropsychological implications. *Dev. Neuropsychol.* 3: 101–112, 1987.

Light, L., Singh, A., and Capps, J. Dissociation of memory and awareness in young and older adults. *J. Clin. Exp. Neuropsychol.* 8: 594–610, 1986.

Llinás, R. and Ribary, U. Coherent 40-Hz oscillation characterizes dream state in humans. *Proc. Natl. Acad. Sci. USA* 90: 2078–2081, 1993.

Locke, J. *An Essay Concerning Human Understanding* (1690) Philadelphia: Kay and Troutman, 1894.

Logothetis, N. K., Pauls, J., Augath, M., Trinath, T., and Oeltermann, A. Neurophysiological investigation of the basis of the fMRI signal. *Nature* 412: 150–157, 2001.

Logothetis, N. K. and Schall, J. D. Neuronal correlates of subjective visual perception. *Science* 245: 761–763, 1989.

Lorente de Nó, R. Cerebral cortex: Architecture, intracortical connections, motor projections. In: *Physiology of the Nervous System*, ed. J. F. Fulton (New York: Oxford University Press, 1938), 291–339.

Löwel, S. and Singer, W. Selection of intrinsic horizontal connections in the visual cortex by correlated neuronal activity. *Science* 255: 209–212, 1992.

Luck, S. J. and Hillyard, S. A. The operation of selective attention at multiple stages of processing: Evidence from human and monkey electrophysiology. In: *The New Cognitive Neurosciences*, ed. M. S. Gazzaniga (Cambridge, MA: MIT Press, 2000), 687–700.

Lund, R. D. Tissue transplantation: A useful tool in mammalian neuroembryology. *Trends Neurosci.* 3: 12–13, 1979.

Luria, A. R. *Higher Cortical Functions in Man* (New York: Basic Books, 1966).

Luria, A. R. *Traumatic Aphasia* (The Hague: Mouton, 1970).

Luria, A. R. and Homskaya, E. D. Disturbance in the regulative role of speech with frontal lobe lesions. In: *The Frontal Granular Cortex and Behavior*, ed. J. M. Warren and K. Akert (New York: McGraw-Hill, 1964), 353–371.

Luria, A. R. and Simernitskaya, E. Interhemispheric relations and the functions of the minor hemisphere. *Neuropsychologia* 15: 175–178, 1977.

Lutzenberger, W., Pulvermüller, F., and Birbaumer, N. Words and pseudowords elicit distinct patterns of 30-Hz activity in humans. *Neurosci. Lett.* 176: 115–118, 1994.

Luu, P. and Tucker, D. M. Vertical integration of neurolinguistic mechanisms. In: *Handbook of Neurolinguistics*, ed. B. Stemmer and H. A. Whitaker (San Diego, CA: Academic Press, 1998), 159–172.

Lynch, G. and Baudry, M. The biochemistry of memory: A new and specific hypothesis. *Science* 224: 1057–1063, 1984.

Mach, E. *Die Analyse der Empfindungen* (Jena: G. Fisher, 1885).

Maffei, L., Berardi, N., Domenici, L., Parisi, V., and Pizzorusso, T. Nerve growth factor (NGF) prevents the shift in ocular dominance distribution of visual cortical neurons in monocularly deprived rats. *J. Neurosci.* 12: 4651–4662, 1992.

Marin-Padilla, M. Dual origin of the mammalian neocortex and evolution of the cortical plate. *Anat. Embryol.* 152: 109–126, 1978.

Marin-Padilla, M. Ontogenesis of the pyramidal cell of the mammalian neocortex and developmental cytoarchitectonics: A unifying theory. *J. Comp. Neurol.* 321: 223–240, 1992.

Marín-Padilla, M. Prenatal and early postnatal ontogenesis of the human motor cortex: A Golgi study: I. The sequential development of the cortical layers. *Brain Res.* 23: 167–183, 1970.

Marina, J. *Teoría de la Inteligencia Creadora* (Barcelona: Anagrama, 1993).

Marr, D. A theory of cerebellar cortex. *J. Physiol.* 202: 437–470, 1969.

Marr, D. A theory for cerebral neocortex. *Proc. R. Soc. Lond. B.* 176: 161–234, 1970.

Martin, A., Ungerleider, L. G., and Haxby, J. V. Category specificity and the brain: The sensory/motor model of semantic representations of objects.

In: *The New Cognitive Neurosicences,* ed. M. S. Gazzaniga (Cambridge, MA: MIT Press, 2000), 1023–1036.

Martin, A., Wiggs, C. L., Ungerleider, L. G., and Haxby, J. V. Neural correlates of category-specific knowledge. *Nature* 379: 649–652, 1996.

Martindale, C. and Hines, D. Creativity and cortical activation during creative, intellectual and EEG feedback tasks. *Biol. Psychol.* 2: 91–100, 1975.

Mateer, C. A., Rapport, R. L., and Kettrick, C. Cerebral organization of oral and signed language responses: Case study evidence from amytal and cortical stimulation studies. *Brain Lang.* 21: 123–135, 1984.

McCasland, J. S., Bernardo, K. L., Probst, K. L., and Woolsey, T. A. Cortical local circuit axons do not mature after early deafferentation. *Proc. Natl. Acad. Sci. USA* 89: 1832–1836, 1992.

McClelland, H. A. and Rumelhart, D. E. *Parallel Distributed Processing* (Cambridge, MA: MIT Press, 1986).

McCulloch, W. S. A recapitulation of the theory, with a forecast of several extensions. *Ann. N.Y. Acad. Sci.* 50: 259–277, 1948.

McGaugh, J. L. and Herz, M. J. *Memory Consolidation* (San Francisco: Albion, 1972).

McLeod, P., Plunkett, K., and Rolls, E. T. *Introduction to Connectionist Modeling of Cognitive Processes* (Oxford: Oxford University Press, 1998).

McNaughton, B. L., Douglas, R. M., and Goddard, G. V. Synaptic enhancement in fascia dentata: Cooperativity among coactive afferents. *Brain Res.* 157: 277–293, 1978.

Merzenich, M. M. and Kaas, J. H. Reorganization of mammalian somatosensory cortex following peripheral nerve injury. *Trends NeuroSci.* 5: 434–436, 1982.

Mesulam, M.-M. A cortical network for directed attention and unilateral neglect. *Neurology* 10: 309–325, 1981.

Mesulam, M.-M. From sensation to cognition. *Brain* 121: 1013–1052, 1998.

Miceli, G., Silveri, M. C., Villa, G., and Caramazza, A. On the basis for the agrammatic's difficulty in producing main verbs. *Cortex* 20: 207–220, 1984.

Michel, A. E. and Garey, L. J. The development of dendritic spines in the human visual cortex. *Hum. Neurobiol.* 3: 223–227, 1984.

Miller, E. K., Li, L., and Desimone, R. Activity of neurons in anterior inferior temporal cortex during a short-term memory task. *J. Neurosci.* 13: 1460–1478, 1993.

Miller, R., Designs for a prototype cerebral cortex. In: *Cortico-Hippocampal Interplay and the Representation of Contexts in the Brain (Vol. 17: Studies of Brain Function),* ed. V. Braitenberg, H. B. Barlow, T. H. Bullock, E. Florey, O.-J. Grüsser, and A. Peters (New York: Springer-Verlag, 1991), 11–32.

Mishkin, M. Memory in monkeys severely impaired by combined but not by separate removal of amygdala and hippocampus. *Nature* 273: 297–298, 1978.

Møllgaard, K., Diamond, M. C., Bennett, E. L., Rosenzweig, M. R., and Lindner, B. Quantitative synaptic changes with differential experience in rat brain. *Int. J. Neurosci.* 2: 113–128, 1971.

Moran, J. and Desimone, R. Selective attention gates visual processing in the extrastriate cortex. *Science* 229: 782–784, 1985.

Mountcastle, V. B. Modality and topographic properties of single neurons of cat's somatic sensory cortex. *J. Neurophysiol.* 20: 408–434, 1957.

Mountcastle, V. B. *Perceptual Neuroscience: The Cerebral Cortex* (Cambridge, MA: Harvard University Press, 1998).

Mrzljak, L., Uylings, H. B. M., Van Eden, C. G., and Judás, M. Neuronal development in human prefrontal cortex in prenatal and postnatal stages. *Prog. Brain Res.* 85: 185–222, 1990.

Mushiake, M., Inase, M., and Tanji, J. Selective coding of motor sequence in the supplementary motor area of the monkey cerebral cortex. *Exp. Brain Res.* 208: 210, 1990.

Mushiake, H., Inase, M., and Tanji, J. Neuronal activity in the primate premotor, supplementary, and precentral motor cortex during visually guided and internally determined sequential movements. *J. Neurophysiol.* 66: 705–718, 1991.

Müller, B., Reinhardt, J., and Strickland, M. T. *Neural Networks* (Berlin: Springer, 1995).

Näätänen, R. *Attention and Brain Function* (Hillsdale, NJ: Erlbaum, 1992).

Neisser, U. *Cognition and Reality: Principles and Implications of Cognitive Psychology* (San Francisco: W. H. Freeman, 1976).

Neville, H. J., Bavelier, D., Corina, D., Rauschecker, J., Karni, A., Lalwani, A., Braun, A., Clark, V., Jezzard, P., and Turner, R. Cerebral organization for language in deaf and hearing subjects: Biological constraints and effects of experience. *Proc. Natl. Acad. Sci. USA* 95: 922–929, 1998.

Neville, H. J., Mills, D., and Lawson, D. Fractionating language: Different neural subsystems with different sensitive periods. *Cerebral Cortex* 2: 244–258, 1992.

Nichelli, P., Grafman, J., Pietrini, P., Alway, D., Carton, J., and Miletich, R. Brain activity in chess playing. *Nature* 369: 191, 1994.

Nicoll, R. A., Kauer, J. A., and Malenka, R. C. The current excitement in long-term potentiation. *Neuron* 1: 97–103, 1988.

Niki, H. and Watanabe, M. Prefrontal and cingulate unit activity during timing behavior in the monkey. *Brain Res.* 171: 213–224, 1979.

Norman, D. A. and Shallice, T., Attention to action. In: *Consciousness and Self-Regulation,* ed. R. J. Davidson, G. E. Schwartz, and D. Shapiro (New York: Plenum Press, 1986), 1–18.

Northcutt, G. and Kaas, J. H. The emergence and evolution of mammalian neocortex. *Trends NeuroSci.* 18: 373–379, 1995.

O'Leary, D. D. M. Do cortical areas emerge from a protocortex? *Trends Neuro-Sci.* 12: 400–406, 1989.

Ogden, J. A. Language and memory fuctions after language recovery periods in left hemispher ectomized subjects. *Neuropsychologia* 26: 645–659, 1988.

Ojemann, G. A. Brain organization for language from the perspective of electrical stimulation mapping. *Behav. Brain Sci.* 6: 189–230, 1983.

Osherson, D., Perani, D., Cappa, S., Schnur, T., Grassi, F., and Fazzio, F. Distinct brain loci in deductive versus probabilistic reasoning. *Neuropsychologia* 36: 369–376, 1998.

Palm, G. *Neural Assemblies* (Berlin: Springer-Verlag, 1982).

Pandya, D. N., Seltzer, B., and Barbas, H. Input-output organization of the primate cerebral cortex. *Neurosciences* 4: 39–80, 1988.

Pandya, D. N. and Yeterian, E. H. Architecture and connections of cortical association areas. In: *Cerebral Cortex, Vol. 4*, ed. A. Peters and E. G. Jones (New York: Plenum Press, 1985), 3–61.

Pantev, C., Oostenveld, R., Engelien, A., Ross, B., Roberts, L. E., and Hoke, M. Increased auditory cortical representation in musicians. *Nature* 392: 811–814, 1998.

Paradis, M., Language and communication in multilinguals. In: *Handbook of Neurolinguistics*, ed. B. Stemmer and H. A. Whitaker (San Diego, CA: Academic Press, 1998), 417–430.

Pardo, J. V., Pardo, P. J., Janer, K. W., and Raichle, M. E. The anterior cingulate cortex mediates processing selection in the Stroop attentional conflict paradigm. *Proc. Natl. Acad. Sci. USA* 87: 256–259, 1990.

Parks, R. W., Loewenstein, D., Dodrill, K., Barker, W., Yoshii, F., Chang, J., Emran, A., Apicella, A., Sheramata, W., and Duara, R. Cerebral metabolic effects of a verbal fluency test: A PET scan study. *J. Clin. Exp. Neuropsychol.* 10: 565–575, 1988.

Partiot, A., Grafman, J., Sadato, N., Wachs, J., and Hallett, M. Brain activation during the generation of non-emotional and emotional plans. *NeuroReport* 6: 1269–1272, 1995.

Paulesu, E., Démonet, J. F., Fazio, F., McCrory, E., Chanoine, V., Brunswick, N., Cappa, S. F., Cossu, G., Habib, M., Frith, C. D., and Frith, U. Dyslexia: Cultural diversity and biological unity. *Science* 291: 2165–2167, 2001.

Penfield, W. and Roberts, L. *Speech and Brain Mechanisms* (New York: Atheneum, 1966).

Peters, A. and Payne, B. R. Numerical relationships between geniculocortical afferents and pyramidal cell modules in cat primary visual cortex. *Cerebral Cortex* 3: 69–78, 1993.

Petrides, M. Monitoring of selections of visual stimuli and the primate frontal cortex. *Proc. R. Soc. Lond. B* 246: 293–306, 1991.

Petrides, M., Alivisatos, B., Evans, A. C., and Meyer, E. Dissociation of human mid-dorsolateral from posterior dorsolateral frontal cortex in memory processing. *Proc. Natl. Acad. Sci. USA* 90: 873–877, 1993a.

Petrides, M., Alivisatos, B., Meyer, E., and Evans, A. C. Functional activation of the human frontal cortex during the performance of verbal working memory tasks. *Proc. Natl. Acad. Sci. USA* 90: 878–882, 1993b.

Piaget, J. *The Origins of Intelligence in Children* (New York: International Universities Press, 1952).

Pinker, S. Rules of language. *Science* 253: 530–535, 1991.

Pitts, W. and McCulloch, W. S. How we know universals: The perception of auditory and visual forms. *Bull. Math. Biophys.* 9: 127–147, 1947.

Plaut, D. C. and Shallice, T. Deep dyslexia: A case study of connectionist neuropsychology. *Cognitive Neuropsychol.* 10: 377–500, 1993.

Ploog, D. W. Neurobiology of primate audio-vocal behavior. *Brain Res. Rev.* 3: 35–61, 1981.

Ploog, D. W. Neuroethological perspectives on the human brain: From the expression of emotions to intentional signing and speech. In: *So Human a Brain: Knowledge and Values in Neurosciences,* ed. A. Harrington (Boston: Birkhauser, 1992), 3–13.

Poliakov, G. I. Some results of research into the development of the neuronal structure of the cortical ends of the analyzers in man. *J. Comp. Neurol.* 117: 197–212, 1961.

Polk, T. A. and Farah, M. J. The neural development and organization of letter recognition: Evidence from functional neuroimaging, computational modeling, and behavioral studies. *Proc. Natl. Acad. Sci. USA* 95: 847–852, 1998.

Pons, T. P., Garraghty, P. E., Ommaya, A. K., Kaas, J. H., Taub, E., and Mishkin, M. Massive cortical reorganization after sensory deafferentation in adult macaques. *Science* 252: 1857–1860, 1991.

Popper, K. *The Logic of Scientific Discovery* (London: Hutchinson, 1980).

Posner, M. I. and Pavase, A. Anatomy of word and sentence meaning. *Proc. Natl. Acad. Sci. USA* 95: 899–905, 1998.

Posner, M. I. and Petersen, S. E. The attention system of the human brain. *Annual Review of Neuroscience* 13: 25–42, 1990.

Prabhakaran, V., Rypma, B., and Gabrieli, J. Neural substrates of mathematical reasoning: A functional magnetic resonance imaging study of neocortical activation during performance of the necessary arithmetic operations test. *Neuropsychology* 15: 115–127, 2001.

Preissl, H., Pulvermüller, F., Lutzenberger, W., and Birbaumer, N. Evoked potentials distinguish between nouns and verbs. *Neurosci. Lett.* 197: 81–83, 1995.

Premack, D. *Intelligence in Ape and Man* (Hillsdale, NJ: Earlbaum, 1976).

Price, C., Indefrey, P., and Van Turennout, M. The neural architecture underlying the processing of written and spoken word forms. In: *The Neurocognition of Language,* ed. C. M. Brown and P. Hagoort (Oxford: Oxford University Press, 1999), 211–240.

Pulvermüller, F. Constituents of a neurological theory of language. *Concepts Neurosci.* 3: 157–200, 1992.

Pulvermüller, F., Birbaumer, N., Lutzenberger, W., and Mohr, B. High-frequency brain activity: Its possible role in attention, perception and language processing. *Prog. Neurobiol.* 52: 427–445, 1997.

Pulvermüller, F., Lutzenberger, W., and Preissl, H. Nouns and verbs in the intact brain: Evidence from event-related potentials and high-frequency cortical responses. *Cerebral Cortex* 9: 497–506, 1999.

Purpura, D. Morphogenesis of visual cortex in the preterm infant. In: *Growth and Development of the Brain*, ed. M. A. B. Brazier (New York: Raven Press, 1975), 33–49.

Purves, D. *Neural Activity and the Growth of the Brain* (Cambridge: Cambridge University Press, 1994).

Quartz, S. R. and Sejnowski, T. J. The neural basis of cognitive development: A contructivist manifesto. *Behav. Brain Sci.* 20: 537–596, 1997.

Quintana, J. and Fuster, J. M. From perception to action: Temporal integrative functions of prefrontal and parietal neurons. *Cerebral Cortex* 9: 213–221, 1999.

Quintana, J., Yajeya, J., and Fuster, J. M. Prefrontal representation of stimulus attributes during delay tasks. I. Unit activity in cross-temporal integration of sensory and sensory–motor information. *Brain Res.* 474: 211–221, 1988.

Raichle, M. E. Images of the mind: Studies with modern imaging techniques. *Annu. Rev. Psychol.* 45: 333–356, 1994.

Rakic, P. Neurons in rhesus monkey visual cortex: Systematic relation between time of origin and eventual disposition. *Science* 183: 425–427, 1974.

Rakic, P. Developmental events leading to laminar and areal organization of the neocortex. In: *The Organization of the Cerebral Cortex*, ed. F. O. Schmitt, F. G. Worden, G. Adelman, and S. G. Dennis (Cambridge, MA: MIT Press, 1981a), 7–28.

Rakic, P. Development of visual centers in the primate brain depends on binocular competition before birth. *Science* 214: 928–931, 1981b.

Rakic, P. Specification of cerebral cortical areas. *Science* 24: 170–176, 1988.

Rakic, P. A small step for the cell, a giant leap for mankind: A hypothesis of neocortical expansion during evolution. *Trends NeuroSci.* 18: 383–388, 1995.

Rakic, P. Neurocreationism—making new cortical maps. *Science* 294: 1011–1012, 2001.

Rakic, P. Bourgeois, J. P., Eckenhoff, M. F., Zecevic, N., and Goldman-Rakic, P. S. Concurrent overproduction of synapses in diverse regions of the primate cerebral cortex. *Science* 232: 232–235, 1986.

Rakic, P., Bourgeois, J. P., and Goldman-Rakic, P. S. Synaptic development of the cerebral cortex: Implications for learning, memory, and mental illness. In: *The Self-Organizing Brain: From Growth Cones to Functional Networks*, ed. J. van Pelt, M. A. Corner, H. B. M. Uylings, and F. H. Lopes da Silva (Amsterdam: Elsevier, 1994), 227–243.

Rapport, R. L., Tan, C. T., and Whitaker, H. A. Language function and dysfunction among Chinese and English-speaking polyglots: Cortical stimulation, Wada testing, and clinical studies. *Brain Lang.* 18: 342–366, 1983.

Raven, J. Standardization of progressive matrices. *Br. J. Med. Psychol.* 19: 137–150, 1941.

Reddy, A. and Reddy, P. Creativity and intelligence. *Psychol. Studies* 28: 20–24, 1983.

Reichle, E., Carpenter, P., and Just, M. The neural bases of strategy and skill in sentence-picture verification. *Cognit. Psychol.* 40: 261–295, 2000.

Rizzolatti, G., Gentilucci, M., Camarda, R. M., Gallese, V., Luppino, G., Matelli, M., and Fogassi, L. Neurons related to reaching-grasping arm movements in the rostral part of area 6 (area 6a). *Exp. Brain Res.* 82: 337–350, 1990.

Rockel, A. J., Hiorns, R. W., and Powell, T. P. S. The basic uniformity in structure of the neocortex. *Brain* 103: 221–244, 1980.

Roland, P. E. Cortical organization of voluntary behavior in man. *Hum. Neurobiol.* 4: 155–167, 1985.

Romo, R., Brody, C. D., Hernández, A., and Lemus, L. Neuronal correlates of parametric working memory in the prefrontal cortex. *Nature* 399: 470–473, 1999.

Rosenberg, D. R. and Lewis, D. A. Postnatal maturation of the dopaminergic innervation of monkey prefrontal and motor cortices: A tyrosine hydroxylase immunohistochemical analysis. *J. Comp. Neurol.* 358: 383–400, 1995.

Rosenzweig, M. R. Experience, memory, and the brain. *Am. Psychol.* 39: 365–376, 1984.

Rubens, A. B. Anatomical asymmetries of human cerebral cortex. In: *Lateralization in the Nervous System,* ed. S. Harnad, R. W. Doty, L. Goldstein, J. Jaynes, and G. Krauthamer (New York: Academic Press, 1977), 503–516.

Rubenstein, J. and Rakic, P. Genetic control of cortical development. *Cerebral Cortex* 9: 521–523, 1999.

Ruiz-Marcos, A. and Valverde, F. Dynamic architecture of the visual cortex. *Brain Res.* 19: 25–39, 1970.

Rumelhart, D. E. and McClelland, J. L. *Parallel Distributed Processing* (Cambridge, MA: MIT Press, 1986).

Sagar, H. J., Cohen, N. J., Corkin, S., and Growdon, J. H. Dissociations among processes in remote memory. *Ann. N.Y. Acad. Sci.* 444: 533–535, 1985.

Sakai, K. and Miyashita, Y. Neural organization for the long-term memory of paired associates. *Nature* 354: 152–155, 1991.

Salamon, G., Raynaud, C., Regis, J., and Rumeau, C. *Magnetic Resonance Imaging of the Pediatric Brain* (New York: Raven Press, 1990).

Sanides, F. Functional architecture of motor and sensory cortices in primates in the light of a new concept of neocortex evolution. In: *The Primate Brain,* ed. C. R. Noback and W. Montagna (New York: Appleton-Century-Crofts, 1970), 137–208.

Sato, K. C. and Tanji, J. Digit-muscle responses evoked from multiple intracortical foci in monkey precentral motor cortex. *J. Neurophysiol.* 62: 959–969, 1989.

Schacter, D. L., Alpert, N. M., Savage, C. R., and Rauch, S. L. Conscious recollection and the human hippocampal formation: Evidence from positron emission tomography. *Proc. Natl. Acad. Sci. USA* 93: 321–325, 1996.

Schacter, D. L. and Curran, T. Memory without remembering and remembering without memory: Implicit and false memories. In: *The New Cogni-*

tive Neurosciences, ed. M. S. Gazzaniga (Cambridge, MA: MIT Press, 2000), 829–840.

Schadé, J. P. and Van Groenigen, W. B. Structural organization of the human cerebral cortex. *Acta Anat.* 47: 74–111, 1961.

Schall, J. D. Neural basis of deciding, choosing, and acting. *Nature* 2: 33–42, 2001.

Scheibel, A. B. Dendritic correlates of higher cognitive function. In: *Neurobiology of Higher Cognitive Function,* eds., A. B. Scheibel and A. F. Wechsler (New York: The Guilford Press, 1990), 239–270.

Schnider, A., Bassetti, C., Gutbrod, K., and Ozdoba, C. Very severe amnesia with acute onset after isolated hippocampal damage due to systemic lupus erythematosus. *J. Neurol. Neurosurg. Psychiatry* 59: 644–645, 1995.

Schuman, E. M. and Madison, D. V. Locally distributed synaptic potentiation in the hippocampus. *Science* 263: 532–536, 1994.

Schwartz, M. L. and Goldman-Rakic, P. S. Callosal and intrahemispheric connectivity of the prefrontal association cortex in rhesus monkey: Relation between intraparietal and principal sulcal cortex. *J. Comp. Neurol.* 226: 403–420, 1984.

Scoville, W. B. and Milner, B. Loss of recent memory after bilateral hippocampal lesions. *J. Neurol. Neurosurg. Psychiatry* 20: 11–21, 1957.

Searle, J. R. Consciousness, explanatory inversion, and cognitive science. *Behav. Brain Sci.* 13: 585–642, 1990.

Selfridge, O. G. Pattern recognition and modern computers. *Proc. 1955 Western Joint Computer Conference* 91–93, 1955.

Sergent, J., Zuck, E., Terriah, S., and MacDonald, B. Distributed neural network underlying musical sight-reading and keyboard performance. *Science* 257: 106–109, 1992.

Shadmehr, R. and Mussa-Ivaldi, F. A. Adaptive representation of dynamics during learning of a motor task. *J. Neurosci.* 14: 3208–3224, 1994.

Shastri, L. and Ajjanagadde, V. From simple associations to systematic reasoning: A connectionist representation of rules, variables and dynamic bindings using temporal synchrony. *Behav. Brain Sci.* 16: 417–494, 1993.

Sidman, R. L. and Rakic, P. Neuronal migration, with special reference to developing human brain: A review. *Brain Res.* 62: 1–35, 1973.

Singer, W. Response synchronization: A universal coding strategy for the definition of relations. I. In: *The New Cognitive Neurosciences,* ed. M. S. Gazzaniga (Cambridge MA: MIT Press, 2000), 325–338.

Singer, W. and Gray, C. M. Visual feature integration and the temporal correlation hypothesis. *Annu. Rev. Neurosci.* 18: 555–586, 1995.

Singh, J. and Knight, R. T. Frontal lobe contribution to voluntary movements in humans. *Brain Res.* 531: 45–54, 1990.

Smith, A. and Fullerton, A. M. Age differences in episodic and semantic memory: Implications for language and cognition. In: *In Aging, Communication Processes and Disorders,* ed. D. Beasly and G. Davis (New York: Grune & Straton, 1981), 139–156.

Spearman, C. *The Abilities of Man.* New York: MacMillan, 1927.

Sperry, R. W. Lateral specialization in the surgically separated hemispheres. In: *The Neurosciences. Third Study Program,* ed. F. O. Schmitt and F. G. Worden (Cambridge, MA: MIT Press, 1974), 5–19.

Sporns, O. and Tononi, G. (Eds.). *Selectionism and the Brain* (New York: Academic Press, 1994).

Spreen, O., Risser, A. T., and Egdell, D. *Developmental Neuropsychology* (New York: Oxford University Press, 1995).

Squire, L. R. Mechanisms of memory. *Science* 232: 1612–1619, 1986.

Squire, L. R. and Kandel, E. R. *Memory* (New York: Scientific American Library, 1999).

Stent, G. S. A physiological mechanism for Hebb's postulate of learning. *Proc. Natl. Acad. Sci. USA* 70: 997–1001, 1973.

Stephan, H., Frahm, H., and Baron, G. New and revised data on volumes of brain structures in insectivores and primates. *Folia Primatol.* 35: 1–29, 1981.

Steriade, M. Central core modulation of spontaneous oscillations and sensory transmission in thalamocortical systems. *Curr. Opin. Neurobiol.* 3: 619–625, 1993.

Sternberg, R. *Beyond IQ: A Triarchic Theory of Human Intelligence* (New York: Cambridge University Press, 1985).

Sur, M., Pallas, S. L., and Roe, A. W. Cross-modal plasticity in cortical development: Differentiation and specification of sensory neocortex. *Trends NeuroSci.* 13: 227–233, 1990.

Swanson, L. W., Teyler, T. J., and Thompson, R. F. Hippocampal long-term potentiation: Mechanisms and implications for memory. *Neurosci. Res. Program Bull.* 20: 613–764, 1982.

Swartz, B. E., Halgren, E., Fuster, J. M., Simpkins, F., Gee, M., and Mandelkern, M. Cortical metabolic activation in humans during a visual memory task. *Cerebral Cortex* 3: 205–214, 1995.

Tallon-Baudry, C., Bertrand, O., Bouchet, P., and Pernier, P. Gamma-range activity evoked by coherent visual stimuli in humans. *Eur. J. Neurosci.* 7: 1285–1291, 1995.

Tanaka, K. Neuronal mechanisms of object recognition. *Science* 262: 685–688, 1993.

Tanzi, E. I fatti e le induzioni nell'odierna istologia del sistema nervoso. *Riv. Sper. Freniatr. Med. Leg. Alienazioni Ment.* 19: 419–472, 1893.

Teuber, H.-L. Unity and diversity of frontal lobe functions. *Acta Neurobiol. Exp.* 32: 625–656, 1972.

Teyler, T. J., Perkins, A. T., and Harris, K. M. The development of long-term potentiation in hippocampus and neocortex. *Neuropsychologia* 27: 31–39, 1989.

Theonen, H. Neurotrophins and neuronal plasticity. *Science* 270: 593–598, 1995.

Tinbergen, N. *The Study of Instinct* (Oxford: Oxford University Press, 1951).

Tomasello, M. and Call, J. *Primate Cognition* (Oxford: Oxford University Press, 1997).

Tomita, H., Ohbayashi, M., Nakahara, K., Hasegawa, I., and Miyashita, Y. Top-down signal from prefrontal cortex in executive control of memory retrieval. *Nature* 401: 699–703, 1999.

Tononi, G. and Edelman, G. M. Consciousness and complexity. *Science* 282: 1846–1851, 1998.

Tononi, G., Sporns, O., and Edelman, G. M. Reentry and the problem of integrating multiple cortical areas: Simulation of dynamic integration in the visual system. *Cerebral Cortex* 2: 310–335, 1992.

Treisman, A. and Gelade, G. A feature-integration theory of attention. *Cognit. Psychol.* 12: 97–136, 1980.

Twain, M. *The Adventures of Huckleberry Finn.* In: The Portable Mark Twain. New York: Viking Press, 1985.

Tucker, D. M. Emotional experience and the problem of vertical integration: Discussion of the special section on emotion. *Neuropsychology* 7: 500–509, 1993.

Tulving, E. and Pearlstone, Z. Availability versus accessibility of information in memory for words. *J. Verbal Learning Verbal Bahav.* 5: 381–391, 1966.

Uexküll, J. V. *Theoretical Biology* (New York: Harcourt, Brace, 1926).

Valverde, F. Apical dendritic spines of the visual cortex and light deprivation in the mouse. *Exp. Brain Res.* 3: 337–352, 1967.

Valverde, F. Rate and extent of recovery from dark rearing in the visual cortex of the mouse. *Brain Res.* 33: 1–11, 1971.

Van Essen, D. C. Functional organization of primate visual cortex. In: *Cerebral Cortex, Vol. 3*, ed. A. Peters and E. G. Jones (New York: Plenum Press, 1985), 259–329.

Van Hoesen, G. W. The parahippocampal gyrus. *Trends NeuroSci.* 5: 345–350, 1982.

Vandenberghe, R., Price, C., Wise, R., Josephs, O., and Frackowiak, R. S. J. Functional anatomy of a common semantic system for words and pictures. *Nature* 383: 254–256, 1996.

Vogel, F. and Schalt, E. The electroencephalogram (EEG) as a research tool in human behavior genetics: Psychological examinations in healthy males with various inherited EEG variants. III. Interpretation of results. *Hum. Genet.* 47: 81–111, 1979.

Von der Malsburg, C. Nervous structures with dynamical links. *Ber. Bunsenges. Phys. Chem.* 89: 703–710, 1985.

Von Frisch, K. *The Dance Language and Orientation of Bees* (Cambridge, MA: Harvard University Press, 1993).

Von Monakow, C. *Die Lokalisation im Grosshirn und der Abbau der Funktion durch korticale Herde.* (Weisbaden: J. F. Bergmann, 1914).

Vygotsky, L. *Thought and Language* (Cambridge, MA: MIT Press, 1986).

Walsh, K. W. *Neuropsychology: A Clinical Approach* (Edinburgh: Churchill Livingstone, 1978).

Waltz, J., Knowlton, B. J., Holyoak, K. J., Boone, K., Mishkin, F., Menezes Santos, M., Thomas, C., and Miller, BL. A system for relational reasoning in human prefrontal cortex. *Psychol. Sci.* 10: 119–125, 1999.

Warrington, E. K. and McCarthy, R. Category specific access dysphasia. *Brain* 106: 859–878, 1983.

Warrington, E. K. and Shallice, T. The selective impairment of auditory verbal short-term memory. *Brain* 92: 885–896, 1969.

Weinrich, M. and Wise, S. P. The premotor cortex of the monkey. *J. Neurosci.* 2: 1329–1345, 1982.

Weiss, P. *Principles of Development* (New York: Henry Holt, 1939).

Weiss, P., Wang, H., Taylor, A. C., and Edds, V. Proximo-distal fluid convection in the endoneural spaces of peripheral nerves, demonstrated by colored and radioactive (isotope) tracers. *Am. J. Physiol.* 143: 521–540, 1945.

Wernicke, C. *Der Aphasische Symptomenkomplex* (Breslau: Cohn and Weingert, 1874).

Wertheimer, M. Laws of organization in perceptual forms. In: *A Source Book of Gestalt Psychology*, ed. W. D. Ellis (New York: Humanities Press, 1967), 71–88.

Westbrook, G. L. and Jahr, C. E. Glutamate receptors in excitatory neurotransmission. *Semin. Neurosci.* 1: 103–114, 1989.

Wharton, C., Grafman, J., Flitman, S., Hansen, E., Brauner, J., Marks, A., and Honda, M. Toward neuroanatomical models of analogy: A positron emission tomography study of analogical mapping. *Cognit. Psychol.* 40: 173–197, 2000.

White, G., Levy, W. B., and Steward, O. Spatial overlap between populations of synapses determines the extent of their associative interaction during the induction of long-term potentiation and depression. *J. Neurophysiol.* 64: 1186–1198, 1990.

Whitehouse, P. J., Price, D. L., Struble, R. G., Clark, A. W., Coyle, J. T., and Delong, M. R. Alzheimer's disease and senile dementia: Loss of neurons in the basal forebrain. *Science* 215: 1237–1239, 1982.

Wickelgren, W. A., The long and the short of memory. In: *Short-Term Memory*, ed. D. Deutsch and J. A. Deutsch (New York: Academic Press, 1975), 41–63.

Wiener, N. *Cybernetics.* New York: Wiley, 1948.

Wiesel, T. N. Postnatal development of the visual cortex and the influence of environment. *Nature* 299: 583–591, 1982.

Wiesel, T. N. and Hubel, D. H. Comparison of the effects of unilateral and bilateral eye closure on cortical unit responses in kittens. *J.Neurophysiol.* 28: 1029–1040, 1965.

Willshaw, D. Holography, associative memory, and inductive generalization. In: *Parallel Models of Associative Memory*, ed. G. E. Hinton and J. A. Anderson (Hillsdale, NJ: Erlbaum, 1981), 83–104.

Winston, P. H. Learning structural descriptions from examples. *AI Laboratory Technical Report 231*, (Cambridge, MA: Massachusetts Institute of Technology, 1970).

Witelson, S. F. Neuroanatomical bases of hemispheric functional specializations in the human brain: Possible developmental factors. In: *Hemispheric*

Communication: Mechanisms and Models, ed. F. L. Kitterle (Hillsdale, NJ: Erlbaum, 1995), 61–84.

Wolpert, S. M. and Barnes, P. D. *MRI in Pediatric Neuroradiology* (Baltimore: C. V. Mosby, 1992).

Wszolek, Z., Herkes, G., Lagerlund, T., and Kokmen, E. Comparison of EEG background frequency analysis, psychologic test scores, short test of mental status, and quantitative SPECT dementia. *J. Geriat. Psychiatry Neurol.* 5: 22–30, 1992.

Yakovlev, P. I. and Le Cours, A. R. The myelogenetic cycles of regional maturation of the brain. In: *Regional Development of the Brain in Early Life,* ed. A. Minkowski (Oxford: Blackwell, 1967), 3–70.

Young, J. Z. Sources of discovery in neuroscience. In: *The Neurosciences: Paths of Discovery,* eds. F. G. Worden, J. P. Swazey, and G. Adelman (Cambridge, MA: The M.I.T. Press, 1975), 15–46.

Young, M. P. and Yamane, S. Sparse population coding of faces in the inferotemporal cortex. *Science* 256: 1327–1331, 1992.

Zacks, J., Rypma, B., Gabrieli, J., Tversky, B., and Glover, G. H. Imagined transformations of bodies: A fMRI investigation. *Neuropsychologia* 37: 1029–1040, 1999.

Zaidel, E. Language function in the two hemispheres following cerebral commissurotomy and hemispherectomy. In: *Handbook of Neuropsychology,* ed. F. Boller and J. Grafman (Amsterdam: Elsevier, 1990), 115–150.

Zaidel, E., Zaidel, D. W., and Sperry, R. W. Left and right intelligence: Case studies of Raven's Progressive Matrices following brain bisection and hemi-decortication. *Cortex* 17: 167–186, 1981.

Zhang, K. and Sejnowski, T. J. A universal scaling law between gray matter and white matter of cerebral cortex. *Proc. Natl. Acad. Sci. USA* 97: 5621–5626, 2000.

Zhou, Y.-D. and Fuster, J. M. Mnemonic neuronal activity in somatosensory cortex. *Proc. Natl. Acad. Sci. USA* 93: 10533–10537, 1996.

Zhou, Y.-D. and Fuster, J. M. Visuo-tactile cross-modal associations in cortical somatosensory cells. *Proc. Natl. Acad. Sci. USA* 97: 9777–9782, 2000.

Zipser, D., Kehoe, B., Littlewort, G., and Fuster, J. A spiking network model of short-term active memory. *J. Neurosci.* 13: 3406–3420, 1993.

Zola-Morgan, S. and Squire, L. R. Medial temporal lesions in monkeys impair memory on a variety of tasks sensitive to human amnesia. *Behav. Neurosci.* 99: 22–34, 1985.

Zola-Morgan, S. M. and Squire, L. R. The primate hippocampal formation: Evidence for a time-limited role in memory storage. *Science* 250: 288–290, 1990.

Zola-Morgan, S., Squire, L. R., Amaral, D. G., and Suzuki, W. A. Lesions of perirhinal and parahippocampal cortex that spare the amygdala and hippocampal formation produce severe memory impairment. *J. Neurosci.* 9: 4355–4370, 1989.

Zurif, E. B., Caramazza, A., and Myerson, R. Grammatical judgments of agrammatic aphasics. *Neuropsychologia* 10: 405–417, 1972.

Index

....

Abstract attitude, 74
Abstraction, 71, 73, 77, 94, 98, 202.
  See also Symbolization
Access to lexicon, 208–210
Acetylcholine, 48, 149
Action
  categorization, 74–80
  future, 131. *See also* Planning
  hierarchical organization, 74–80
  schemas, 128, 130, 208
Adaptive resonance theory, 151
Agnosia, 94, 192–193
Agraphia, 73
AI, 9, 225
Amnesia, 45–46, 113–114, 118, 133
  anterograde, 134
  global, 134
  psychogenic, 133
  retrograde, 134
Amygdala, 137
  emotional memory, 47–48
  memory acquisition, 115
Analogical mappings, 232

Angular gyrus. *See* Wernicke's
  area
Animal intelligence, 214–215
Anomia, 192
Anterior cingulate cortex
  attention, 167
  intelligence, 222
  language, 194, 207
Aphasia, 73, 190–195, 206
  conduction, 191
  frontal dynamic, 194
  global, 191
  motor, 191. *See also* Broca's
  aphasia
  semantic, 94, 191. *See also*
  Wernicke's aphasia
Aplysia
  learning, 48
Artificial intelligence. *See* AI
Association, 8, 10, 14, 45, 50, 72,
  107, 113. *See also* Binding
Attention, 143–175
  anterior cingulate, 167

285

Attention *(continued)*
  biology, 144–149
  brain stem, 149
  consciousness, 252–253
  disorders, 154, 167, 175
  exclusionary component, 86, 110,
    146, 148, 151–152, 164,
    173–175, 217, 228, 241
  executive, 164–175
  inclusive component, 86, 148,
    151–152. *See also* Focus of
    attention
  inhibition, 146, 148, 164, 173–175
  limbic system, 149–150
  neurotransmitters, 149
  orbital prefrontal cortex, 167,
    175, 241
  perceptual, 149–155
  spatial, 167, 172
  top-down control, 51, 84–85, 116,
    144, 146, 150–151
Attractors, 100–103, 161, 209
Axons, 27, 29, 31, 40. *See also*
  Cortical structure

Binding, 72, 95–96, 161, 226. *See
  also* Association
  perceptual, 60–61, 99–106
  temporal, 61
Blind sight, 97
Bottom-up processing, 50, 67,
  150–151
Broca's aphasia, 191, 195, 207
Broca's area, 78, 191–192, 207
  syntax, 207, 210

Categorization, 38, 59, 81
  action, 74–80
  knowledge, 59–62
  perception, 60–61, 84–87,
    89–99, 101, 105–106
Central motor aphasia. See Frontal
  dynamic aphasia
Cholinergic system
  attention, 149
  learning and memory, 48

Classification. *See* Categorization
CNV, 79, 169
Cognits, 14–16, 55–82, 72, 81–82,
  112. *See also* Networks;
  Representation
  categorical, 193
  cognitive functions, 15–16
  conceptual, 74
  cross-modal, 193
  executive, 61–62, 74–80, 166
  lexical, 193, 203–206
  perceptual, 67–74, 91–99
Coherence, 100–102
Coincidence detectors, 100
Columnar structure, 62–64
Complexity, 36, 53, 72, 82–83,
  89, 91, 109, 131, 166–167,
  194, 206, 212, 232–233, 236,
  243
Conceptual memory, 80–81, 125
Connectionism, 4–5, 9–10, 56–59
Connectionist models, 56–59
  distributed representation, 56
  learning, 57
  neurons, 56
  nodes, 56
  synapses, 57
  units, 56
Connectivity
  convergence, 50–51, 57, 67, 76, 93
  corticocortical, 11, 49–51, 67–80,
    106–110
  divergence, 51, 57, 67, 76, 93
  evolution, 22
  heterarchical, 107
  interhemispheric, 107
  limbic, 46–47, 67, 69, 75, 78, 94
  methods of study, 11
  modes, 50–51
  recurrence, 50–51, 93. *See also*
    Reentry
  strength, 82, 126, 204, 209. *See
    also* Synaptic strength
Consciousness, 85, 132–133,
  138–139, 249–256
  attention, 251–253

binding, 250
creative intelligence, 251
delusions, 256
dreaming, 256
dynamic core, 255
focus of attention, 251–252,
    254–255
Gestalt psychology, 250
high-frequency oscillations, 250
network activation, 252–254
phenomenology, 249–250, 253
prefrontal cortex, 251, 255–256
psychosis, 256
reentry, 250–251, 255
split brain, 253
stream of consciousness, 249, 254
temporal continuity, 250–251
temporal integration, 251,
    253–254
threshold, 255
unity, 250, 252–253
working memory, 251, 253–256
Constructivism, 37, 39
Contingent negative variation. *See*
    CNV
Convergence zones, 97
Corollary discharge, 129, 144, 174
Correlation, 7, 38, 42, 44, 50, 71, 100.
    See also Coherence; Synchrony
Cortical damage
    cognitive vulnerability, 72, 74, 98,
        117, 126, 131
    recovery, 36, 117, 133, 183, 189
Cortical structure, 62–67
Creative intelligence, 242–247, 251
    divergent thinking, 245–246
    EEG synchrony, 245
    inputs from limbic system, 246
    inputs from mesencephalon,
        246
    inputs from sensory systems, 246
    language, 242
    monoamines, 246
    network formation, 245–247
    planning, 242
    prefrontal cortex, 242–245, 247

reward systems, 246–247
    right hemisphere, 243–244
    role of other cognitive functions,
        243
    value systems, 246–247
Creativity/logical thinking
    dissociation, 245
Critical periods, 35–36, 49
Cross-modal integration, 129
Cross-modal representation, 50, 68
Cross-temporal contingency, 159,
    167–168, 211–212
Cross-temporal integration, 129

Decision making, 236–242
    emotional influences, 238, 240
    free will, 236, 240–242
    frontal cortex, 237–238,
        240–242
    perception-action cycle, 237–238,
        240
    role of perception, 237–238, 240
    social influences, 238
    values, 238–240
Declarative memory, 45, 115, 134
    hippocampus, 46, 114, 134
Degeneracy, 9, 39, 82, 92, 94, 117
Delay tasks. *See* Working memory
Delusions, 256
Dementia
    cholinergic system, 48
    paraphasia, 209
Dendrites, 22–23, 27, 29, 40. *See also*
    Cortical structure
Development of cortex. *See*
    Ontogeny of cortex
Development of intelligence. *See*
    Intellectual development
Development of language. *See*
    Language development
Disconnection syndromes, 74, 191
Distributed representation, 5–8, 15,
    56–57, 67, 96, 163, 187
Dopamine, 34
Dysexecutive syndrome, 165
Dyslexia, 202, 210

Efferent copy, 76, 128, 174
Emotional memory, 72
  amygdala, 47–48, 137
  orbital prefrontal cortex, 138
Entorhinal cortex
  memory, 47
Episodic memory, 125, 141–142
Evolution of cortex. *See* Phylogeny
  of cortex
Evolution of intelligence, 215
Evolution of language, 178–181
  cortical coonectivity, 180–181
  limbic system, 179–180
  motor skills, 180
  neocortex, 179–180
  primates, 180
  symbolic communication, 180
Executive attention, 164–175
  prefrontal cortex, 165–166
Executive memory, 127–132, 139
  hippocampus, 46–47
Executive networks, 74–80, 110
Explicit memory, 139

Face representation, 72, 94, 124
False memory, 117, 138
Feedback, 9, 57, 108–110, 140,
  144–146, 211–212. *See also*
  Reentry
Feedforward, 57, 108, 146
Focus of attention, 145, 148,
  158–159, 161, 172, 251–252,
  254
Forgetting. *See* Amnesia
Frontal cortex in decision making,
  237, 240–242
  inhibitory control, 240–241
  inputs from limbic system, 240
  inputs from sensory areas, 240
  perception-action cycle, 237–238,
  240
Frontal dynamic aphasia, 194, 207

GABA, 48
Gamma-aminobutyric acid. *See* GABA
Genetic factors, 27, 35, 38,
  181–183, 201–202, 216

Gestalt
  principles, 88–89, 100
  psychology, 6, 87–91, 101, 250
Gilles de la Tourette syndrome, 138,
  179
Glutamate, 48
Graceful degradation, 59
Group selection theory, 9, 38–39

Hebbian principles, 42–45, 57, 116
Heterarchical representation, 61,
  80–82, 96, 106, 122, 124, 136,
  141, 173
Hierarchical organization, 51, 53,
  59, 67–74, 106–110, 124, 128
  executive knowledge, 61
  executive networks, 74–80
  language, 193–196, 202–207
  perceptual categories, 60, 91–99
  perceptual networks, 67–74
  Piagetian stages of development,
  217–218
High-frequency oscillations,
  99–103, 161, 250
Hippocampus
  amnesia, 45–46, 113–114, 118
  connections with cortex, 46–47.
  See also Connectivity, limbic
  declarative memory, 46, 113,
  134
  executive memory, 46–47
  LTP, 42
  memory acquisition, 45–46, 48,
  113–115
  memory consolidation, 45–46
  memory retrieval, 134
  NMDA, 48–49
  short-term memory, 118
Holography, 90

Iconic memory, 71
Illusory contours, 97
Imagery, 93, 106, 251
Implicit memory, 114–115, 139, 237
Inference, 225–226
Inferotemporal cortex, 98, 151–154
  associative properties, 64–65

attention, 151–154
  working memory, 158–160
Inhibition, 173–175, 241
  memory consolidation, 115
  working memory, 164
Inhibitory control, 173–175,
  217–218, 241
Integration, 57, 59–60, 67, 72, 76,
  81, 217–219, 250, 252
  cross-modal, 129
  cross-temporal, 129
  interhemispheric, 81
  sensory-motor, 106–110
  temporal, 61, 77–79, 92, 97,
    108–109, 129, 235–236
Intellectual development, 213–
  247
  genetic factors, 216
  hierarchical organization,
    217–218
  inhibition, 217
  integration, 217–219
  language, 217
  network formation, 215
  numerical system, 217
  perception-action cycle, 218
  Piagetian stages, 216–217
  prefrontal cortex, 217–219
Intelligence, 213–247
  analytical, 220. See also Reasoning
  animal, 214–215
  anterior cingulate, 222
  artificial. See AI
  cortical structure, 220–224
  creative, 221, 242–247
  decision making, 236–242
  development. See Intellectual
    development
  EEG coherence, 222
  EEG synchrony, 222, 243
  evolution, 215
  fluid, 221
  general, 222–223. See also
    Spearman's g-factor
  language, 217
  practical, 220–221, 232. See also
    Problem solving

prefrontal cortex, 217–218,
  222–224
problem solving, 231–236
quotient. See IQ
reasoning, 224–231
role of attention, 221–222
tests, 221
Intelligence tests, 215
  Raven's Progressive Matrices
    (RPM), 221, 232–233
  Stanford-Binet, 221
  Wechsler-Bellvue, 221
IQ, 221
  EEG synchrony, 222
Isocortex, 19, 62
Isomorphism cortex-mind, 3–4,
  88–89

Knowledge, 55–82. See also Cognits;
  Memory; Networks
  categorization, 59–62

Language, 177–212
  access to lexicon, 208–210
  anterior cingulate, 194, 207
  bilinguals, 188–189
  cerebellum, 198
  cortical asymmetry, 184–185
  cortical dissociation
    function/content words,
      196–197
  cortical dissociation verbs/nouns,
    194–196
  distributed representation, 187
  dyslexia, 202, 210
  frontal linguistic hierarchy, 194,
    206, 211–212
  hemispheric lateralization,
    184–190
  hierarchical organization,
    193–196, 202–207
  left cortical dominance, 184–187,
    200
  lexical-semantic system, 203–
    205
  module, 187
  music, 190

Language *(continued)*
  planum temporale, 185
  polyglots, 188–189
  prefrontal cortex, 194, 207–208, 210–212
  premotor cortex, 194, 207–208
  prosody, 181, 188, 206–207
  right hemisphere, 188
  schemas, 208
  semantics, 195–206
  sign language, 189, 199–200
  syntax, 206–212
Language development, 181–183
  genetic factors, 181–183, 201–202, 207
  intelligence, 217
  motor skills, 183
  plasticity, 182–183
  universal grammar, 181–183
Language neurobiology, 178–184
Language neuropsychology, 190–195
Learning. *See also* Memory
  Aplysia, serotonin, 48
  language, 182
  supervised, 57
  unsupervised, 10, 57
Localizationism, 5
Long-term memory, 118. *See also* Cognits; Networks, cognitive
Long-term potentiation. *See* LTP
LTP, 42–43, 49

Memory, 111–142. *See also* Knowledge
  acquisition, 45, 48, 112–117
  associative aspects, 113, 132, 136
  conceptual, 80–81, 125
  consolidation, 45–46, 112–117, 119–121
  declarative, 45, 114–115, 134
  emotional, 47–48, 72, 137–138
  episodic, 125, 141–142
  executive, 127–132, 139

explicit, 139
  hemispheric lateralization, 125–126
  heterogeneity, 121–122, 141. *See also* Heterarchical representation
  iconic, 71
  implicit, 114–115, 139, 237
  long-term, 118. *See also* Cognits; Networks, cognitive
  perceptual, 121–126
  phyletic, 8, 49–50, 60, 66, 113, 124, 128
  procedural, 114–115, 131
  rehearsal, 117, 130
  retrieval. *See* Memory retrieval
  role of attention, 115
  semantic, 125, 130
  short-term, 7, 44, 117–121
  temporal aspects, 112–113, 123, 141–142
  two-store model, 118–119, 121
Memory cells, 79, 156, 158–161, 171, 254
Memory retrieval, 113, 132–142
  emotional inputs, 137–138
  false memory, 138
  heterarchical, 133, 139
  internal inputs, 136–137
  overretrieval, 133
  prefrontal cortex, 140
  priming, 139
  sensory inputs, 135–136
  visceral inputs, 137
Mental age. *See* IQ
Mental models of reality, 227
Middle temporal (MT) visual area, 238
Migration of executive cognits, 79, 130
Mirror units, 77, 128, 166–167
Mnemonic strategies, 136
Modules, 6, 20, 27, 35, 50, 62–67, 76
Monitoring, 172–175, 211
  prefrontal cortex, 174, 211

Motor cortex, 74–80, 128
Movement representation, 77. *See*
    also Executive networks
Music, 190

Neglect, 154, 167
Network
    activation, 99–106, 132–142, 155,
        158–159, 209. *See also*
        Consciousness; Memory
        retrieval; Working memory
    formation, 17–53, 215, 245–247
    structure, 49–82
Networks, 53
    cognitive, 4–5, 7–9, 11, 112. *See*
        also Cognits
    emergent properties, 53
    executive, 74–80, 110
    hierarchical organization, 51, 53,
        59–80
    language development, 182
    layered, 51–52, 57
    nodes, 10, 14, 56–57, 70, 72,
        96–97, 106, 124, 187
    perceptual, 67–74
Neural Darwinism, 35
Neurotransmitters
    acetylcholine, 48, 149
    dopamine, 34
    GABA, 48
    glutamate, 48
    memory acquisition, 48, 115–116
    memory consolidation, 48,
        115–116
    monoamines, 34, 48, 149, 246
    norepinephrine, 34
    serotonin, 34, 48
NMDA, 48–49, 116
N-methyl-D-aspartate. *See* NMDA
Nonsynaptic contacts, 43
Norepinephrine, 34
Numerical system, 205–206, 217,
    225

Obsessive-compulsive disorder, 138,
    179

Ontogeny of cortex, 24–36
    cortical layering, 27
    cortical plate, 25
    critical periods, 35–36, 49
    dendrites, 27, 29
    elimination of structure, 28–29,
        33–34
    exuberant growth, 28–29, 34
    genetic factors, 27, 35
    modules, 35
    myelination, 29, 31–33
    neuron migration, 25–27
    neurotrophins, 31
    order of areal maturation, 34
    prefrontal cortex, 32–34
    proliferative zone, 25
    recurrent axons, 27
    synaptogenesis, 27, 29–31, 33
    thyroxine, 30
Orbital prefrontal cortex
    attention, 167
    attention disorders, 175
    emotional memory, 138
    inhibitory control, 175, 241
Oscillations
    high-frequency, 99, 100–103, 161,
        250

Parallel processing, 10, 52, 57, 67,
    76, 85, 91–93, 151–152,
    173–174, 225
Parietal cortex, 67–68, 73, 97, 151,
    180, 202, 234
    spatial attention, 145, 158, 254
    working memory, 158–159
Patient H.M., 113, 115, 134
Pattern recognition, 59
Pattern representation, 94
Perception, 83–110
    categorization, 60–61, 84–87,
        89–99, 101, 105–106
    cortical dynamics, 91–99
    hierarchical organization, 67–74,
        91–99
    role of affect, 86
    role of attention, 84–86

Perception *(continued)*
  role of memory, 84, 85–87,
    91–99
  role of values, 86
  segmentation, 88
  segregation, 88
Perception-action cycle, 74,
  106–110, 129, 140, 144, 151,
  168, 212, 218–219, 247
Perceptual attention, 149–155
Perceptual constancy, 39, 90,
  98
Perceptual memory, 121–126
Perceptual networks, 67–74
Perirhinal cortex
  memory, 47
Phyletic memory, 8, 49–50, 60, 66,
  113, 124, 128
Phylogeny of cortex, 18–23
  amphibians, 19
  connectivity, 22, 180
  cortical maps, 21
  dendrites, 22–23
  homology, 19–20
  isocortex, 19
  layered cortex, 19, 21
  modules, 20
  neopallium, 18
  ontogenetic sequence, 22
  primates, 19, 180
  radial columns, 20
  sensory areas, 22
  specialized areas, 21
  ventricular ridge, 19
  white matter, 23
Planning, 76, 78–79, 127, 165,
  169–170
Planum temporale, 185
Plasticity, 36, 39, 49, 93, 182–183
Practice, 130
Preattentive processing, 151
Prefrontal cortex
  attention, 110, 130, 152–154,
    165–167
  creative intelligence, 242–245,
    247
  emotional memory, 138

executive attention, 165–167
executive networks, 74–80
frontal dynamic aphasia, 194, 207
inhibitory control, 175, 241
intelligence, 217–218, 222–224
language, 194, 208
memory retrieval, 140
monitoring, 174, 211
perception-action cycle,
  109–110, 140, 168, 211–212,
  219
preparatory set, 169, 170–172
problem solving, 234–236
reasoning, 228
syntax, 207–208, 210–212
temporal integration, 110, 129,
  168, 211, 235–236
temporal organization of
  behavior, 110, 140, 207
working memory, 110, 155–161,
  208, 211–212, 255
Premotor cortex, 74–80, 128
language, 194, 207–208
syntax, 207–208
Preparatory set, 77, 79, 146,
  167–172. *See also* Executive
  attention
prefrontal cortex, 169–172
readiness potential, 169
Primacy effect, 118–119
Priming, 139, 209–210
Problem solving, 231–236
prefrontal cortex, 234–236
Procedural memory, 114–115, 131.
  See also Executive memory
Prospective memory. *See* Planning
Psychophysics, 85, 88, 238, 250
Psychosis, 256

Raven's Progressive Matrices test.
  See RPM test
Reasoning, 224–231
analogical, 232, 234
deductive, 226–227
inductive, 231–236
inference, 224
inhibitory control, 228–229

left cortical dominance, 227
logical bias, 230
perceptual bias, 230
prefrontal cortex, 228
reflexive, 225
spatial, 234
Reasoning models
computational, 226
connectionist, 224–225
symbolic, 224–225
Recall. *See* Memory retrieval
Recency effect, 118–119
Reciprocal innervation, 147–148
Recognition. *See* Memory retrieval
Reentry, 9, 38, 44, 57, 98, 100, 160, 161–163. *See also* Feedback
Relational complexity, 232
Relational representation, 87–91, 116, 117, 232. *See also* Association; Binding
Remembering. *See* Memory retrieval
Representation. *See also* Memory
animals, 73
cross-modal, 50, 68
faces, 72, 94, 124
goals, 76, 128
movements, 77. *See also* Executive networks
patterns, 94
plans, 76. *See also* Planning
semantic, 105. *See also* Semantic memory; Symbolization
sequences, 76–77, 127–128
tools, 73
trajectory, 76, 128
words, 73, 194–206
Reticular formation, 149
Right hemisphere
creative intelligence, 243–244
language, 188
reasoning, 227
RPM test, 221, 232–233

Scaling, 13
Scientific logic, 232
Segregation, 61, 88
Selectionism, 37–39

Self-organization, 10, 50, 57, 113
Semantic memory, 105. *See also* Symbolization
executive, 130
perceptual, 125
Semantics of language, 195–206
abstraction, 202
cortical dissociation function/content words, 196
cortical dissociation verbs/nouns, 196
dyslexia, 202
lexical system, 203–205, 211
sign language, 189, 199–201
syntax, 196
words, 195–199
written words, 198–199
Sensory deafferentation, 39
Sensory deprivation, 40
Sensory qualia, 60, 205, 252
Sensory stimulation
enriched environment, 40
Sequence representation, 76–77, 127–128
Serial processing, 52, 76, 85, 91–93, 151–152, 173–174, 212, 234
Serotonin, 34, 48
Short-term memory, 7, 44, 117–121
hippocampus, 118
Sign language, 189, 199–201
Sleep, 256
SMA, 77–78, 128, 172
language, 194
Spatial attention, 167, 172
Spearman's *g-factor*, 221–223
Split brain, 188, 253
Stream of consciousness, 249, 254
Supervisory attentional system, 165
Supplementary motor area. *See* SMA
Symbolization, 90–91, 94–98, 101–102, 218
words, 195–196, 202–203
Synapses, 27, 29–31, 33, 38, 40, 42, 44
Synaptic modulation, 113, 115–116

Synaptic strength, 8, 38, 42, 115, 126, 133, 225
Synaptic weight. *See* Synaptic strength
Synchronous convergence, 43–44, 59, 116
Synchrony, 43–44, 222, 243, 245. *See also* Coherence; High-frequency oscillations
Syntax, 206–212
  access to lexicon, 208–210
  Broca's area, 207, 210
  function words, 207
  grammar, 210
  hierarchical organization, 207
  monitoring, 211
  perception-action cycle, 211
  prefrontal cortex, 207–208, 210–212
  premotor cortex, 207–208
  working memory, 208, 210–211
Syntax of action, 180, 207

Taxonomy of memory, 123
Temporal code, 100, 226
Temporal coincidence, 7, 42, 44, 59. *See also* Synchronous convergence; Temporal correlation
Temporal correlation, 38. *See also* Correlation; Synchronous convergence; Temporal coincidence
Temporal gestalts, 89
Temporal integration, 61, 77–79, 92, 97, 108–109, 168, 251
  language, 62, 78–79
  prefrontal cortex, 110, 129, 211, 251
Temporal organization of behavior, 106–110
  prefrontal cortex, 110, 140, 207
Thalamic projections
  cortical specificity, 11, 31, 45

Theory of mind, 238
Thinking. *See* Reasoning
Tool representation, 73
Top-down control, 51, 67, 76, 84–85, 93, 106, 116, 136, 144, 150–151, 255

Unitary theory of memory, 121
Universal grammar, 181–183, 207

Voluntary action, 78, 236–238, 240
  free will, 240–242
  frontal cortex, 237–238, 240

Wernicke's aphasia, 191–192, 195
Wernicke's area, 73, 97–98, 191–193
Will. *See* Voluntary action
Word representation, 73, 194–206
Working memory, 79, 98, 121, 155–164
  auditory, 156
  consciousness, 251, 253–254
  cortical cooling effects, 159–160
  definition, 155
  inferotemporal cortex, 158–160
  long-term memory, 155, 163
  mechanisms, 160, 161–163
  memory cells, 156, 158–161, 171, 254
  parietal cortex, 158
  prefrontal cortex, 155–164, 208, 211–212, 255
  prefrontal-inferotemporal interaction, 159–160
  recurrent computational model, 160–161
  reverberating circuits, 160–163
  spatial, 156, 158, 254
  syntax, 208, 210–211
  tactile, 158
  verbal, 159
  visual, 158–159